RADIOLOGY
DIGEST

Kenneth C. Eze

authorHOUSE®

AuthorHouse™
1663 Liberty Drive
Bloomington, IN 47403
www.authorhouse.com
Phone: 1-800-839-8640

Published by AuthorHouse   04/23/2015

ISBN: 978-1-4969-5805-1 (sc)
ISBN: 978-1-4969-5806-8 (e)

Library of Congress Control Number: 2014922106

Print information available on the last page

DEDICATION

To a great teacher of teachers, for his development
of Radiology in Nigeria and Africa.
Professor Benjamin. C. Umerah (1935-2012), Professor of Radiology,
Department of Radiation Medicine, College of Medicine,
University of Nigeria, Enugu Campus and Consultant
Radiologist, University of Nigeria Teaching Hospital, Enugu, Nigeria

ACKNOWLEDGEMENT

The message in the light was to strive for the truth and to always struggle to improve as well as to pass on the knowledge and light to younger generations. This light is manifested in this small work. Ugwueze Augustine Onwuamaeze, my loving brother, father-figure, mentor and exciting friend showed me this light of how to live right. Thank you. I am also exceedingly grateful to your loving wife, Nneoma Joan Nkechinyere Eze and your wonderful nuclear family for the lavish love, great understanding, bonding, and readiness to accept fault and correction, and extreme charity sometimes to a fault. To ChukwuEmeka Augustine Eze, Ikenna Eze, Chinyere Eze, Chigozie Eze and Amarachukwu Eze, I say thank you for your support and love and living to quickly forgive so that the family love may flourish.

My deep gratitude goes to Professor R. O. Ofoegbu of the Department of Surgery, University of Benin, Benin City for creating the culture of determination to achieve perfection in quality of work and output, his lovely wife Professor Mrs Felicia I. Ofoegbu and children, Bibian, Chichi, Hadrain, Stephany, Theresa and Chizoba. Thank you for your steadfast love, loving kindness and support even in the face of many of my shortcomings.

My love for Radiology was motivated by the excellent work of Dr Nwaka and Dr LBO Benka-Coker both of St. Bridget X ray centre, Benin City and Dr Akamagwuna of Benin Radiological Services, Benin City for supporting creativity in radiology. All these had earlier worked at the Department of Radiology, University of Benin, Benin City, Nigeria. Professor S.O. Mgbor of Hansa Clinic, Enugu and Department of Radiology, University of Nigeria, Enugu Campus/University of Nigeria Teaching Hospital (UNTH), Enugu encouraged me to venture to the exciting world of Radiology. He made it clear that radiology is the field of medicine where academics is on fire! To you all I will ever remain grateful.

As a resident, the fire of academic radiology was ignited by Dr U.S Enukegwu, Dr T.T Marchie, Dr A.A Adeyekun, Dr A. O. Akhigbe, Dr V. Ajiduah (nee Bekederemo) and late Professor Odita, all of the University of Benin Teaching Hospital, Benin City. This fire was kindled by Professor SB Lagundoye of the Department of Radiology University of Ibadan/ University College Hospital, Ibadan and Professor Umerah of the Department of Radiology, University of Nigeria, Enugu Campus during the uncountable times we as residents, have been made to sit round them and be taught radiology in the most exposing and exciting manner. Other teachers of whom I remain indebted are: Professor D.A Nzeh of the University of Ilorin, Ilorin, Professor Adetiloye of the Obafemi Awolowo University Teaching Hospital, Ile-Ife; Professor SO Mgbor and Professor Ifeoma Okoye, both of the University of Nigeria/UNTH, Enugu; Professor A.O Ogunseyinde, Professor Obajimi and Dr Adeyinka, all of the University College Hospital, Ibadan, Professor G.O.G Awosanya of the University of Lagos/ Lagos University Teaching Hospital (LUTH), and others too numerous to mention in this small space. Professor AA Tahir of University of Maiduguri Teaching Hospital, Maiduguri, Nigeria. I remain grateful to you all.

I wish to thank my colleagues, Professor Obiora C. Okpala, Dr (Mrs) Chisolum Okafor, Dr Michael Aronu, Dr EO. Ajekwenu, Dr Ukamaka Ebubedike and Dr Eric Umeh all of the Department of Radiology, Nnamdi Azikiwe University Nnewi campus/Nnamdi Azikiwe University Teaching Hospital, Nnewi for their encouragements and constructive criticisms.

I wish to thank present Vice Chancellor of Nnamdi Azikiwe University, Awka, Professor Joseph Ahaneku for creating conducive atmosphere for academic activities in the University. I acknowledge the past and present principal officers of our University and College for also creating conducive atmosphere for academic activities at Nnamdi Azikiwe University, Nnewi Campus. Among these are the following Professors; Boniface Egboka, Ilochi Okafor, Okey Ikpeze, Clement C. Ezechukwu, Joseph IB Adinma, Stanley Anyanwu, Joseph Ikechebelu, Sabastine NN. Nwosu, MC Nwosu, Ebele F. Ugochukwu, Andrew N. Osigwe, Richards Uwakwe, Alexander Nwofor, Anthony Igwegbe, SNN Nwosu, Robinson Ofiaeli, JC Orakwe, Christian C. Ibeh, Amobi Linus Ilika, P.U. Ele, Felix E. Emele, Prince C. Unekwe, Nworah J.A. Obiechina, Obiora. C Okpala and Gerald O. Udigwe and other important persons but too numerous to enter in this small space.

My colleagues who have shown challenging interest in radiology and who in one way or the other made us to go the extra mile in Radiology practice, I say thank you. Some of them whom I find it difficult not to mention their names are Drs Egbue, KC Oranusi, JKC Emejulu, Titus O. Chukwuanukwu and Anthony I. Ugezu of Department of Surgery, Drs John Chukwuka, Thomas O. Ulasi, Wilson C. Igwe and Joy C. Ebenebe of Department of Paediatrics, Drs IV Onyirioha, Comfort N. Akujobi, Daniel C.D. Anyiam and Dr CO Ukah of Department of pathology, Drs Betrand Obi Nwosu, Charles I. Okafor of Department of Obstetrics and Gynaecology, Drs Echendu Adinma, F.O. Emelumadu, Simon A. Nwabueze and ACN. Okaro of Department of Community Medicine, Drs Kingsley C. Chilaka, John O. Ogamba, O.J. Afonne, O.J. Elo C. Ilo of Department of Pharmacology, Dr. Godswill A. Nnaji of Department of Family Medicine, Drs O. Kalu, G. Ahaneku, E.I. Onwubuya, Arthur Ebelenna Anyabolu, O.C. Oguejiofor, C.U. Osuji, M.N. Nwosu, C.U. Odenigbo and Lasbrey Asomugha of the Department of Medicine of the Department of Medicine all of Nnamdi Azikiwe University Teaching Hospital, Nnewi, Anambra State.

I also wish to thank the staff of Institute of Diagnostic and Interventional Radiology, University Hospital, Zurich, Switzerland, for their support during the period that I was there, particularly Professor Juerg Hodler, Professor Thomas Pfammatter and Professor Hatem Alkhadi.

To the Radiology Residents and medical students whom I have taught at the University of Benin/ University of Benin Teaching Hospital, Benin City, Ambrose Alli University, Ekpoma/ Irrua Specialist Teaching Hospital, Irrua, Nnamdi Azikiwe University/ Nnamdi Azikiwe University Teaching Hospital, Nnewi Campus and at update courses for Residents in Nigerian Nigerian postgraduate medical college the West African sub-region, I thank you for being "yourselves" that encouraged me to labour hard to find out how to make the understanding of Radiology easier.

I am also very grateful to the resident doctors in the Radiology at the Department of Nnamdi Azikiwe University Teaching Hospital, Nnewi, for their prompt and accurate corrections of typographical errors in the manuscript and their useful suggestions and they include Dr Obi Adaeze C, Dr Okam Ikenna, Dr Obilo Kingsley, Dr Obieje Kanayo, Dr Anajuba Odira, Dr Uzukwu Ifenayi, Dr Elendu Collins, Dr Umeokafor Chijioke, Dr Ike Chinelo and Dr Brenda Nwammuo.

I thank Dr Darlington Obi of Department of Community Health, Nnamdi Azikiwe University Teaching Hospital, Nnewi, for his love at difficult times. To the loving staff of the Radiology Department, NAUTH, Nnewi, I say thank you and the unforgettable of these are Mrs Ikegwuonu NC, Mrs Oranye Virginia, Mrs Mgboji Mary, Mr Onyedikachi Chukwuma, Mr Adejo Thomas, Eze Precious, and others too numerous to mentioned in this small space. I am also grateful to Mr Eze Cletus of College of Medicine, University of Lagos, Dr Christian C Nzotta and Anthony Ugwu of Department of Radiography, Nnamdi Azikiwe University, Nnewi Campus for their steadfast love.

Sir Anthony and Lady Medline Nwabueze and family, Mr Isaac and Mrs Esther Asomgba, Madam Christiana Oyidiya Eze, Engr and Mrs Fabian Anyaogu, I remain indebted to your love and sacrifices. I also thank my brothers and sisters who one way or the other missed my love and sometimes responsibilities to them while I laboured to write this book and these include Anayo Hyginus Eze, Ozoemenam Ugochukwu and Theresa Eze, Mrs Adaobi Mmaduabuch (nee Eze), Chinedu Anthony Nwabueze, Chigozie Ndubisi Asomgba, Tobechukwu Anyaogu, Obianuju Anyaogu, Chibuike Mgbor, Mr and Mrs Cosmos Nwosu and their lovely triplets, Paulina Alaneme, Ifechukwu Ojukwu, Onyinyechukwu Obidiro, Miss Ijeoma Janeth Okafor, Ijeoma Beatice Ezeanyaoha and others too numerous to include in this small space, I am grateful for your sacrifices while I laboured to write this book. I thank Rev. Fr Joseph Alaekwe, Rev. Fr. Oberenwa Jesus of Abbah town, Rev. Fr. Cyril Duru for always remembering me at the masses. I am also grateful to Pastor Isaac, Pastor Basil and Pastor John for their spiritual assistance at various times when they had interactions with my family through my sister, Evangelist Esther Asomgba.

My late father, Nze Anthony Ezeagwula Ezerioha, my late mother, Mrs Angelina Mgbeke Eze, and late aunt, Mama Nkeukwu Chiekasi Ezerioha, I thank you for your lavish love to us, our friends and visitors and for teaching us that the only thing worthy of dying for is love for the human person. You thought us how to treat people as human beings and as kings! Thank you for teaching us how to build people and not houses! Thank you for teaching us how to feed people and not how to feed the bank and bankers!

I thank Professor SB. Lagundoye for critically reviewing the book and taking me back to the drawing board many times. To Professor GOG Awosanya, who spared his time at odd hours to go through the book and write the forward, I am ever grateful for your faith in me and your bridge-building rather than digging holes! I thank Dr S.U. Eluehike for painstakingly going through the manuscript many times and making many critical corrections and Miss Hope Oneshevwe Ufuoma for typing the manuscript.

My loving wife Ijeoma and children, Chisom, Ifeoma, Blessing and Ebuka, I remain encouraged by your extreme humility, love and support when I kept late at night in the office or had to cut short your due share of affection and agape love while writing this book. Thank you.

Kenneth C. Eze

PREFACE

The backbone of this book was written to teach enthusiastic and knowledge-hungry Resident Doctors in Radiology at different levels of training whom I could not resist their continuous calls for detailed and yet simplified materials for preparation for seminars and examinations. The search to provide a guide that could help Residents in preparing for examination in order to reduce my trip to various centres where I travelled to discuss with Resident Doctors on tutorials was the critical impetus to write this book.

The aims of this book are:
1. To provide a simple compact book for the study and preparation for the various postgraduate fellowship examinations in radiology.
2. To provide a guide to residents in radiology and residents from other departments on clinical posting to various Radiology Department for their early understanding of radiology.
3. To provide a brief summary of radiological features of common diseases for teachers and examiners in radiology who need quick reference for radiological features of diseases both for teaching purposes and examinations.

All attempts have been made to keep the book simple, concise and straight to the point. Topics which are unavailable in this book may be available in other titles by the author. The book will be updated periodically. Comments and observations are welcome from students, residents and their teachers.

KC Eze

FOREWORD

The scope of imaging continues to widen so much so that concerted efforts should be made at guiding radiology residents in training. The aims of the book are to guide radiology residents in their approach at answering questions, increase their information base and to assist in film reporting. This effort has been in conception for over ten years. This guidebook is concise and descriptive. The author's style is smooth.

As radiology cuts across all the fields of medicine, this book is also a vital tool for residents in all the clinical departments. It is hoped that the information contained therein will be of immense benefit for residents in their preparation for the Fellowship Examinations and in passing down radiology information to medical students.

Teachers and examiners in radiology and clinical departments will also find the book very useful for their marking scheme for the discussed hot topics.

This book is also recommended for all those who are seeking for accurate understanding of the field of Radiology. The medico-legal aspects will be of great interest to emergency room clinicians, pathologists, paediatricians, physicians, surgeons, gynaecologists, forensic practitioners in all fields, administrators and the legal profession!

Professor G.O.G. Awosanya
Provost, College of Medicine,
Lagos State University, Ikeja, Lagos.
Formerly, Head of Department of Radiology,
Lagos State University Teaching Hospital and Lagos State University, Ikeja, Lagos
Formerly, Head of Department of Radiodiagnosis,
Lagos University Teaching Hospital (LUTH), Idi-Araba,
and University of Lagos, Lagos, Nigeria

CONTENTS

CHAPTER 1

MUSCULOSKELETAL SYSTEM

1.1   RADIOLOGY OF RICKETS

Definition
Rickets is a disease caused by lack of vitamin D in children (the immature or growing skeleton) leading to failure of mineralization of the bone (addition of calcium and phosphate to the bone).

Sources of Vitamin D
1.   Direct exposure to sunlight
Direct exposure of the skin to sunlight, particularly ultraviolet rays of wavelength (l) in the range of 296 – 310 nm, that is present in the sunlight. The rays are too weak to pass through house window glass, tree shade, car window glass and protective clothing of even thin fabrics.
Pigmentation of skin of black-skinned children also leads to inadequate penetration of ultraviolet rays. Therefore, to be effective, the exposure of skin must be *direct* to the sunlight; and for adequate effect, the exposure should be for a sufficient length of time.

2.   Diet: Especially fatty meat.

Pathogenesis
Cholecalciferol (vitamin D) absorbed from the gut or derived from the result of effects of *direct sunlight on skin* is transported to the liver where it is hydroxylated to 25–hydroxycholecalciferol (25– HCC). This is transported to the kidney where, in the proximal convoluted tubules in the cortex of the kidney, it is further hydroxylated to 1, 25-dihydroxycholecalciferol (1, 25-DHCC). The 1, 25-DHCC produced in the kidney is called vitamin D3 and is the active metabolite of vitamin D.

Actions of vitamin D (D$_3$) in bone metabolism
Vitamin D acts both as a hormone and as a vitamin.

Major Functions
Mobilization of calcium and phosphorus from the bone
This requires the presence of both 1, 25-DHCC (D$_3$) and parathormone. The aim is to maintain normal serum calcium level. The calcium in the breast milk is independent of maternal dietary calcium and vitamin D.
Promotion of mineralization and maturation of the bone

1

Minor Actions

Absorption of calcium and phosphorus is promoted in the intestines by 1, 25-DHCC.

It affects the kidney function directly (on proximal convoluted tubules of the renal cortex) or indirectly (by stimulating the production of 24, 25-Dihydroxycholecalciferol (24, 25-HCC) which has a negative feedback effect. These limit the production of 1, 25-DHCC.

It acts on receptors in other organs like the pituitary gland, placenta and breast causing them to reflect the increased demand for calcium that may occurs during pregnancy, lactation and growth.

Causes of Rickets

Note that various *causes of Rickets* have been separately classified as separate diseases. Deficiency of vitamin D results only when there is both a lack of adequate direct exposure to sunlight and dietary deficiency from inadequate intake, malabsorption and other causes. This is because the body can produce an adequate amount of vitamin D from the action of ultraviolet light on skin alone.

A. Abnormality in the metabolism of vitamin D

This is also associated with hyperparathyroidism.

1. Vitamin deficiency
   a. Lack of adequate dietary intake of vitamin D
   b. Lack of direct exposure to sunlight
   c. Malabsorption of the vitamin. This is seen in pancreatic disease, biliary disease, steatorrhoea, Coeliac disease, inflammatory bowel disease such as ulcerative colitis and Crohn's disease, post-gastrectomy and scleroderma
   (Note that these three factors listed above cause over 95 percent of the cases of rickets. The others are rare).

2. Defective hydroxylation
   i. Liver diseases
      Hepatitis, cirrhosis of the liver, metastasis and carcinoma
   ii. Anticonvulsant therapy
      There is induction of enzymes that promote increased degradation of the active metabolite of vitamin D. such drugs include phenytoin and dilantin. (Rifampicin and glutethimide also have the same effect).

3. Defective hydroxylation in the kidney
   i. Chronic renal failure
   ii. Nephrosclerosis
   iii. Vitamin D-resistant rickets (now separately classified as a disease entity).

B. Abnormality in the metabolism of phosphates

This is not associated with hyperparathyroidism.
   1. Deficiency of phosphate
      i. Severe malabsorption states
      ii. Parenteral hyperalimentation
      iii. Ingestion of aluminium salts (especially antacids) that form insoluble complex with phosphates
      iv. Malabsorption of phosphates in the intestines

2. Disorder in renal tubular reabsorption of phosphates
3. Hypophosphatasia
4. Hypophosphataemia in some non endocrine tumours

C. Calcium deficiency
1. Malabsorption
2. Intake of substances forming chelates with calcium
3. Milk-free diet (rare)

Clinical Features
Irritability, bone pain, tenderness, swelling of wrists, knees and ankles, delayed dentition, delayed crawling and walking, rickety / rachitic rosary (ribs), bowlegs, knock-knees, windswept deformity, craniotabes, pectus carinatum/excavatum and breathing difficulty.

Areas of the body most affected
Areas of rapid growth and weight bearing are most commonly affected and thus should be the first to be examined radiologically. These include the knees, wrists and ankles.

Necessary Tests
Plain x-ray, serum phosphatase, serum calcium and serum alkaline phosphatase.

Radiological Features
This is the same in all types of rickets but it may vary in severity and location. The findings include:

Changes at the growth plate and cortex
Reduction in the thickness and density of the zone of provisional calcification: The earliest changes as bone calcification starts reducing is reduction in the thickness and density of zone of provisional calcification, which is the zone where calcium is preferential laid down in the bone by the action of vitamin D.
Loss of zone of provisional calcification: As the condition progresses, the density of the zone of provisional calcification will be lost completely. Still this is at the early changes of rickets.

Fraying: Thread-like shadows like brushes extending from metaphysis to epiphysis. It represents irregularly arranged and irregularly calcified osteoids and trabecullae (figure 1.11).
Small underdeveloped and osteopaenic epiphysis: This represents further effect of lack of calcium on the bone, which makes it appear osteopaenic and small because the full extent of the bone cannot be seen by the unaided eye due to marked osteopaenia in a part of bone that was not normally very dense.
Cupping: Increased weight-bearing results in depression of the metaphysis due to the effect of weight on weak uncalcified osteoids that make up the metaphysis.
Splaying: Widening of the metaphysis due to weight bearing and cupping (figure 1.11).

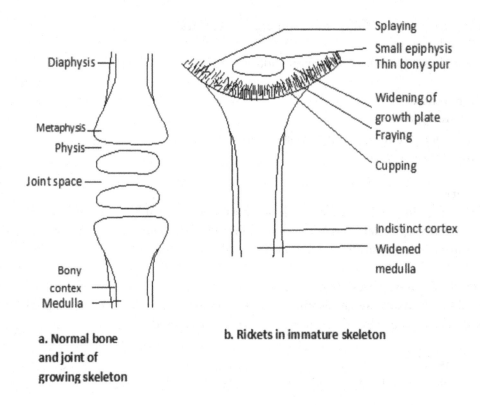

Figure 1.11: Diagram of bone ends around a joint illustrating in **a**. Normal growing skeleton and **b**. Rickets.

Apparent widening of the growth plate (physis): Lack of calcification of metaphyseal bone most adjacent to radiolucent growth plate (zone of provisional calcification) and the presence of excess uncalcified osteoids at the metaphysis render it to appear radiolucent and in continuity with the radiolucent growth plate cause it to then appear widened.

Thin cortical bony spurs at metaphyseal margins: These extend from the metaphysis to surround the excess uncalcified asteroids.

Lack of distinctiveness or poor definition of the cortex: It is caused by irregular calcification of the cortex and presence of excess unqualified sub-periosteal osteoids.

Loss of corticomedullary junction: Lack of distinctiveness of cortex also due to excess uncalcified osteoid of cortex adjacent to the medulla leads to loss of corticomedullary distinction.

Looser's zone (uncommon). This is fracture that is incompletely healed by uncalcified osteoids. This appears as area of lucency with sclerotic margin.

Haziness of cortical margin of epiphysis: This is due to irregular calcification of the cortex.

Rickety or rachitic rosary: Excess accumulation of uncalcified osteoids at the ribs where the cortical bones meet the cartilaginous part of the rib leading to abnormally enlarged costochondral junctions appearing like beads of rosary.

Changes due to bone softening

Bowing of long bones: This occurs at the diaphysis of long bones especially tibia, fibula and femur.

Genu valgum deformity: It is also known as knock-knee. This is a K-shaped appearance of the knees due to the fact that one knee is normal and straight while there is lateral angulation of the tibia, fibula and occasionally the femur of the other lower limb at the knee.

Genu varum deformity: The lower limb is bowed with the apex of the curvature at the knees (bowleg).

Windswept deformity: Medial bowing of one knee with lateral bowing of the other knee. This appears as a limb bend by blowing wind at the position of the knees.

Changes in the chest

Harrison's Sulcus: Softened ribs lead to in-drawing of lower part of the chest wallby respiratory muscles of the chest. It may contribute to respiratory difficulty.

Rickety or rachitic rosary: This is accumulated excess uncalcified osteoids at the costochondral junctions forming bead-like masses.

Biconcave vertebral bodies (codfish vertebrae): This is grooved depression of the vertebral end plates (margins of the vertebra) above and below giving it a biconcave appearance. It is equivalent to cupping of metaphysis as the vertebral end-plate (inferior and superior margins of vertebra) is the equivalence of the metaphysis. The effect is due to severe osteopaenia of the vertebrae making the incompressible intervertebral discs to put pressure of the vertebral margins and depress the weak porous bones.

Vertebral alignment deformities: Thoracic scoliosis, kyphosis and kyphoscoliosis, wedge collapse, multiple vertebral fracture and vertebral plana.

Deformities of the sternum and chest: These are *pectus carinatum* (pigeon chest) or *pectus excavatum* (funnel chest). In serious cases, these leads to respiratory difficulty as age advances.

Changes in the skull

Craniotabes: Thin skull bone with accumulation of excess uncalcified osteoid in frontal and parietal bones as a result of flattening of the occiput.

Platybasia or basilar invagination: This is due to the weak skull bones at the base of the skull, the weight of the head as a load presses the skull on atlas and axis. The softened skull bone invaginates at the foramen magnum.

Frontal bossing: Excess piling of osteoid at frontal bone.

Parietal bossing: Excess piling of osteoids at parietal bone.

Closing up of basal foramina: This is seen at the calvarium and base of the skull caused by excess uncalcified (soft) osteoid. This leads to cranial nerve entrapments with resultant deafness, blindness and nerve paralysis.

Widening of sutures in infants: Severe osteopaenia leads to real and apparent widening of sutures in infants with delay in their fusion.

Dental abnormalities: This is seen with malocclusion.

Changes at the pelvis

Coxa vara deformity, triradiate pelvis and pelvic asymmetry

Slipped femoral capital epiphysis (other epiphyses may rarely slip)

General changes

Generalised osteopaenia: Decreased bone density. This is uncommon.

Retarded bone maturation: There is delay in appearance and late fusion of ossification centres.

Coarse trabecular pattern: There is resorption of secondary trabeculae laving behind the coarse-appearing trabecullae of the bone due to osteopaenia.

Spontaneous fractures in low birth weight infants (<1000g at 28 weeks gestation)*:* This presents with respiratory difficulty due to weak, painful and tender ribs. It must be differentiated from birth injury, non-accidental injury (battered baby syndrome) and osteogenesis imperfecta.

Fractures in long-standing cases: This is seen in older infants and may present with bony deformities.

Changes due to treatment

Patchy sclerosis of metaphysis: This occurs when there is incomplete or inadequate treatment as calcium deposition of the bone becomes incomplete.

Dense transverse white line: This appears at zone of provisional calcification due to its re-appearance.

Periosteal reaction: This could be irregular.

Differential diagnosis

Scurvy, hypophosphatasia, vitamin D-resistant rickets (familial type, acquired type and the type associated with renal tubular disorder), fibrogenesis imperfecta ossium, familial hyperphosphataemia metaphyseal dysplasia, osteogenesis imperfecta (tarda) and battered baby syndrome.

(Adam & Dixon, 2008; Dahnert, 2011; Sutton, 2003; Swischuk, 2004; Palmer & Reeder, 2001).

References

1. States LJ. Imaging of rachitic bone. Endocr Dev 2003;6:80-92.
2. Ecklund K, Doria AS, Jaramillo D. Rickets on MR images. Pediatr Radiol 1999;29:673-5.
3. Rauch F. The rachitic bone. Endocr Dev 2003;6:69-79.
4. Gilchrest BA. Sun exposure and vitamin D sufficiency. Am J Clin Nutr 2008; 88:570S-577S.
5. Rennie LM, Beattie TF, Wilkinson AG, Crofton P, Bath LE. Incidental radiological diagnosis of rickets. Emerg Med J 2005; 22:534-7.
6. Ward LM, Gaboury I, Ladhani M, Zlotkin S. Vitamin D-deficiency rickets among children in Canada. CMAJ 2007;177:161-6
7. Haworth JC, Dilling LA. Vitamin-D-deficient rickets in Manitoba, 1972-84. CMAJ 1986;134237-41.
8. Nagi NA. Vitamin D deficiency rickets in malnourished children. J Trop Med Hyg 1972;75:251-4.
9. el Hag AI, Karrar ZA. Nutritional vitamin D deficiency rickets in Sudanese children. Ann Trop Paediatr 1995;15:69-76.
10. Opie WH, Muller CJ, Kamfer H. The diagnosis of vitamin D deficiency rickets. Pediatr Radiol 1975;3:105-10.

1.2   OSTEOMYELITIS

Definition: This is defined as inflammation of the bone and osteoid as a result of infection. The infection is at the marrow cavity.

Why osteomyelitis?
The importance of inclusion of osteomyelitis in this book stems from the fact that it is very difficult to diagnose at the early stages when treatment is promising and very difficult to treat at late stages when diagnosis is unproblematic. Even with the present era of antibiotics and improved surgical techniques, the infectious organisms are frequently very difficult, and sometimes impossible to eradicate. Also, even though it is a benign condition, its chronic stages could connote an impression of incurable disease. Therefore, early diagnosis and adequate treatment of acute stages when treatment is possible is critical in dealing with this disease.

Which bones are affected?
1. Lower limbs 70% (Femur 25%, tibia 32%, fibula 7%, bones of the foot 3%, knee joint 1%.
2. Upper limbs 20% (affecting humerus 11%, radius and ulna 8%, bones of the hand 1%.
3. Other bones (Pelvis including sacroiliac joints 5%, ribs 2.5%, jaw 0.5%, clavicle 0.5%, other sites 3.5%).

Where in the bone?
1. Metaphysis due to rich blood supply with slow-flowing sinusoids of metaphyseal spongiosa leading to foci of haematogenous infections in this area.
2. In sickle cell disease, diaphysis of the long bones is affected by Salmonella infection due to repeated bone infarction.

Disc spaces are involved in the spine with disc oedema and disc fluid collection.

Route of Spread
This is from:
1. Haematogenous spread from distant foci from the skin, genitourinary lung and soft tissue infection (monomicrobial). Patients with diabetes mellitus due to vascular compromise and patients with HIV/AIDS due to immune compromise have increased propensity to develop osteomyelitis.
2. Direct invasion from infected wound or fracture site (polymicrobial).
3. Spread from infected joint (this is less than haematogenous spread).

Offending bacterial organisms
Adult: *Staphylococcus aureus* (60%-90%) more common in adults.
Children: *Streptococci, Staph aureus, Escherichia coli*, pneumococci, etc.
Sickle cell anaemia: Salmonella species.
Drug addicts: *Pseudomonas, Klebsiella, Enterobacteriaceae.*
Metallic prosthetic implants: This is caused by indolent organisms particularly Staphylococci (coagulase-negative), *propionibacterium*
Other organisms such as fungus, virus and tuberculosis could be involved but the infections from these agents are slower and less destructive. Fungal infections simulate malignancies while tuberculous

infections have a varying pattern from slow to aggressive but with frequently recurrence pattern. However laboratory identification of the organism is the final arbiter.

Types of Osteomyelitis:
1. *Acute osteomyelitis*
2. *Chronic osteomyelitis*
3. *Subacute osteomyelitis*

Blood supply to the bones
1. *Nutrient artery.* It supplies the marrow and inner cortex and is the major blood supply throughout life.
2. *Periosteal artery. It* supplies the outer cortex
3. *Metaphyseal, epiphyseal arteries and transphyseal arteries. They supply* the epiphysis and metaphysis. Anastomosis between them occurs and that with the other vessels occasionally occurs.

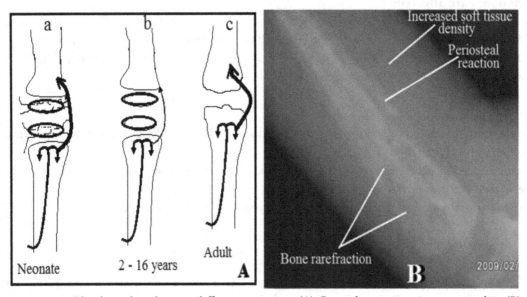

Figure 1.21: Blood supply to bone in different age groups (A). Bone changes in acute osteomyelitis (B).

In Infants
Vessels from the different arteries penetrate the epiphyseal plate in both directions. Metaphyseal infection can spread to the epiphysis and then to the joint leading to septic arthritis. The periosteum is loosely bound and pus can elevate it and extend to the shaft of bone or the joint space, (figure 1.21A).

In Childhood: Between 2 – 16 years, very few vessels cross the epiphyseal plate. The periosteum is still loosely bound relative to the adult. Very few or no metaphyseal vessels cross the growth plate. Osteomyelitis does not frequently lead to septic arthritis or vice versa. This is nature's way of preservation of joints against septic arthritis since osteomyelitis which is common in this age group will not frequently lead to septic arthritis, (figure 1.21A).

Adult: After epiphyseal plate has fused, metaphyseal and epiphyseal vessel once again become connected with each other. Osteomyelitis of the metaphysis frequently leads to septic arthritis and vice versa. The periosteum is well bound and infection of the bone through metaphyseal vessel is reduced, (figure 1.21A).

Imaging of osteomyelitis

Radiographic findings lag behind clinical symptoms and pathological findings by 10 – 14 days. Radiographic findings lag behind ultrasound finding by several days.

However, colour Doppler flow detection of abscess lags behind clinical symptoms by 4 days. Subperiosteal abscess appears as spindle-shaped fluid collection along the cortex of bone and has either decreased or increased echogenicity. In colour Doppler flow studies, this area of pus collection will be seen as avascular periosteal mass with peripheral hyperaemia. Imaging features lag behind clinical improvement when treated with appropriate and sensitive antibiotics.

Radiological Features of Acute Osteomyelitis
Plain radiography

1. *Increase in soft tissue density due to deep soft tissue swelling* or oedema (3-10 days). This is adjacent to the bone and site involved by the osteomyelitis.
2. *Blurring of adjacent fat planes.* Soft tissue swelling and oedema may also appear as blurring of fat planes.
3. *Osteopenia.* This is due to permeative osteolysis usually involving the affected metaphysis but also lysis of medullary trabeculae (10 – 14 days) of other affected bones. (often metaphyseal in children).
4. Cortical irregularities or *bone rarefaction*: These are areas of focal loss of cortex due to multiple small cortical lytic changes. *Bony rarefaction* is due to hyperaemia causing intracortical fissuring and multiple small cortical lucencies.
5. *Endosteal erosions.* In the acute osteomyelitis cortical irregularities affecting the endosteal bones appear as endosteal erosions and are caused by lysis of adjacent trabecular to the medulla where the osteomyelitis is seated.
6. *Periosteal reaction.*
   This is observed as variable degrees and types of opacities superficial to and paralleling the cortex of the bone. In acute pyogenic osteomyelitis it is due to periosteal elevation by fluid which tracked from the medulla, traversing the cortex via the Haversian canal. The fluid results from the initial oedema following medullary inflammation. The elevated periosteum is only visualised in the plain radiograph when it has ossified after about 10 to 14 days and for this reason there is a time lag before its identification using plain radiography but it could be visualised with ultrasound before its ossification. There are various appearances of periosteal reaction in osteomyelitis.
   i. *Thread-like, pencil-like or superficial thin line:* This is close to and paralleling the outer cortex and is the commonest type of periosteal elevation. It is an elevated periosteum due to subperiosteal fluid collection and denotes osteomyelitis in the presence of infection. This is thin and fine in adult. When seen bilaterally in neonates it is usually physiological due to rapid growth with elevation of loosely attached periosteum (figure 1.21 B).
   ii. *Exuberant periosteal reaction*: This is abundant periosteal new bone most commonly observed in neonates and young children. It is also seen is Caffey's disease, scurvy due to intermittent subperiosteal bleeding and in bone metastasis from bladder carcinoma.
   iii. *Fluffy periosteal reaction:* Periosteal reactions can also appear as fluffy appearance at the outer cortex. It is due to subacute, inadequately or low virulence pyogenic infections such as salmonella spp., shigella spp., campylobacter spp., Chlamydia trachomatis or Neisseria

gonorrheae. It is observed in chronic infections such as fungal infection or it may also be due to repeated trauma, psoriatic arthropathy and Reiter's syndrome.

iv. *Radiating periosteal reaction: Spiculated, 'Sun-ray', 'sunburst' or hair-on-end appearance* types of periosteal reaction may also be observed and are caused by rapid bone destruction within a small area. This may also be seen in osteosarcoma or Ewing's sarcoma.

v. *'Laminated', 'multilaminar', 'lamellar' or onion-peel periosteal reaction:* Laminated', 'multilaminar' and 'lamellar' appearances are due to repetition of interval of rapid destructive process with period of quiescence occurring in pyogenic or other bone infections. For this reason they are also called *interrupted periosteal reaction.* They are also observed in sickle cell disease associated with increased bone destruction. Tumours, vitamin A toxicity, leukaemia, eosinophilic granuloma, healing stage of Langerhans cell histiocytosis and neuroblastoma could have similar appearance. Lamella appearance could be physiologic in younger children. When osteomyelitis remains untreated, there may be 'onion-peel' appearance of periosteal reaction. It is also observed in Ewing's sarcoma and osteosarcoma.

vi. *Solid periosteal reactions:* Solid and thick periosteal reaction is observed in chronic infections such as tuberculosis or fungal infections. Other causes are eosinophilic granuloma, osteoid osteoma and low grade chondrosarcoma.

vii. *Codman's triangle:* This is caused by interruption of periosteal reaction by rapid bone destruction or abscess. It may also be seen in osteosarcoma, Ewing's sarcoma, and due to haemorrhage or metastases.

viii. *Solid cloaking periosteal reaction:* This is observed in chronic infections such fungal and tuberculous infection. It is also observed in storage diseases such as mucolipidosis type II and venous stasis.

ix. *Disorganised periosteal reaction:* This is commonly seen in chronic osteomyelitis. It is also seen in inadequacy stabilised fracture, pathological fracture, resolving haematoma and lymphoma.

x. *Dense periosteal reaction.* This is thick and dense periosteal reaction simulating extensive sclerosis observed in subacute and chronic infections such as chronic granulomatous disease of the childhood and sclerosing osteomyelitis of Garé. It is also observed in osteoid osteoma and in osteosarcoma.

7. *Increase in density of adjacent joint:* Due to joint effusion and haemorrhage within the joint.

8. *Cellulitis:* This is soft tissue infection with inflammation, oedema, microabscess, haemorrhage and sometimes abscess formation. It is a pointer of osteomyelitis and could be the point of entry of the infection.

MRI Findings

1. Alteration of the normal marrow signal intensity due to inflammatory oedema (earliest finding). This becomes low or intermediate on T1-weighted sequence and high on fat-suppressed T2-weighted sequence.

2. Hyperintense halo close and contiguous to the cortex signify subperiosteal infective inflammation.

3. Periosteal reactions: This is seen earlier than in plain films.

4. High signal occurring from reactive oedema on T2-weighted sequences often overestimates the extent of the infection.

CT Findings
1. Increased density of medullary cavity as the fat becomes replaced by oedema.
2. Blurring of adjacent fat planes.

Sonography

Subtle permeating changes of the cortex permit the passage of sound waves into the bone marrow even through what appears to be an intact cortex allowing for sonographic imaging of the bone in osteomyelitis. Sonography is highly useful in children and infants as it can localise the seat and extent of the disease in the affected site.
1. One of the earliest findings is subperiosteal echo-free lines beneath the line that denotes the reflective periosteum signifying periosteal oedema and periosteal thickening.
2. Local soft tissue oedema/swelling may also be demonstrated especially when comparison is made with the contralateral side. The whole circumference of the bone must be examined and thus involves turning the patient or putting in a position where this is possible.
3. Other sonographic findings in children in acute osteomyelitis include subperiosteal fluid or abscess collection.
4. Sonography will also demonstrate abscess within the muscle or soft tissue which acts as a pointer to osteomyelitis.
5. Ultrasound will demonstrate intra-articular fluid collection when osteomyelitis is adjacent to an infected joint particularly the knee or elbow joint. Ultrasound however will not differentiate between transudate, exudates, blood or pus and joint aspiration is required for this confirmation and to exclude infection, microscopy culture and sensitivity is the arbiter.

Doppler sonography

Findings elicited by Power Doppler sonography include:
1. Hyperaemia around subperiosteal abscess
2. Congestion of vessels around the area of inflammation
3. Affectation of small vessels by thrombosis caused by abscess formation.

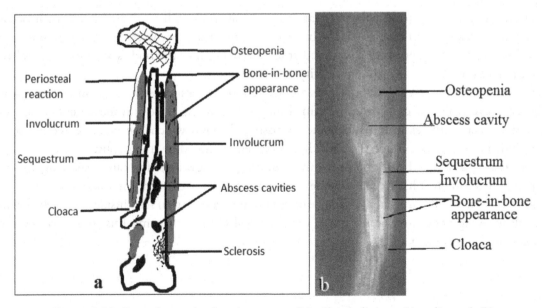

Figure 1.22: Bone changes in chronic osteomyelitis. Sketch diagram (a), radiograph (b).

Radiological Features of Chronic Osteomyelitis

1. *Periosteal reaction* observed (after 10 – 14 days).

   Thread-like, superficial thin line: This is close to and paralleling the outer cortex and is the commonest type of periosteal elevation. It is an elevated periosteum due to subperiosteal fluid collection and denotes osteomyelitis in the presence of infection. Periosteal reaction is thin and fine in adult but exuberant in neonates and children. Periosteal reactions can also appear as fluffy appearance at the outer cortex.

   Radiating periosteal reaction: Spiculated, 'Sun-ray' or 'sunburst' appearance of periosteal reaction may also be observed and are caused by rapid bone destruction within a small area. This may also be seen in osteosarcoma or Ewing's sarcoma.

   Onion-peel periosteal reaction: When osteomyelitis remains untreated, there may be 'onion-peel' appearance of periosteal reaction. In sickle cell disease there is 'laminated' or 'multilaminar' or 'lamellar' periosteal reaction associated with increased bone destruction. Tumours, vitamin A toxicity, leukaemia and neuroblastoma could have similar appearance. This appearance could be physiologic in younger children.

   Solid periosteal reactions: This is observed in chronic infections such as tuberculosis or fungal infections.

   Codman's triangle: This is caused by interruption of periosteal reaction by rapid bone destruction. It may also be seen in osteosarcoma, Ewing's sarcoma, and due to haemorrhage.

2. *Involucrum* (observed after 3 weeks). This is healthy new bone at the outer cortex. It is abundant, prolific or aggressive in infants and children. It is formed by the elevated periosteum (figure 1.21 a and b).

3. *Sequestrum.* Dead, devitalised bone due to vascular compromise especially involving cortical bone. It is surrounded by the involucrum. It is denser than surrounding healthy living bone or the involucrum. This is because it is no more vascularised and its calcium is not available for mobilization by the body.

4. *Abscess cavities.* Pus collecting in pockets surrounds pieces of dead cortical bone. Abscess is found close to the sequestrum. Pus also helps involucrum formation by elevating the periosteum.

5. *Cloaca.* This is a gap, rent, defect, or tear in the involucrum with corticated margins. It occurs in area of dead periosteum. Cloaca is in reality a sinus tract in the cortex. Cloaca allows pus and sequestra to escape and be extruded from the bone. It is the body's attempt to expel the sequestrum out from the medullary cavity.

6. *Sinus tract/fistula in the soft tissue.* This is a line of communication between the medullary cavity where there is abscess cavity and the skin through the cortical bone and the subcutaneous soft tissue. Tract in the skin and subcutaneous tissues through which the pus and sequestra are extruded or escape to outside the body. It can be demonstrated by sinography.

7. *Sclerosis.* Areas of dead cortical bone with weak irregular new bone formation showing attempt at healing. Usually it has increased bone density than other areas of normal bone.

8. *Bone-in-bone appearance.* The appearance of dead bone (sequestrum) seen inside the newly formed healthy living bone (involucrum). It is diagnostic of chronic osteomyelitis in the evidence of infection (figure 1.22a and b).

9. *Defective modelling of the bone.* When there are areas of bone expansion the bone lose its normal shape and appearance and this is indicative of osteomyelitis. It is frequently caused by bone sclerosis.
10. *Cellulitis and soft tissue abscess.* Areas of cellulitis due to osteomyelitis may progress to soft tissue necrosis, haemorrhage and soft tissue abscess formation. This may lead to affectation of adjacent joints and structure.
11. *Soft tissue calcification.* This may occur at the margins of abscess. Necrotic or haemorrhagic tissues could also calcify.
12. *Joint involvement.* This includes joint effusion, haemorrhage within the joint, destruction of articular cartilage and destruction of juxta-articular bones sometimes with bone ankylosis.

CT scan
1. Periosteal reaction is well demonstrated particularly at later stages of the disease.
2. Small focal areas of loss of cortex.
3. CT is invaluable at defining the full extent of bone cortex destruction
4. CT is invaluable at showing the existence of sequestrum which is critical at classifying the state of osteomyelitis.
5. Areas of soft tissue gas are also shown

MR Imaging
1. On T1 spin echo images, during the interval between acute and chronic osteomyelitis or in subacute infection, the abscess cavity has a low signal core region surrounded by granulation tissue appearing as a peripheral fairly high signal halo giving a typical 'penumbra sign'. Eosinophilic granuloma and chondrosarcoma may have similar appearance and thus are important differential diagnosis.
2. This will also show abscess cavities in soft tissues and muscles which may be pointer to adjacent bone or joint involvement.

Sonography
1. When small abscess cavities coalesce, they may be significant as to be identified by ultrasound.
2. Graded ultrasound compression, Doppler ultrasound and occasionally venography are used for diagnosis of deep venous thrombosis.
3. Radiological and surgical drainage are employed for the treatment of conventional abscesses. While MR or CT studies may be engaged at the planning stages, ultrasound is unsurpassed for guiding percutaneous drainage. Area of bone necrosis should particularly be searched for near the abscess at imaging, and when present should favour open surgical drainage as against radiological aspiration.

Radionuclide studies
Radionuclide scanning is useful as a screening tool for identifying the location and extent of disease. However, technetium monodiphosphonate (^{99m}Tc-MDP) imaging displays high sensitivity but low specificity for osteomyelitis. Other agent may have just the opposite such ^{111}In-labelled white cell which is shown to exhibit high specificity but low sensitivity. However, ^{18}F-FDG PET imaging is believed by many to possess high sensitivity and specificity. Imaging with more than one agent may be the solution to arrive at the best result.

Scintigraphy
This will help in the detection of multifocal osteomyelitis

Subacute (Special Forms of) Osteomyelitis

These are sometimes called subacute osteomyelitis

1. **Brodie's abscess**

   This is a localized form of osteomyelitis, found in the metaphysis. It is a well-defined spherical lucent lesion due to bone destruction and has sclerotic margin. It may have accompanying periosteal reaction. Tunnelling which are finger-like extensions into epiphysis or surrounding bone is the hallmark of infection as opposed to tumour. Brodie's abscess may contain cortical sequestrum within it. The sequestrum of Brodie's abscess enhances on delayed isotope scan and may persist for several months. In subacute infection such as Brodie's abscess, the abscess cavity has a low signal core region surrounded by granulation tissue appearing as a peripheral fairly high signal halo giving a typical 'penumbra sign'. On T2 and STIR images a "double-line sign" is observed representing hyperintense granulation tissue surrounded by low signal sclerosis.

2. **Sclerosing Osteomyelitis of Garre**

   This shows extensive sclerosis without bone destruction. There is focal bulge of thickened sclerotic cortex. The mandible is most commonly affected. The infection is mainly sterile and non-purulent. There is absence of necrosis and the extensive sclerosis is mostly due to low grade and slow aggression of the offending agent. The disease may simulate osteosarcoma or osteoid osteoma but there is absence of frank bone destruction or area of nidus formation within the cortex.

3. **Chronic Granulomatous Disease of Childhood**

   In this inherited immunodeficiency disorder, leucocytes (phagocytes) engulf offending organisms (bacilli) but cannot completely destroy them so that the organisms are weakened but not killed and toxins are still produced. This leads to purulent low grade infection which extensive but slow inflammatory response. Chronic inflammatory process with granuloma formation ensues and brings about widespread small areas of osteolysis (bone destruction) which do not cross the epiphyseal plate. Lesions heal with florid and extensive new bone formation both endosteally and superficially with the end result of the appearance of marked and widespread sclerosis within the involved bone and bone expansion. Many organs are affected in the process in different types but bones (especially long bone) are commonly affected, followed by the spine, ribs and metatarsals. There are purulent collections in skin and subcutaneous tissues as well as suppurative lymph node involvement. It is more common and more severe in boys. There is a recessive X-linked inheritance in 60% while about 40% is inherited as autosomal inheritance.

Complications of Osteomyelitis

1. Pathological fracture
2. Septic embolisation to distant organs/soft tissue abscess.
3. Fistula formation
4. Amyloid disease(secondary amyloidosis).
5. Septic arthritis
6. Growth shortening because of destruction of epiphyseal plate
7. Malignant change (latent period 20 – 30 years).
   - Epithelioma/fibrosarcoma of sinus tract
   - Osteosarcoma
8. Severe deformity when treatment is delayed
9. Loss of a limb through amputation

Differential Diagnosis of Osteomyelitis
Ewing's sarcoma
This is a malignant bone disease, occurring in children with an aggressive medulla-based process that eat away cancellous and cortical bone and producing moth-eaten and permeative changes with wide transition zone. There is onion-peel periosteal reaction and adjacent soft tissue swelling and oedema. Since the patient has fever, the differentiation from osteomyelitis is difficult but the presence of fat globules within the bone marrow or at subperiosteal location on MRI indicates osteomyelitis as opposed to tumour.

Osteosarcoma
This is an aggressive malignant bone tumour characterised by wide transition zone, radiographic cloud-like density around the lesion due to bone formation within the soft tissue, lytic bone destruction, moth-eaten appearance, ossification/calcification within the soft tissue and 'sun-ray'/sunburst' spiculation. Sclerotic and lytic changes exist in the same area of bone. There is absence of sequestra and involucrum and cavitating pulmonary metastases or pneumothorax (due to cavitative and subpleural metastases) is important differentiation criteria from osteomyelitis.

Osteoid osteoma
This is a benign bone lesion characterised by dull pain which later progresses to severe localized pain, which is on and off for several weeks or months, more marked at night. The pain wakes the patient at night and causes sleep deprivation and is relieved by activity and aspirin or other non-steroidal anti-inflammatory drugs. Radiographically, there is a nidus which is a round or oval or spherical area of radiolucency with sclerotic margin. However, extensive sclerosis of the cortex may obscure identification the nidus. There is also a central radiodensity within the oval lucency. There is also sclerotic margin around the oval radiolucency. This is minimal if the tumour is in spongy bone or close to the joint and more marked at the diaphysis of long bones

Cellulitis
Cellulitis is infection of the soft tissues. It is often caused by pyogenic organisms but tuberculosis and fungal agents could also be the offending organisms. In cellulitis, there is soft tissue swelling with increased density of the soft tissue in plain radiography. There is also blurring of fat planes and soft tissue planes. There could be gas in the soft tissue. Bone osteitis as reactive changes may occur. Since the earliest changes of acute osteomyelitis include these soft tissue changes, cellulitis is an important differential diagnosis of osteomyelitis.

Chronic recurrent multifocal osteomyelitis
This is a non-bacterial, noninfectious inflammation of bone characterized by nonspecific auto-inflammatory disease. Findings in radiographs usually include osteolysis and sclerosis involving multiple sites and some of the radiographically diagnosed sites are asymptomatic. On MRI, bone marrow oedema, periostitis and soft tissue inflammation are identified. Treatment is by the use of anti-inflammatory drugs. Metaphyses of the long bones, clavicles, spine and pelvis are more commonly involved as well as mandible, scapula, ribs, sternum, hands and feet. Synovial inflammation, joint effusion and erosion of cartilage and subchondral bone are also seen. However, abscess formation, sequestra, cloaca formation and sinus tracts are more frequently observed in bacterial osteomyelitis. Other deferential diagnoses of osteomyelitis are neuropathic joint, Langerhan cell histiocytosis, non accidental injury and Caffey's disease.

(Adam & Dixon, 2008; Dahnert, 2011; Sutton, 2003; Swischuk, 2004; Hodler et al, 2009; Palmer & Reeder, 2001).

References
1. Cardinal E, Bureau NJ, Aubin B, Chhem RK. Role of ultrasound in musculoskeletal infections. Radiol Clin North Am. 2001;39(2):191-201.
2. Robben SG. Ultrasonography of musculoskeletal infections in children. Eur Radiol. 2004;14 Suppl 4:L65-77.
3. Kothari NA, Pelchovitz DJ, Meyer JS. Imaging of musculoskeletal infections. Radiol Clin North Am. 2001;39(4):653-71.
4. Chau CL, Griffith JF. Musculoskeletal infections: ultrasound appearances. Clin Radiol. 2005;60(2):149-59.
5. Santiago Restrepo C, Giménez CR, McCarthy K. Imaging of osteomyelitis and musculoskeletal soft tissue infections: current concepts. Rheum Dis Clin North Am. 2003;29(1):89-109.
6. Bureau NJ, Chhem RK, Cardinal E. Musculoskeletal infections: US manifestations. Radiographics. 1999;19(6):1585-92.
7. Pugmire BS, Shailam R, Gee MS. Role of MRI in the diagnosis and treatment of osteomyelitis in pediatric patients. World J Radiol 2014;6(8):530-7.
8. Hatzenbuehler J, Pulling TJ. Diagnosis and management of osteomyelitis. Am Fam Physician 2011;84(9):1027-33.
9. Schillaci O. Hybrid imaging systems in the diagnosis of osteomyelitis and prosthetic joint infection. Q J Nucl Med Mol Imaging 2009;53(1):95-104.

1.3   OSTEOSARCOMA

Definition: Osteosarcoma is defined as primary malignant tumour of bone that seeks to form new bones.

It is the second most common primary malignant tumour occurring in bone after multiple myeloma.
It accounts for 15 – 25% of all primary malignant bone tumours.

Other name: Osteogenic sarcoma, bone-forming malignant bone tumour.

Characteristic Feature/Pathology
1. The tumour is of mesenchymal origin with the malignant tumour cells directly forming osteoids or bone without cartilaginous ancestor. The tumours occur in sites of fast bone growth as fast bone production makes osteoblastic cells to acquire mutations that could lead to transformation.
2. It may rarely arise from the soft tissue.
3. Abundant alkaline phosphatase is found within the tumour cells.

Epidemiology/Age of Affectation
It is second to multiple myeloma in primary malignant bone tumour occurrence.
It is the most common malignant primary bone tumour in people aged 10 – 30 years. About 75% occurs in those aged 15 – 25 years.
It comprises 15-20% of all malignant bone tumours and 0.2% of all malignant tumours.
It is made of approximately 3-5 cases per million populations per year in the USA.
Bimodal distribution with peaks at 10 – 25 years (70% - 85% between 10 – 30 years). The other peak incidence is above 60 years but rare.
The tumour is very rare in the very young (below 5 years) and the very old (above 80 years).

Sex Distribution: Male to female ratio ranges from 1.5:1 to 3: 2.

Predisposing factors/associations
1. Hereditary retinoblastoma particularly, the bilateral familiar type.
    Due to a defect in the RB gene (close to 1000 fold increase).
2. Defect in p53 gene (Li-fraumeni syndrome).
3. Abnormalities in INK 4a which encodes p16 and p14 genes.
4. Radiation exposure (2%); this is dose related and in patients above 60 years.
5. Rothmund-Thompson syndrome.
6. Electrophilic chemotherapeutic agent.
7. Paget's disease (in patients above 60 years).
8. Chondrosarcoma (dedifferentiated chondrosarcoma).
9. Viral origin or involvement has also been implicated.
10. Chronic osteomyelitis (those lasting above 20 years).

Tumour markers
1. High level of serum alkaline phosphatase (ALP).
2. High level of lactate dehydrogenase (LDH).
Increased bone formation is responsible for high level of alkaline phosphatase in osteosarcoma.

High level of serum alkaline phosphatase is observed in:
1. Heavy tumour burden
2. Poor prognostic cases
3. Poor response to therapy
4. Presence of metastasis
5. Tumour recurrence/ residual tumour after therapy.

Classification of osteosarcoma (according to WHO)
This is based on anatomical sites and behaviours which are prognostic criteria (table 1.31).

Table 1.31: WHO classification of osteosarcoma[1-3]				
Types	Description, division and subtypes			
Type 1.	**Primary osteosarcoma**			
	Intramedullary /central osteosarcoma			
		a	Conventional/ high grade (75% – 90%)	
			i	Osteoblastic (50%)
			ii	Chondroblastic (25%)
			iii	Fibroblastic (25%)
		b	Small cell (round cell) type	
		c	Telangiectatic osteosarcoma	
		d	Low grade central osteosarcoma	
		e	Unusual forms of osteosarcoma (rare)	
	Surface osteosarcoma			
		a.	Parosteal	
		b.	Periosteal	
		c.	High grade surface	
Type 2.	**Secondary osteosarcoma** (Paget's disease, radiation therapy, etc)			

Behaviours according to different parameters
Type of bone: Long bones are generally more affected, long tubular bones 80%-90%.
Where in the bone? Metaphysis of long bones 90%, diaphysis of long bone 2-11%.
Where in the skeleton: Around the knees 50% – 75% (area with greatest longitudinal growth); followed by upper end of humerus and upper end of the femur. Axial skeleton is rarely affected.
Which bones are involved: Femur, tibia and humerus accounts for 80-90%; less than 1% is found in hands and feet.
Changing pattern with age: Flat bones including pelvis, ilium and spine are affected mostly among those aged over 50 years. Also the involvement of non-long bone increases with age. Secondary type involves flat bones and those aged above 50 years.
Primary osteosarcoma: This occurs mostly in patients aged 10-30 years, typically in metaphyseal region of long bones with a striking predilection for around the knee region.

Unusual forms of osteosarcoma: Gnatic, osteosarcomatosis (multicentric), extraskeletal/ soft tissue and intracortical osteosarcoma are rare.

Secondary osteosarcoma: This occurs in Paget's disease, develops from sites after irradiation, from dedifferentiated chondrosarcoma, sites of osteonecrosis, fibrous dysplasia, chronic osteomyelitis, osteogenesis imperfect and associated with familiar bilateral retinoblastoma. Secondary osteosarcoma has a higher incidence in flat bones, especially pelvis (where the incidence of Paget's disease is high) and those aged above 50 years and the elderly (due to malignant degeneration of Paget's disease).

Diagnosis

Radiology is essential in diagnosis as most of the tumour exhibits characteristic appearance.

Biopsy for histology is the final definitive diagnosis. There will be demonstration of osteoids directly formed by malignant cells. Mode of obtaining biopsy and site of biopsy and experiences of biopsy surgeon and pathologist are critical to accurate diagnosis and prognosis.

Site in the Bone

1. Metaphysis (within medullary cavity) 90 – 95%.
2. Diaphysis 2 – 11%.

Metastatic Spread

1. Haematogenous especially to the lungs
2. Lymphatic spread may occur but is uncommon.
3. Spread to other bones is from the metastases that had spread to the lungs

Clinical Features

Bone pain, soft tissue swelling, palpable mass, fever (frequent), elevated alkaline phosphatase (slight), tenderness, history of trauma may exist, pathological fracture, anorexia, diabetes mellitus (paraneoplastic syndrome, etc.)

Radiological Features
Plain film

1. Moth-eaten or permeative pattern bone destruction. This is an area of bone destruction in the metaphysis especially around the knee.
2. Cortical bone destruction with medullary sclerosis.
3. Lytic destructive lesion with mixed sclerotic and lytic appearance of the affected area.
4. Soft tissue mass often symmetric and extensive between 2 – 10 cm in length and up to 5 cm in width with wide zone of transition with new bone formation in the soft tissue.
5. Cloud-like density or appearance, due to irregular new bone formation (figure 1.41 a and b)
6. Sun-ray / sunburst spiculation or appearance, (figure 1.31 a and b)
7. Codman's triangle: Periosteal elevation due to erosion of the cortex with formation of Codman's triangle.
8. Entirely lytic type of bone destruction 1-5%.
9. Osteolysis and bone expansion in telangiectatic form.
10. The physis frequently acts as barrier to the spread of the tumour but not always.
11. Canon ball or multiple nodules of pulmonary metastasis
12. Spontaneous pneumothorax due rupture of cavitating subpleural lesions
13. Calcified metastases particularly in the lung or rarely in the brain.

14. Sclerotic and lytic areas in the same area of bone
15. Periosteal reaction (often aggressive)
16. Codman's triangle. Periosteal elevation (periosteal reaction) caused by fast-growing tumour cells, forming a triangle with the parent bone)
17. Cavitating pulmonary metastases with or without the formation of pneumothorax.

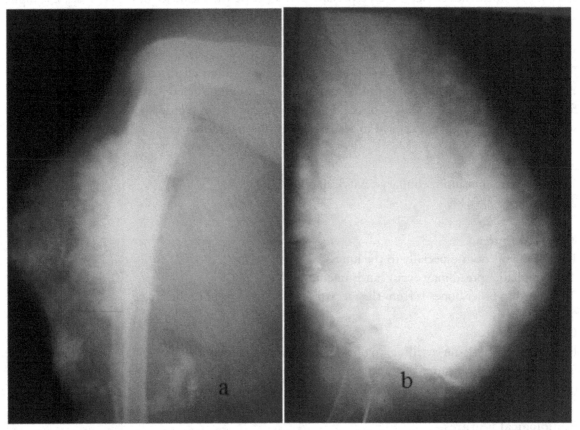

Figure 1.31: Plain radiographs of osteosacoma. **a.** Involvement of the humerus, and, (**b**). involvement of the distal femur. Note the sun-ray (sun-burst) spiculations and gross destruction of the bone with increased density and extensive soft tissue component (**a** and **b**). Also note ossification within the soft tissue in (**a**).

Computed tomography
1. This detects all the radiological features that are evident on plain films.
2. In addition, it can detect pathological fracture at an early state.
3. CT scan can define the full extent of the tumour including permeative bone infiltration and metastasis.
4. CT can assess ossification and calcification more clearly than plain films
5. CT can also assess skip metastasis which are metastasis occurring in the same bone as the primary.
6. CT can detect smaller metastasis than plain films
7. There is replacement of fatty bone marrow by soft-tissue density
8. Areas of low attenuation within bone are due to bone destruction, haemorrhage or necrosis.
9. Areas of very high density due to high attenuation are areas of highly mineralized bone substance

MR Imaging
1. It is the best modality for assessing the full extent of soft tissue and bone involvement of the tumour particularly in T1WI.
2. The tumour show intermediate signal intensity on TlWI and high signal intensity on T2WI
3. It can identify skip lesions
4. MRI identifies the tumour crossing of the growth and neurovascular encasement.
5. MRI can also monitor the effects of therapy
6. Decrease of neovascularisation; tumour necrosis and shrinking with better capsulation is noted with MRI following chemotherapy.
7. MRI findings are usually correlated with x-ray finding for improved assessment.

Radionuclide scan
This detects osseous metastasis and is the best method for detection of osseous metastasis. The agent used is technetium-99 methylene diphosphonate (Tc-99 MDP). It detects osteoblastic activity and highly vascular area when metastasis has occurred.

Findings on Radionuclide studies are:
1. There is strongly increased activity on blood pool phase and delayed images because the tumour is hypervascular with new bone formation.
2. There is demonstration of soft-tissue extension of the tumour and skip lesions by showing activity within the soft tissue and in separated bone segments.
3. There is demonstration of multiple areas of high activities due to metastasis

PET/CT and PET/MRI
These combine images that show anatomical structure as well as function. The advantage of PET/MRI is reduced radiation dose compared to PET/CT. Agent of the PET component of the hybrid imaging is ^{18}Fluorodeoxy glucose (FDG).

Uses of PET/CT
1. It is used in selecting the region of tumour most likely to yield diagnostic information for biopsy.
2. It is used for staging of the tumour.
3. To monitor the effects of therapy.
4. To monitor and assess the cause of suspected recurrence observed in other modalities.
5. To detect tumour recurrence in the presence of elevated tumour marker.
6. For guiding radiation therapy.
7. It is used for searching for unknown primary tumour of unknown origin.

Biopsy for histology
Biopsy should best be carried out after full history, physical examination and radiological investigations. This is because it may interfere with these assessment methods if done before they are completed. It should best be done by the surgeon who would carry out the operation. It is a major step in the diagnosis and treatment and adequate representative sample and tissues with good pathologists are necessary to avoid both false positive and false negative diagnosis with associated increased morbidity and mortality.
Advantages of biopsy: Confirms the diagnosis, reveals specific type of the tumour and provides the grade of the tumour.

Methods
Open or incisional method
Advantage: Adequate sample ideal for histopathology, immunohistocytochemistry (IHC) and genetic studies obtained.

Disadvantage: Time consuming, entails an equipped operation theatre, infection, morbidity from wound healing, tumour cells seeding into normal soft tissues through any resultant hematoma and it is more expensive to the patient.

Closed method or Core needle biopsy (using Jamshidi needle)
Advantage: This is a better, safe and accurate method, less extensive and quicker procedure and can be done with local anaesthesia at a much cheaper cost. When done under image assistance or guidance such as CT, MRI and ultrasound the sensitivity is improved.

Fine needle aspiration cytology (FNAC) (not advised).

Disadvantages: Inadequate and unrepresented sample may be obtained.

Table 1.32: Staging of osteosarcoma (Enneking system)[1-3]

Stage	Grade	Site	Metastasis
IA	Low	Intracompartment	No
IB	Low	Extracompartment	No
IIA	High	Intracompartment	No
IIB	High	Extracompartment	No
III	Any	Any	Regional/distant metastases

Treatment
This consists of surgical excision, chemotherapy and radiotherapy depending on immunohistocytochemistry, genetic studies and the stage of the tumour (table 1.32).

Complications
1. Pathological fracture
2. Osteosarcoma after irradiation
3. Pneumothorax due to cavitory metastasis
4. Solitary metastasis to the lung
5. Pulmonary metastasis in childhood

Prognosis
Five year survival rate is 50 – 80%

Monostotic osteosarcoma of the extremities without metastases, treated with combined neoadjuvant therapy has a cure rate of 60-70%.

Those of the axial skeletal has cure rate of 30% with therapy.

Predictors of prognosis
A number of factors determine the survival of the patient before and after treatment. These factors include:
1. Presence of metastases at initial presentation; this reduces the survival outcome and prognosis.

2. Localisation of tumours to one anatomical site or monostotic disease pattern.
3. Anatomic site of tumour location (extremity or axial) due to monostotic disease.
4. Histological response to preoperative chemotherapy. This is measured by histological cell differentiation of resected specimen.
5. Level of biomarker particularly serum levels of alkaline phosphatase and lactate dehydrogenase. These are the most powerful predictors of survival for patients with osteosarcoma as they predicts tumour burden, metastasis after treatment, recurrence after treatment and completeness of tumour resection following treatment.
6. The degree of tissue necrosis in post surgical resection specimen after chemotherapy is currently proposed as the best predictor. There is about 90% survival with tumour necrosis more than 90%, and about 14% survival with less than about 90% of tumour necrosis.
7. The most important prognostic factor for recurrent osteosarcoma is the ability and possibility of achieving a complete resection of metastatic lesions.

Biochemical makers

Serum alkaline phosphatase (ALP) and Lactate dehydrogenase (LDH) are raised in osteosarcoma due to increased osteoblastic activity. Very high levels before treatment are associated with heavy tumour burden and poor prognosis. Persistent high level after treatment is associated with residual disease, tumour recurrence or untreated or unresected metastases.

Differential Diagnosis: 1. Myositis/pyomyositis/cellulites, osteomyelitis, 2. Myositis ossificans. 3. Osteoid osteoma, 4. Chondrosarcoma. 5. Ewing's sarcoma, 6. Fibrosarcoma, 7. Metastasis.

(Adam & Dixon, 2008; Dahnert, 2011; Sutton, 2003; Swischuk, 2004).

References

1. Picca P. Osteosarcoma (Osteogenic sarcoma). Orphanet Journal of Rare Diseases 2007; 2:6:
2. Kundu ZS. Classification, imaging, biopsy and staging of osteosarcoma. Indian J Orthop. 2014; 48(3): 238–246.
3. Fletcher CD, Bridge JA, Hogendoorn PC, Mertens F,(eds). World Health Organization, classification of tumours: Pathology and genetics of tumors of soft tissue and bone. Lyon: IARC Press; 2013.
4. Yarmish G, Klein MJ, Landa J, Lefkowitz RA, Hwang S. Imaging characteristics of primary osteosarcoma: nonconventional subtypes. Radiographics 2010;30(6):1653-72.

1.4   MULTIPLE MYELOMA

Definition
Multiple myeloma is defined as a tumour of the B-cells within the bone marrow. It occurs by means of monoclonal proliferation of the plasma cells within the bone marrow producing monoclonal immunoglobulins. Plasma cells are mature B-cells that produce antibodies.

Blood and urine findings that define the disease
There is elevation of total serum protein due to abnormally elevated immunoglobulins produced by the monoclonal proliferated plasma cells. There is elevated ESR often above 100 mm per hour. Bence-Jones protein and TammHorsfall protein casts occur in renal tubules (20-50%) with eventual impairment of renal function. These are precipitated in the urine as casts. There is amyloidosis in 10-15% of cases. Hypercalcaemia occurs but phosphate and serum alkaline phosphatase levels are not elevated. Amyloidosis may precede the development of multiple myeloma.

Epidemiology
This disease occurs in those aged 40 years and above but particularly in those aged 60 years and above and is rare in those aged less than 30 years. Male to female (M: F) ratio = 3:1. This is the most common malignant bone tumour occurring in the bone marrow. It is the second most common haematological malignancy after non-Hodgkin's lymphoma. It accounts for 10% of haematological malignancy and constitute 1% of all malignancies. It is the most common neoplasm in adults.

Associations
POEM syndrome, amyloidosis (10-15%).

Symptoms
There may be localised bone pain, back pain, fever, unexplained fatigue and weakness of the body, reduction in height, unexplained recurrent infection, and unexplained peripheral neuropathy (carpal tunnel syndrome being a common type). About 30-34% of the patients are asymptomatic at presentation but the disease is detected by elevated plasma cells in bone marrow aspirate. Other symptoms are anorexia, nausea, polydipsia, compression fractures, osteoporosis, destructive bone lesion, arterial infarction due to hyper viscosity states and pathological fracture (up to 25%). There is anaemia, renal insufficiency and hypercalcaemia.

Investigations
Full blood count, other blood tests and serum electrophoresis
Bone marrow biopsy and histology of aspirate
Skeletal radiographic survey
CT, MRI, PET, PET/CT (including complete body scanning with these imaging modalities where techniques guarantee safety of the procedure).

Diagnosis
1. Bone marrow containing more than 10% of plasma cells (normal < 4%).
2. Blood serum containing an abnormal protein. Abnormal serum electrophoresis (serum M protein level equals to 3 g per dl (30 g per litre) or greater.
3. Generalized osteopaenia /or lytic bone changes on plain films with typical punched out lesions.

4. Blood serum and /or urine containing an abnormal protein (usually a monoclonal M-protein in blood and Bence-Jones proteins in urine (excretion of k- or λ- light chain)
5. Positive bone marrow result and absence of radiographic evidence occurs in one third of the cases.
6. There are anaemia with haemoglobin level of less than 10 g per dl (100 g per litre), renal insufficiency resulting in serum creatinine level more than 2 mg per dl (180 μmol per litre) and hypercalcaemia with serum calcium level higher than 11 mg per dl (2.75 mmol per litre), as other supporting evidences.

Pathology

The diseases results from abnormal proliferation of monoclonal plasma cells. Myeloma cells attach to osteoblast by vascular cell adhesion molecules-1 (VCAM-1). This leads to the stimulation of osteoclastogenesis. Myeloma cells inhibit osteoblastic differentiation into mature osteoblasts. This inturn inhibits osteoblastogenesis. Myeloma cells also secret substances that inhibit osteoblastogenesis. The effect of all these is to cause increased bone destruction and osteopaenia. Histologically, the plasma cells may be pleomorphic and in those with diffuse changes, the plasma cells are thoroughly mixed up with haematopoietic cells. In areas where there are solitary tumour masses the haematopoietic cell are completely displaced by a bunch of myeloma cells.

Smouldering multiple myeloma is defined by serum M protein equal to or more than 3 g/dL or bone marrow plasma cells equal to or more than 10%, in addition to absence of anaemia, hypocalcaemia, lytic bone lesions, or renal failure that are as a result of the plasma cell proliferative disorder.

Aims of radiology

1. Initial staging of the tumour
2. Detection and characterization of complications
3. Evaluation of patient's response to treatment
4. The traditional role of radiology as adjunct to diagnosis by means of skeletal radiographic survey is being gradually relegated.

Radiological features

1. *Generalized osteopaenia.* This is reduction in bone density. The axial skeleton is more affected. It is seen in about 10-20% of the cases.
2. *"Rain–drop"* or *"Moth-eaten"* or *"Punched–out" radiolucent lesion.* Characteristic small spherical lucencies or circular defects due to osteolysis with endosteal scalloping in bone of varying diameter from a few millimetres reaching 2 – 3 cm. The average size is 2 cm. There is absence of sclerotic margins in these lesions. The skull, spine and the inner surfaces of long bones are affected (figure 1.41).
3. *"Pepper-pot appearance".* These are diffuse small lytic lesions in the skull with the well-defined margins of each lesion contrasting in the skull and giving the appearance of pepper spread in a pot (figure 1.41).
4. *Erosion of outer ends of clavicles.*
5. *Pathological fracture.* This occurs in up to 50% of the cases. This often heals with massive or exuberant callus formation. Any unexplained fracture in the affected age group should raise the suspicion of the disease.
6. *Sternal expansion which could be gross and sometimes with distorted appearance is frequent and associated soft tissue component of the mass may be area of extremedually haematopoiesis.*

7. *Soft tissue mass adjacent to area of bone destruction. The CT density is similar to muscle and the mass enhances following contrast IV injection. This could be a site for extramedullary haematopoiesis.*

8. *Vertebral compression* with destruction appearing as solitary or multiple collapsed vertebrae. Vertebral collapse is observed in between 50-70% of the cases at some stages in the disease. Benign fracture from osteopaenia accounts for two third of the cases while pathological fractures from diffuse tumour infiltration into the bone accounts for one third of cases of the vertebral fracture.

9. *Soft tissue mass adjacent to area of bone destruction* especially paraspinal area and around the ribs. Paraspinal soft-tissue mass may have an extradural extension

10. *There could be scalloping of anterior margin of vertebral bodies.* This is usually due to osseous pressure from adjacent enlarged lymph nodes.

11. *Expansile osteolytic lesion or ballooning of ribs,* long bones and pelvis.

12. Paraspinal mass adjacent to area of bone destruction. *This could also be a site for extramedullary haematopoiesis*

13. *Diffuse osteolysis* of sacrum and pelvis

14. *Sclerotic changes occur in* 1-4% of untreated cases. It appears as periosteal reaction similar to osteosarcoma or chalky lesions of prostatic carcinoma. It is associated with peripheral neuropathy. It may also be seen after radiotherapy or chemotherapy in which cases the overall cases may reach 10%.

15. *Rarely, periosteal reaction* appearing as periosteal elevations may be seen.

16. *Mandibular* involvement. When multiple moth-eaten lesions are seen in the mandible, this is almost diagnostic of the disease as the involvement of metastases is very rare.

Imaging findings
Plain radiography
Types of radiological involvement:
a. Solitary deposit (plasmacytoma).
b. Diffuse involvement of the skeleton (multiple myelomatosis).
c. Generalized osteopaenia.
d. Sclerosing myeloma (1-4%). There could be solitary sclerotic lesion which is often observed in the spine. Diffuse sclerosis is also occasionally seen.

Common sites of involvement
Vertebrae 66%, ribs 45%, skull 40%, shoulder 40%, pelvis 30%, bones 25%.

Advantages of plain radiography
1. Skeletal survey. This involves the important views of the body to identify areas of bone affectation.
2. Radiography is superior to bone scintigraphy in multiple myeloma lesion identification because the lesion is basically osteolytic.
3. Pain radiography detects cortical bone destruction which is not available with MRI or radionuclide imaging.
4. About 80-90% of multiple myeloma has radiographic evidence of involvement and up to 80% of the anatomical site affected by the disease is identified by plain radiography.
5. It is cheap, cost effective, readily available and easy to interpret.
6. About 30% of the lesions are demonstrated only on radiography
7. Even with MRI studies, plain radiography studies are required for comparison for accurate interpretation.

Disadvantages of radiography

1. Poor diagnosis and high rate of under-staging of multiple myeloma (table 1.41). This is due to high false negative findings of 20 – 70% depending on the stage of the disease and method of skeletal survey and radiological interpretations (figure 1.41).
2. There is the inability to identify diffuse bone marrow involvement (table 1.41).
3. Failure to detect early myeloma since lytic lesions are only visualized when up to 30 – 50% of bone mineral density is lost (table 1.41).
4. Diffuse osteopaenia due to multiple myeloma in an elderly could be erroneously diagnosed as osteoporosis (senile or post-menopausal).
5. In patients with multiple myeloma, positioning for radiography could be painful, difficult and uncomfortable in the elderly as they may also have pathological fracture.
6. The disease history and activity status cannot be estimated by this method.

Computed tomography

CT detects cortical breaches or erosion earlier than plain radiography.

Advantages

1. It detects small lytic lesions better than radiography
2. It is fast without the need to change patient's position.
3. It is the imaging modality of choice in imaging-guided spinal and pelvic biopsy of focal lesion identified by MRI.
4. There is no need to use iodinated contrast medium for bone imaging in multiple myeloma since the lesions are basically osteopaenic.

Disadvantages

1. It cannot be done for whole body scanning due to high radiation dose.
2. It shows persistent bone lesion through the course of the disease.
3. It cannot assess continued activity in multiple myeloma that has bone destruction unlike MRI and PET/CT.

Whole body MRI (using multiple sequences)

1. *Myeloma tumour has low signal intensity on T1-weighted images*
2. *It has high signal intensity on T2-weighted images.*
3. *The lesion shows enhancement with IV gadolinium contrast injection.*
4. Abnormal MRI patterns in patients with smouldering multiple myeloma possibly will justify the commencement of systemic treatment.

Advantages

1. It is the best modality for detecting diffuse spine and extraskeletal involvement (table 1.41).
2. It is the best modality for detecting focal spine and extraskeletal involvement.
3. It is the best imaging modality for evaluating the bone marrow as it lacks radiation exposure.
4. MRI finding is prognostic as the number and pattern of lesion tends to correlate excellently with treatment outcome and survival.
5. MRI is superior, more sensitive and specific than radiographic skeletal surveys in detecting disease.

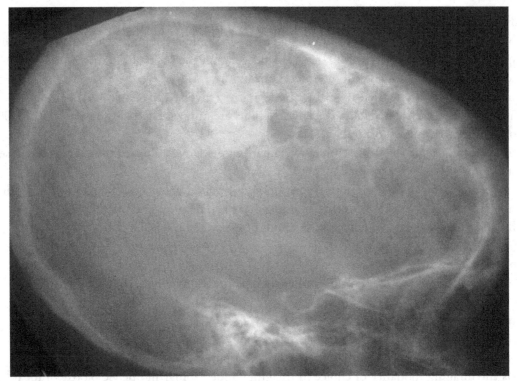

Figure 1.41. Plain skull radiograph showing multiple small round lucent lesions due to Multiple myeloma.

Disadvantages

1. Normal pattern of bone marrow appearances for different age groups must be known before hand for accurate interpretation.
2. MRI lacks specificity and has variable non-predictable response.
3. MRI can show false negative findings as multiple myeloma can show normal bone marrow appearance.
4. Focal and diffuse pattern may represent pathological or physiological process.
5. MRI abnormalities reverse 9-12 months after successful and effective treatment meaning that it cannot be used to monitor therapy before 9 months after therapy.
6. MRI findings must be compared with plain radiography for accurate interpretation.
7. MRI is unable to view specific bones such as the skull, clavicle or ribs and these bones are not reliably investigated by MRI due respiratory movements or small size resulting to false-negative results and disease under-staging.

Radionuclide studies
Bone scintigraphy
This is identification of bone involvement using technetium-99 labelled diphosphonate.

1. It detects osteoblastic response to compression/fracture.
2. It is used in evaluation of areas not well demonstrated on radiography such as ribs and sternum.

PET/CT imaging
This is tomographic nuclear medicine imaging using labelled radiopharmaceutical. Intravenous injection of ^{18}Fluoro-deoxy glucose (^{18}F-FDG) is carried out followed by tomographic scanning after

10-40 minutes of the injection. Tumour cells have high metabolic rate with associated high demand for oxygen and this enables them to be differentiated from normal cells.

Advantages
1. It is superior to radiography in detecting rib lesion since associated fractures are easily detected with bone scan.
2. It detects bone involvement in solitary plasmacytoma better than magnetic resonance imaging (MRI) or technetium-99 sestamibi (MIBI) studies.
3. It detects extra-medullary involvement.
4. It is used to assess the extent of active disease.
5. It can differentiate active myeloma from monoclonal gammopathy of undetermined significance (MCGUS). MCGUS is negative in PET/CT while active myeloma is positive. This is due to absence of diffuse uptake and absence of focal disease in bone marrow.
6. Active myeloma is positive for focal disease and diffuse abnormalities.
7. It can identify new sites of disease at the same time areas of unsuspected extramedullary spread.

Disadvantages
The following gives false positive:
1. Inflammation from active infection gives false positive findings.
2. Chemotherapy within the last 4 weeks gives false positive findings.
3. Radiation therapy within 2-3 months of PET/CT studies.
4. There is alterations of FDG activity due to therapy and are normally limited to a 1-month interval after discontinuation of treatment.

Table 1.41. Durie – Salmo PLUS staging system[1,2]	
Stage	**Imaging findings (using MRI, PET and FDG)**
Stage I clinical criteria	<5 focal spine lesion ± mild diffuse spine disease
State II clinical criteria	1-20 focal lesions ± moderate diffuse spine disease
State III clinical criteria	> 20 focal lesions ± severe diffuse spine disease

MIBI studies
This uses technetium-99 sestamibi (MIBI) also written as ^{99}Tc-MIBI. This is ^{99m}Tc-labelled hexakis-2-methoxyisobutylisonitrile, a radiopharmaceutical that selectively builds up in tissues with high cellular density and mitochondrial activation. These are the parameters found in malignant tissues such as multiple myeloma.

Advantages
1. It is superior to PET/CT in identification of diffuse disease.
2. It can detect very low level multiple myeloma not detected by PET/CT.

Disadvantages
1. It is limited in detecting focal lesions.
2. It underestimates the extent of bone marrow infiltration in the spine when compared to MRI.
3. It has enhanced uptake by drug-resistant myeloma cells. Where as in FDG scanning, it is metabolically active myeloma cells that have enhanced uptake allowing for effective therapy.

Treatment follow up
1. Punched-out lesions do not change with effective treatment.
2. New vertebral compression fracture on plain radiography or other imaging does not necessarily signify relapse or disease progression.
3. Sclerosis in radiography and CT may occur after chemotherapy, radiotherapy, fluoride administration but may not be prognostic.
4. CT scan done as a follow up of treated disease may demonstrate the resolution of extramedullary disease.
5. There may be the reappearance of a continuous cortical outline on CT.
6. There may be replacement of marrow contents by fatty marrow in areas with prior lytic changes in treated cases demonstrated on CT.
7. FDG uptake reduces very fast after effective therapy.
8. Persistent FDG signify early relapse.
9. There is poor prognosis if abnormal FDG uptake is present after high-dose drug therapy or stem cell transplantation.

Imaging findings in the kidneys
1. Nephrocalcinosis develops from hypercalcaemia
2. Normal or smoothly enlarged kidneys which may later become small with time due to reduced renal blood flow from increased viscosity of blood and associated amyloidosis.
3. Increasingly dense nephrogram is observed in IVU in patients with acute oliguric renal failure. Dehydration is avoided and low osmolar contrast medium is used.
4. The echogenicity of the kidney can be normal or show increased echogenicity depending on the stage of the disease.
5. Renal amyloidosis

Plasmacytoma
This is a solitary deposit of plasma cell tumour and occurs in about 2% of plasma cell tumours. It may remain localized and, asymptomatic for many years but may present with local pain and up to 30% proceed to multiple myeloma after an average latent period of five to ten years. Serum electrophoresis and ESR may be normal and it is found in younger age group than multiple myeloma. Radiological studies show in general, a lytic destructive medullary-based lesion with frequently well-defined margins due slow growth. There is bony expansion which can be rather marked with cortical thinning and prominent peripheral trabeculation forming a network often with soap-bubble appearance. There is absence of sclerotic margins. Vertebral lesions which are common in the thoracic and lumbar regions do not cross the disc spaces and there may be associated vertebral collapse. The pelvis is the next most commonly affected site. Very rarely, purely sclerotic lesions have been observed. Differential diagnosis includes aneurismal bone cyst, solitary metastasis, chordoma, fibrous dysplasia, lymphoma, hyperparathyroidism

Differential diagnosis
1. Osteopaenia due to senile osteoporosis.
2. Osteopaenia due to post menopausal osteoporosis
3. Other forms of monoclonal gammopathy
4. Hyperparathyroidism
5. Metastasis
6. Renal osteodystrophy
7. Othere are Lymphoma, Myelosclerosis and Amylodosis

Complications of multiple myeloma
1. Renal involvement with resultant acute or chronic renal failure.
2. Secondary amyloidosis in about 10%.
3. Recurrent chest infection due to chronic leukopaenia.
4. Pathological fracture.
5. Sepsis due to bacterial infection resulting from neutropaenia.
6. Thromboembolism from increased viscosity of blood and rouleaux formation.

(Adam & Dixon, 2008; Dahnert, 2011; Sutton, 2003; Swischuk, 2004).

References
1. Lütje S, de Rooy JW, Croockewit S, Koedam E, Oyen WJ, Raymakers RA. Role of radiography, MRI and FDG-PET/CT in diagnosing, staging and therapeutical evaluation of patients with multiple myeloma. Ann Hematol 2009; 88(12): 1161–1168.
2. Konrad CN, William DL. Multiple Myeloma: Diagnosis and Treatment. Am Fam Physician 2008;78(7):853-859.
3. Derlin T, Bannas P. Imaging of multiple myeloma: Current concepts. World J Orthop 2014;5(3):272-82.

Chapter 2

CHEST

2.1 DIFFERENTIAL DIAGNOSIS AND RADIOLOGICAL FINDINGS IN A PATIENT PRESENTING WITH HAEMOPTYSIS

Definition

Haemoptysis is defined as coughing up of blood or blood-spitting. The bleeding usually originates from the lower respiratory tract and its coughing up, heralds life-threatening thoracic disease condition requiring urgent investigations.

The blood is usually small and mixed with sputum. However, in certain conditions like bronchiectasis, the blood may be mouthful.

The following must be excluded before diagnosis is made:

Haematemesis and factitious disorder
Bleeding from the nose, pharynx, nasopharynx and larynx.
Epitaxis from trauma, hypertension and nasal tumours
Bleeding from the mouth, dental caries, gingivitis or oral tumours
Aspirated or inhaled blood or blood components

Classification of haemoptysis

Mild haemoptysis: Blood loss is less than 50 ml per 24 hours. It could also be streaks, stain, or flecks of blood in the sputum.
Moderate haemoptysis: Blood loss is 50 ml to less than 200 ml per 24 hours;
or three or more episodes of haemoptysis measuring 100 ml within one-week period.
Severe haemoptysis: Blood loss is from 200 ml to 300 ml per 24 hours; or a maximum of 600 ml in 48 hour
Massive haemoptysis: The blood loss is more than 300 ml per 24 hours or any amount of blood loss that resulted to haemodynamic instability.

Definition of terms

Frank haemoptysis is said to occur where there is expectoration of blood without any accompanying sputum.
One episode of haemoptysis is recorded when there has been one incident of bleeding lasting up to 7 days.

Recurrent haemoptysis is recorded when there is a break of 2-3 days in continuity of the bleeding within one week or when the duration of bleeding is longer than 7 days.

Origin of blood in haemoptysis

1. Mostly from the bronchial artery (> 90%). The blood is in high tension since it is systemic blood and this frequently results to more amount of blood loss.
2. Pulmonary artery and non-bronchial systemic arteries (< 10%). Only small amount of blood is lost when bleeding is from any of these vessels since the blood is in low tension of pulmonary circulation.

Causes of Haemoptysis

A. Vascular lesions

Pulmonary venous hypertension (commonest), (cardiac failure, mitral stenosis, and pulmonary oedema, Pulmonary embolism with infarction), Chronic bronchitis, bronchiectasis, Arteriovenous malformation (many different types), Rupture of aneurysm of pulmonary artery. This occurs in vasculitis (Behcet disease, Takayasu arteritis), neoplasm due to neovascularisation (leaky vessels), trauma, tuberculosis (Rasmussen aneurysm), lung abscess, septic emboli, long indwelling catheter, Hughes-Stovin Syndrome and Osler-Weber-Rendu Syndrome, Rupture of aneurysm of the bronchial artery/pulmonary artery (tuberculosis, necrotising fungal infection).

A. **Tumours**

Bronchogenic carcinoma, bronchial carcinoids, bronchial adenoma, Hodgkin's disease and other carcinomas

B. **Infections/infestations:**

Bronchiectasis, tuberculosis (rupture of Rasmussen aneurysm), lung abscess, chronic bronchitis, pneumonia (rusty sputum), histoplasmosis, aspergillosis, amoebiasis, blastomycosis, paragonimiasis and viral haemorrhagic fever

In the tropics, pulmonary tuberculosis is common as a cause of haemoptysis

C. **Injury to the bronchial wall or iatrogenic**

Erosion from foreign body (inhaled or foreign body), bronchoscopy, pulmonary artery inflation devices, anticoagulant therapy, biopsy (lung biopsy) and trauma (History is significant for accurate diagnosis)

D. **Pneumoconiosis**

Silicosis: This is from the breakdown of vascular nodules of progressive massive fibrosis due to rapid growth, Haemosiderosis (idiopathic type), etc.

E. **Idiopathic/cryptogenic** (No cause was found)

F. **Congenital disorders**

Pseudosequestration, Pulmonary artery artresia/stenosis, Pulmonary artery malformation, Endometriosis or catamenial haemoptysis

Note: The most common identifiable causes on radiological investigations in over 95% of cases are: Bronchiectasis, pulmonary tuberculosis or fungal infections, chronic bronchitis and bronchial carcinoma.

Role of radiology
The roles of radiology are to determine:

1. The source of the bleeding
2. The importance of the bleeding
3. The primary cause of the bleeding
4. The volume of haemoptysis
5. The effects of the haemoptysis on cardiorespiratory functions
6. Recognition of sentinel bleeding which could herald major bleeding episodes

In about 15% to 30% of haemoptysis, the cause cannot be diagnosed.

Problems of haemoptysis
Death from asphyxia, death from excessive hypovolaemic shock, anaemia from recurrent bleeding, social problems of bleeding in the public and risk of cancer, pneumonectomy if the cause is not quickly treated.

Radiological Assessment
The main problem of haemoptysis is airway compromise or obstruction from aspiration of the blood. Accurate history is taken to assess the possible cause of the bleeding; the quantity of blood coughed up, the duration of patient's illness, and to exclude any sign of infection like Lassa fever or other viral haemorrhagic fevers. The possible cause and the quantity of blood will determine the order of radiological assessment.

Table 2.11: Investigative modalities

Plain chest radiography	Pulmonary arteriography
Conventional tomography	Bronchial arteriography
Computed tomography	Radionuclide study
Ultrasonography	Ventilation scan
Echocardiography	Perfusion scan
Angiography	Magnetic resonance imaging

Ventilation-Perfusion Scan
This will confirm pulmonary embolism as area of perfusion defect without matching ventilation defect. Chronic obstructive pulmonary disease will be confirmed as an area of ventilation defect without perfusion defects. Technetium-99m pertechnetate is used for perfusion. Krypton-81m may be used in the ventilation (table 2.11).

Angiography
The advantage of angiography is ability to carry out interventional studies to stop the bleeding at the same time (table 2.11).

Differential diagnosis of haemoptysis
Bronchiectasis
Bronchiectasis is the commonest cause of massive haemoptysis. A great number of diseases end up with bronchiectasis in their pathogenesis so that the underlying primary disease may be masked by changes of bronchiectasis. Anastomosis between the pulmonary and bronchial circulations from chronic inflammation and tissue necrosis resulting in vascular engorgement, aneurysm formation and rupture of vessels is implicated as the main cause of the haemoptysis. In bronchiectasis or mycetoma, when the bleeding is severe, recurrent and life threatening, and when surgery is contraindicated, the bleeding artery can be embolised by injection of a sclerosant or gelfoam into it to obliterate it. However, the site of the bleeding must be confirmed and highly selective embolization done to avoid occluding the spinal artery of Adamkiewicz arising from the bronchial, intercostal or intercostal-bronchial arteries and supplying parts of the spinal cord.

Pulmonary tuberculosis
Necrosis of pulmonary parenchyma or rupture of Rasmussen aneurysm which is a dilated terminal branch of pulmonary artery in the wall of a tuberculous cavity as a result of inflammatory necrosis of the wall of the vessel is responsible for the haemoptysis. The bleeding is from bronchial artery after bronchial-pulmonary artery anastomosis or bronchial-pulmonary vein fistula or anastomosis with blood coming mainly from bronchial artery derived from the high-pressure systemic circulation. Chest radiography will identify fibrocystic changes and cavitary lesions. Sputum examination for acid and alcohol fast bacilli testing will prove the diagnosis in active cases.

Bronchogenic carcinoma
The tumour mass will be seen as an opacity often with irregular or spiculated margins. Hoarseness, chest pain, brachial plexus neuropathy and Horner's syndrome (Pancoast's tumour), superior vena caval obstruction, dysphagia and problems of pericardial tamponade frequently indicate invasion of the mediastinum or chest wall by the tumour and therefore, a poorer prognosis. CT scan will show and diagnose tumour mass but histology of biopsy specimen is required for confirmation. Necrosis of lung parenchyma or outgrowing the tumour blood supply with resultant tumour necrosis or bronchial mucosal invasion is responsible for the haemoptysis.

Bronchitis and obstructive pulmonary disease
The haemoptysis appears as streaks of blood in the sputum and there may be a history of chronic smoking, tuberculosis, chronic sinusitis, irradiation or exposure to lung irritants. The tendency for bleeding is higher in the presence of bacterial colonization of chronic bronchitis lesions. In a great majority of the cases, the lung is normal in a chest radiograph. Lung collapse due to mucous plugging, pneumothorax or areas of consolidation may be seen in both chronic bronchitis and asthma. Emphysematous bullae with crowding of vessels at their margins are observed in pulmonary emphysema.

Aspergillus infection
It is usually caused by *Aspergillus fumigatus*. Aspergillus mycetomas colonize a pre-existing cavity in the lung with little or no invasion of the cavity wall or surrounding lung. The radiological diagnosis is based on finding a dense solid mass within a cavity and formation of an air-crescent within the cavity. Vascular granulation tissue within the cavity is responsible for the bleeding and haemoptysis. A freely moving fungus ball may be shown by changing the patient's position on imaging. Embolization

of supplying bronchial or intercostal artery or surgical excision of a lobe may be required to treat massive haemoptysis.

Bronchial adenoma

If this is within or outside the lumen of the bronchi, CT will confirm it as a nodular mass with location properly defined. It presents as chronic haemoptysis, usually in a young healthy female. Radiological findings on the plain chest radiographs include bronchial obstruction resulting in collapse and/or consolidation of a lung, lobe or segment. Other imaging features are compensatory emphysema, obstructive emphysema due to incomplete obstruction by a ball-valve adenoma and well-defined nodular opacities that are seen in both plain film bronchoscopy and CT scan.

Foreign body

Chest CT may identify small unsuspected aspirated objects within an area of consolidation. There are signs of volume loss or segmental or lobar collapse. There are consolidations due to recurrent pneumonia as well as intrabronchial mass formation due to chronic inflammatory reaction around the foreign body. CT and MRI can also diagnose radiolucent foreign body. Bronchoscopy is often diagnostic and therapeutic as free intraluminal objects can be retrieved, though open lobectomy may be required in some cases. Bronchial mucosal erosion or inflammation triggered by the foreign body attachment are responsible for the haemoptysis.

Congestive cardiac failure

This appears as blood-tingled white, frothy sputum. On plain chest radiography there will be cardiomegaly, upper lobe blood diversion, pulmonary oedema, full, bilateral hilar regions and pleural effusion, which is often right-sided. Rupture of the pulmonary capillaries as a result of increased pulmonary venous pressure is responsible for the haemoptysis.

Mitral valvular disease

Different types of mitral valvular diseases may present as a sudden massive haemoptysis. They may also manifest in mild form appearing as blood-stained sputum. It is thought that shunting of blood from congested pulmonary veins to non-congested bronchial veins but which have a tendency to bleed easily is responsible for the massive haemoptysis in mitral valvular disease. Massive haemoptysis also occurs when the pulmonary venous pressure increases suddenly without prior development of high pulmonary resistance that acts as protection against bleeding in advanced mitral valve disease. This has been termed *paroxysmal pulmonary haemorrhage*. Other implicated mechanism of haemoptysis in this condition include pulmonary infarction, pneumonia, pulmonary oedema, and acute heart failure. Echocardiography will demonstrate the stenosis of mitral valve. Haemoptysis from pulmonary bleeding during intercourse in patients with mitral stenosis has also been described.

Lung abscess

Lung abscess can be defined as necrosis of lung tissue and development of large holes or cavities containing necrotic fragments or fluid caused by microbial infection. Pyogenic organisms such as streptococcus and anaerobic organism and fungal infections such as actinomycosis and blastomycosis are responsible for most of the lung abscesses. Disruption of hyperaemic granulation tissues that line the abscess cavity is responsible for the haemoptysis. An area of consolidation with a large cavity, thick wall and air-fluid level often in the right middle or lower lobe is typical of lung abscess when seen in plain chest radiography. The abscess will be confirmed by CT scan as a consolidation with thick-walled cavity with air-fluid level inside it. CT scan will also excluded mass lesions but not in all cases. Examination of surgical specimen after lobectomy is the final arbiter.

Pulmonary oedema
On plain chest radiography, there is middle and lower lobe fluffy opacities with bilateral hilar fullness. Peribronchial and perivascular cuffing are observed. There will also be irregularity and lack of distinctiveness of the margins of the hilar vessels. The haemoptysis results from increased congestion and rupture of very small pulmonary veins occasioned by external pressure from oedematous lung.

Anticoagulants
The use of anticoagulant drugs to prevent the formation of blood clots in patients at risk of deep vein thrombosis and pulmonary embolism has been associated with haemoptysis. Massive endobronchial bleeding following heparin therapy for pulmonary embolism occurs and is frequently fatal. These drugs also cause direct pulmonary haemorrhage. Injury to the spinal cord due to anastomosis of the bronchial artery with the artery of Adamkiewicz, which supplies the spinal cord, is a major drawback if this arterial supply is not first identified during interventional angiography procedures in the treatement of life-threathening massive haemoptysis caused by anticoagulant therapy.

Drugs
Many types of drugs can injure the pulmonary and bronchial vessels or the lung itself and cause haemoptysis. These drugs cause haemoptysis through a wide range of mechanisms including diffuse alveolar damage, nonspecific interstitial injury, bronchiolitis obliterans, organizing lung inflammation, oesinophilic lung inflammation and pulmonary haemorrhage. Such drugs include cytotoxic drugs amphotericin B, cyclophosphamide, mitomycin, high-dose cytarabine (ara-C), D-penicillamine and methotrexate. Other drugs include aspirin, cocaine, anticoagulants, amiodarone, nitrofurantoin, as well as lipiodol used in lymphangiography. On chest radiography, there may be pulmonary oedema, diffuse non-specific lung shadowing and heterogeneous opacities particularly at the bases. Withdrawal of the drug or drastic reduction in dose is the first treatment option.

Lung contusion
Contusion of the lung causes exudation of blood and fluid into the alveoli leading to the production of rusty-coloured non-purulent sputum. History of trauma to the lung is very important. The injury can be from sports, fire arm, road traffic accidents, fall, occupation-related or assault. Pulmonary haematoma from trauma also causes haemoptysis. The opacity may enlarge within one to three days and in some cases there could be its clearance within the same period depending on the degree of injury. However, in most cases there is complete resolution within a month. This will appear as a hyperdense lesion on CT scan and there may be adjacent rib fracture. History of trauma will be beneficial.

Pulmonary embolism or pulmonary infarction
There is a great disparity between clinical diagnosis and true incidence as proven by autopsy. Collapsed lung due to embolism may get infarcted and produce haemoptysis. The haemoptysis is variable, ranging from blood-streaked sputum to copious blood-staining of sputum. Plain chest radiography may show lung consolidation, pulmonary oedema and areas of collapse. Ischemic lung necrosis is responsible for the haemoptysis. CT can diagnose the embolus as a hypodense area with peripheral wedge-shaped consolidation. Angiography will shown the embolus as intravascular filling-defect and

interventional studies can be used to lyse or remove the embolus and re-establish circulation. Tumour embolism also occurs and presents with haemoptysis as well as fainting attacks, unfortunately the diagnosis is almost always missed until at autopsy.

Pyogenic pneumonia and other haemorrhagic pneumonia.

Some organisms cause infection with blood vessel invasion resulting to infarction, formation of vascular granulation tissue with hyperaemia and symptoms of haemoptysis. The haemoptysis appears as rusty-coloured purulent sputum. Some types of pyogenic pneumonias especially in immunocompromised patients are associated with haemoptysis because most often they are necrotizing pneumonia with cavitations. They may also be complicated by bronchiectasis. Several organisms are implicated. Plain radiography often shows consolidation with air-bronchogram. Laboratory examination of sputum or bronchioalveolar lavage will identify the offending organism.

Candidiasis pneumonia

Candidiasis pneumonias usually derive from aspiration and haematogenous dissemination of gastrointestinal tract disease and is seen particularly in patients with lymphoreticular malignant disease. Persistent fever, cough and haemoptysis are usual presentations. Chest radiography may show patchy pulmonary consolidation in lower lobes with interstitial pattern and diffuse micro- or macro-nodular opacities.

Amoebic pneumonia

Pneumonia may also be associated with underlying amoebic liver abscess, which may or may not be diagnosed with plain film and liver ultrasound as its drainage into the lung through a rupture diaphragm may lead to marked reduction of the liver abscess. Hepato-bronchial fistula (47%) is the commonest association. In others, pleural effusion and empyema (29%), lung abscess (14%), and consolidation (10%) have been associated with amoebic liver abscess that presented with haemoptysis and pulmonary pyogenic infection. Plain radiography often shows consolidation with air-bronchogram. CT scan will demonstrate consolidation and air-bronchogram better and show any other associated condition such as bronchiectasis, lung abscess, tumour or pleural effusion. Laboratory examination of sputum or bronchioalveolar lavage will identify the offending organism.

Viral pneumonia

The haemoptysis initially appears as rusty-coloured which later often leads to frank haemoptysis. The implicated organisms are usually those that cause viral haemorrhagic fever and in some of them, haemoptysis is an important diagnostic criterion. They include yellow fever, hansa fever, q-fever, lassa fver, ebola disease, etc. Other viruses such as *cytomegalovirus, herpes simplex virus,* infectious mononucleosis and Rocky Mountain spotted fever also cause haemoptysis.

Bronchopulmonary sequestration syndrome

This is a mass of non-functioning lung tissue that fails to communicate with the normal bronchial tree. It receives its vascular supply from aberrant arterial branches from the thoracic or abdominal aorta and venous drainage is into the left atrium through the pulmonary vein, or the right atrium or azygos vein. They are classified as intralobar or extralobar. Antenatal sonography will display a solid, well-defined intrathoracic echogenic mass but its anomalous systemic arterial supply is difficult to visualize even in colour flow Doppler due to its small size and abnormal position. Some cases involute before birth. Most presentations occur after birth and at an older age. This is because recurrent focal infections, recurrent pneumonia, bronchiectasis, tuberculosis, aspergillus infection with resulting haemoptysis are frequently what draw attention to the disease. It can be asymptomatic or presentation may also be in adulthood. Contrast CT, MRI or angiography of the chest and upper abdomen are effective diagnostic modalities.

Bronchial carcinoids

This is an uncommon disease and appears as well-circumscribed nodules or masses, which are usually of solitary locations on chest radiographs. Calcification may be seen with CT scan and the tumour enhances following contrast administration. Carcinoids are neuroendocrine tumours and are derived from bronchial *amino precursor uptake decarboxylation* (APUD) cells. These are the same cells that give rise to small cell carcinoma. Bronchial carcinoids are classified as either typical or atypical. Typical carcinoids are relatively benign, grow slowly and metastasize infrequently. They make up 90% of carcinoids. Atypical carcinoids are relatively more malignant and about 50% will eventually metastasize. About *80%* of carcinoids arise in lobar or main segmental bronchi and growth of tumour into the lumen is responsible for bronchial obstruction and lung collapse. Partial bronchial obstruction may result in recurrent segmental pneumonia, bronchiectasis or abscess formation, or air-tapping and haemoptysis. Carcinoids may produce different types of hormones such as kallikreins, insulin, serotonin, histamine, ACTH and gastrin.

Cystic fibrosis

Haemoptysis seen in this condition may be due to bronchiectasis. Sudden massive haemoptysis occurs due to arterial bleeding from an infected cavity or secondary to bronchial arterial hypertrophy due to cor pulmonale. Selective bronchial arteriography and embolisation are frequently life-saving and should be considered where facility and technical competence are available. Early radiographic features of cystic fibrosis include air- trapping and bronchial wall thickening. Diffuse interstitial opacities, bronchiectasis, and cyst formation occur as the disease progresses. The lung disease progresses at a variable rate to an 'end-stage lung' in early adult life. Serial radiography at yearly intervals is often used to monitor progression of the pulmonary disease. Pneumothorax is uncommon, but is often life-threatening.

Eosinophilic pneumonia haemoptysis

It can be acute or chronic eosinophilia but is the general pathway for many parasitic infections such as Ascariasis lumbricoidis, hydatid infection, malaria and others. In plain radiography, there are characteristic patchy, nonsegmental areas of consolidation in the middle and upper zones. 'Photographic negative of pulmonary oedema' is observed which represent peripheral opacities paralleling the chest wall. This is better revealed on CT scan.

Wegener's granulomatosis

This is a multisystem disease with variable clinical expression characterized by necrotizing granulomatous inflammation of the upper and lower respiratory tracts, (pulmonary involvement in about 90% of cases); focal necrotizing glomerulonephritis; and a small vessel vasculitis affecting arteries, capillaries and veins. Multiple nodules or masses are the most common findings seen with plain film or CT scan. Nodules are bilateral in over 70% of cases. They are often diffuse and those up to 2 cm in diameter usually show cavitations which may lead to erroneous diagnosis of tuberculosis. Airspace consolidation and appearance of ground-glass opacities also occur with or without the presence of nodules. Diffuse bilateral areas of ground-glass opacities are often due to pulmonary haemorrhage, which can also present with haemoptysis.

Alveolar proteinosis

Alveolar proteinosis also known as alveolar lipoproteinosis or alveolar phospholipoproteinosis is a rare disease of unknown aetiology. There is overproduction of proteinaceous lipid-rich material by type II pneumocytes to the extent that the capacity of the lung to remove it is overwhelmed.

The chest radiographic changes are non-specific, both lungs are usually involved, and airspace opacification is most pronounced in the central lung. Plain film appearance is similar to pulmonary oedema, with small bilateral acinar and perihilar opacities, which may coalesce. On thin-section CT images, a 'crazy-paving' pattern which is a striking geographical distribution of ground-glass appearance, consolidation and thickened interlobular septa is the characteristic feature but not specific. Diagnosis is by histology of lung biopsy or bronchoalveolar lavage specimen. About a quarter of cases die within 5 years.

Kaposi's sarcoma

Abnormalities seen on Chest radiograph and CT are poorly defined peribronchovascular nodular opacities which typically measure 10–20 mm in diameter. Solitary nodular lesion occurs but bilateral multiple lesions are typical. Coarse linear opacities scattered diffusely in both lungs, particularly in the perihilar and lower lobes also occur. The lung opacities tend to coalesce together differentiating it from the nodules seen with lymphoma. Unilateral or bilateral pleural effusion is observed in less than 50% of patients and lymphadenopathy has been reported in less than 30%. Unusual radiographic features include pericardial fluid, intratracheal or endobronchial nodular masses and cavitations.

Broncholithiasis

Broncholithiasis is defined as the presence of calcified or ossified material within the bronchial lumen. Broncholithiasis is usually formed by erosion and extrusion of calcified adjacent lymph node into the bronchial lumen and is frequently associated with long-standing foci of necrotizing granulomatous lymphadenitis. On chest radiographs, there are calcified hilar or mediastinal nodes, bronchial obstruction with collapse and lobar consolidation with features of bronchiactesis. CT findings of broncholithiasis are calcified nodules that are either endobronchial or peribronchial associated with atelectasis, obstructive pneumonitis, or bronchiectasis. Both broncholithiasis and its obstructive changes are more common on the right lung.

Paragonimiasis

In plain chest radiograph, there are nodular and cystic lesions within the lung. The cysts measure 5-30 mm in diameter and are located in the apical part of the upper lobe, appear, and disappear rapidly. Homogenous reactive pneumonia that heals with fibrosis may occur. There may be hilar lymphadenopathy, ring shadows and calcification. Lung parenchymal changes in lower lobes simulating bronchiectasis, and in the upper lobes, tuberculosis are usual. Peripheral linear opacities believed to be worm migration tracks are seen in CT. Pleural effusion occur in 50% of cases. In CNS affectation there may be signs of raised intracranial pressure, hydrocephalus and intracranial calcification. Intracranial abscess may develop. Biopsy of pulmonary lesion or cerebral lesion is required for confirmation. If the above cannot be done, detection of anti-paragonimus antibody in blood or ova in sputum also confirms the diagnosis.

Diffuse pulmonary haemorrhage syndrome

Following pulmonary haemorrhage, lung fibrosis develops leading to alveolar thickening. Components of this syndrome include idiopathic pulmonary haemosiderosis and antibasement membrane antibody disease also known as Goodpasture's syndrome. Patchy alveolar infiltrates which may be initially focal and unilateral but may become more diffuse with time are seen on plain chest radiography. Recurrent disease may have a background of chronic interstitial opacities or fibrosis. Kerley B lines suggest mitral stenosis or pulmonary veno-occlusive disease as the cause of alveolar haemorrhage. The extent of the lesion and its alveolar nature are confirmed by CT scan. Histology of lung biopsy specimen shows blood and intra-alveolar haemosiderin-laden macrophages as the cardinal findings. Destruction of the alveolocapillary basement membrane by the antibasement membrane antibody or intra-alveolar bleeding from severe anaemia is responsible for the haemoptysis.

Bronchogenic carcinoma

The tumour mass of the carcinoma will be shown within the lung as an area of opacity. Areas of rib destruction, phrenic nerve involvement or involvement of other vital structures such as bronchus with collapse may be identified. This is one of the most identifiable causes of haemoptysis. Lymphadenopathy due to bronchogenic carcinoma will be shown by CT scan and the pulmonary tumour mass lesions associated with the lymphadenopathy will help in accurate diagnosis. Embolisation of vessls supplying the tumour may reduce the vascular nature of the tumour before surgery as well as help to stop any acute bleeding. In some cases, embolisation of vascular supply may be the definitive treatment. Endobronchial presentation of metastasis or Hodgkin's disease also causes haemoptysis. Perfusion CT studies can identify aneurysmal or bleeding vessels and thrombus in the arteries. With CT scan any tumour mass hidden in a consolidated lung or collapsed and distorted lung can be diagnosed.

Angiomatous malformation

This is usually arteriovenous malformations which is present from birth. This will appear as an area of inhomogeneous opacity with nodular appearances. Contrast enhancement will show the lesion better with early and intense contrast enhancement on CT studies. These lesions can be embolised by injection of sclerosant or gelfoam to cause occlusion of the angiomatous malformation-feeding vessel and destroy the malformation. It is difficult to differentiate haemoptysis caused by this from factitious haemoptysis unless accurate history is volunteered in the later or relevant imaging studies is performed in the former.

Pulmonary venous varix

This is abnormal tortuous dilatation of pulmonary vein occurring just before its entrance into left atrium. It is often symptomless but haemoptysis may develop in some cases. The condition is *congenital* although some cases are associated with pulmonary venous hypertension. These lesions are typically located in the perihilar regions at about medial one-third of both lungs often below the hilar region close to left atrium. It presents as well-defined round, oval or lobulated mass that change in size during Valsalva manoeuvre. On contrast CT, it tends to opacify at the same time with the left atrium. It is a major source of cerebral emboli and it causes cardiac failure. Its rupture is catastrophic.

Laryngeal adenoid cystic carcinoma

This is a malignant laryngeal tumour composed of uniform small basal cells, which shows large oval-shaped nuclei that are arranged in anastomosing cords or islands pattern. These tumours are usually seen at subglottis region of the larynx at its junction with trachea in most cases. However, widespread submucosal tumour spread of the whole larynx *and its invasion* of cricoid cartilage, thyroid gland and the oesophagus may occur. This tumour is noted by its tendency to invade nerves and thus is characteristically associated with recurrent laryngeal nerve paralysis. The tumour presents with episodic cough, wheeze and haemoptysis. It is diagnosed using bronchoscopy.

Laryngo-pulmonary papillomatosis

This is squamous papillomas in the larynx and lung caused by human papilloma virus types 6 and type II. It occurs equally in both sexes but those occurring in patients aged less than 10 years show diffuse involvement while those occurring in older patients of 21-50 years of age are usually single. It results in thickened lumpy vocal cord. There is subglottic extension and it may occur in the uvula, palate and the pulmonary tissue. The symptoms are hoarseness of voice, aphonia, cough, recurrent pneumonia, haemoptysis, asthma-like symptoms and respiratory distress.

Hughes-Stovin syndrome

This is a rare and fatal autoimmune condition seen in boys. It is caused by recurrent deep peripheral vein thrombosis, which is frequently associated with haemoptysis resulting from ruptured aneurysm particularly from the segmental pulmonary artery or bronchial artery. Other presentations are cough, dyspnoea, fever and chest pain. Its aetiology is unknown but considered a clinical variant of Behçet disease. The supplying artery can be identified on angiography and embolised using interventional techniques.

Osler-Weber-Rendu syndrome

It is also known as hereditary haemorrhagic telangiectasia. In this condition, there are arterovenous fistulae in the lung with abnormal communications with the skin and other organs such as the lung, brain, liver and gastrointestinal tract. Large fistulae present as round homogenous masses with enlarged serpentines vessels radiating to the hilar and are diagnosed with CT or MRI. There are frequently multiple lesions in the lung. They are usually asymptomatic but some may present with cyanosis, finger clubbing, polycythemia and haemoptysis. They can also be embolised to stop the bleeding during angiography.

Thoracic splenosis

This is caused by seeding of splenic tissue to pleural space subsequent to thoracoabdominal trauma. It is usually discovered about 10 to 30 years after the precipitating trauma. The patients present with recurrent haemoptysis but in most cases, it is asymptomatic. On chest radiography or CT, it appears as single or multiple pulmonary opacities measuring about few millimetres to 6 cm in diameter located in the left pleura or fissure. Radionuclide studies shows positive Tc-99m sulfur colloid scan. Other studies using indium-111-labeled platelets and Tc-99m-labeled heat-damaged red blood cells are also positive.

Catamenial haemoptysis

It is also called *chest endometriosis syndrome*. This is defined as cyclical haemoptysis associated with menses in a woman of childbearing age when all other causes of recurrent haemoptysis has been excluded. It is usually caused by pulmonary endometriosis. The diagnosis is based on clinical history of haemoptysis, pleuritic chest pain associated with menses and radiological evidence of a pulmonary mass lesion whose size, and character changes with menses. There could also be history of pneumothorax and haemothorax. Plain films may show right-sided nodules and effusions. Lesions are caused by lymphatic or vascular micro seeding of tissues into the chest or peritoneal-pleural migration through a diaphragmatic defect. Angiography with embolisation of the supplying vessel is the treatment of choice. More recently uterine fibroid and pulmonary arteriovenous malformation have also been implicated in catamenial haemoptysis. The influence of cyclical changes of oestrogen on the blood, blood volume or the masses has been forwarded as possible mechanism of occurrence of this type of haemoptysis.

Iatrogenic haemoptysis

Many different diagnostic or surgical procedures used by clinicians in the course of management of the patient may injure the bronchial or pulmonary vessels and result in haemoptysis. The important procedures that results in haemoptysis are lung biopsy, bronchoscopy, angiography, vascular interventional procedures and dislodgement of stents and filter material or fracture of catheter tips. Many of these cases are mild and require little or no imaging or simple chest radiography for diagnosis. However, occasionally some of them may result to severe haemoptysis requiring angiography with vascular interventional procedures to stop the bleeding.

Amyloidosis

In this disease, there is extracellular deposit of proteinaceous twisted B-pleated sheet fibrils of immense chemical diversity. These materials are immunoglobulin proteins or *polysaccharide* complex with affinity for Congo red stain. Those that have lung involvement are mostly primary amyloidosis in over 65% to 70% of case. The tracheobronchial type, which is the commonest type present with haemoptysis, cough, stridor, difficulty with breathing, wheeze and hoarseness. In chest radiography or CT, the lesion at this site is composed of multiple protruding nodules from the tracheal or large bronchial wall. There may be narrowing and rigidity of an involved tracheal segment. The bronchovascular markings are accentuated and there is also destructive pneumonitis. Multiple parenchymal nodules at subpleural locations may be seen with or without pleural effusion. Calcification may be observed. Histology of biopsy specimen will conclusively diagnose the lesion.

Tracheal tumours

These are made of benign or malignant lesions. Among the malignant tumours, squamous-cell carcinoma is the commonest primary accounting for about 50% of all malignant tracheal lesions. Other malignant lesions include adenoid cystic carcinoma, metastasis, mucoepidermoid carcinoma, carcinoid, lymphoma and plasmacytoma. The benign tumours are cartilaginous tumour (a hamartoma), haemangioma, squamous cell papilloma, granular cell myoblastoma, fibroma, lipoma, tuberculoma, sarcoidosis, Wegener granulomatosis, amyloid tumour and gossypiboma. They present with wheeze, cough, hoarseness, and haemoptysis. They are usually diagnosed with bronchoscopy and histology of biopsy specimen.

Cryptogenic haemoptysis

This is a condition in which no identifiable cause is discovered but is often limited by available facilities, and expertise from centre to centre. As much as 15% to 30% of haemoptysis may not have diagnosable underlying cause. This is true even after extensive diagnostic tests, including a bronchoscopy. This type of haemoptysis is usually mild and non-specific bronchial inflammation is believed to be the cause of the haemoptysis. Most patients in this group have good prognosis.

Post-coital haemoptysis

Haemoptysis following coitus is a rare condition seen in adults with equal frequency among the sexes. Most patients have underlying cardiac pathology as the predisposing factors. Such conditions often result in cardiac decompensation before causing the post-coital haemoptysis and they include hypertension, left ventricular failure, pulmonary embolism, rheumatic heart disease, coronary artery disease, left atrial tumour, mitral stenosis and mitral regurgitation.

Other reported non-cardiac predisposing factors include amyloidosis, lymphangioleiomyomatosis, tuberous sclerosis, pulmonary hypertension and Takayasu arteritis. There may be a combination of two or more of the predisposing conditions in the same patient. The haemoptysis results when physical exertion associated with sexual stimulation and coitus causes momentary elevation of pulmonary capillary pressure with rupture of capillaries and bleeding into the pulmonary alveoli and tracheobronchial tree. The role of radiology is to exclude other causes of haemoptysis as well as diagnose the predisposing condition and if possible treat these conditions using interventional studies where applicable.

Factitious haemoptysis

This is a pulmonary manifestation of Munchausen syndrome. This condition describes a category of patients who intentionally put up symptoms, signs or disabilities. There are both physical and psychological components and in severe cases, the sufferer may undergo repeat invasive procedure; and surgeries and jump from one hospital to the other to avoid being detected. The patient may use multiple names, social security numbers, identity cards and birth dates to avoid discovery. Reported self-inflected wound sites for the haemoptysis include injury to posterior pharynx with a piece of glass, self-inflicted injury to posterior part of the tongue, trauma to trachea with cotton swab, self venesection, biting the inside of the lip and self administration of dicoumarol (a type of anticoagulant). The patients are often aged 21 to 47 years and many are health care workers. The goal of the patient is to involuntarily gain many varieties of benefits such as attention, nurturance, sympathy, financial gain, and leniency that are perceived as impossible through any other means. Radiology only excludes organic causes.

(Adam & Dixon, 2008; Dahnert, 2011; Sutton, 1998 and 2003, Palmer & Reeder 2001).

References

1. Bruzzi JF, Rémy-Jardin M, Delhaye D, Teisseire A, Khalil C, Rémy J. Multi-detector row CT of hemoptysis. Radiographics 2006; 26:3-22.
2. Ofoegbu RO, Anah OO, Jarikre LN, Ojogwu LI. Changing significance of haemoptysis in the tropics: experience from Benin City, Nigeria. Trop Doct 1984;14:188-9.
3. Yoon W, Kim JK, Kim YH, Chung TW, Kang HK. Bronchial and nonbronchial systemic artery embolization for life-threatening hemoptysis: a comprehensive review Radiographics 2002; 22:1395-409.
4. Lee KS, Kim Y, Han J, Ko EJ, Park CK, Primack SL. Bronchioloalveolar carcinoma: clinical, histopathologic, and radiologic findings. Radiographics 1997; 17:1345-57.
5. Yoon YC, Lee KS, Jeong YJ, Shin SW, Chung MJ, Kwon OJ. Hemoptysis: bronchial and nonbronchial systemic arteries at 16-detector row CT. Radiology 2005; 234:292-8.
6. Andersen PE. Imaging and interventional radiological treatment of hemoptysis. Acta Radiol 2006; 47:780-92.

7. Makanjuola D, Adeyemo AO. Lower lungfield tuberculosis in a rural African population. West Afr J Med 1991;10: 412-9.

8. Nwafor DC, Egbue MO. Intrathoracic manifestations of amoebiasis. Ann R Coll Surg Engl 1981;63:126-8.

9. Ibadin MO, Oviawe O. Trend in childhood tuberculosis in Benin City, Nigeria. Ann Trop Paediatr 2001;21:141-5.

10. Elesha SO, Bandele EO. Primary pulmonary carcinoma in Lagos, Nigeria: a clinicopathological study. East Afr Med J 1995;72:276-9.

11. Awotedu AA, Igbokwe EO, Akang EE, Aghadiuno PO. Pulmonary embolism in Ibadan, Nigeria: five years autopsy report. Cent Afr J Med 1992; 38:432-5.

2.2 RADIOLOGICAL MANIFESTATIONS OF INDUSTRIAL LUNG DISEASES

Industrial lung diseases are also known as occupational lung diseases or pneumoconioses.

Definition
Pneumoconioses are diseases that result from inhalation of fine subdivisions of particulate matter with the consequence that the lungs become dust-trapped, causing loss of elasticity and function. The diagnosis depends on:
1. History of exposure to dust
    a. Living near a mine, factory or house where such dust exists.
    b. Living with an exposed worker
    c. Working directly with the dust in the factory or occupation
2. Appropriate time interval or duration between exposure and detection of disease.
3. Abnormal chest radiograph or CT scan
4. Abnormal respiratory function test
5. Restrictive pattern of lung disease with improvement after removal from source of exposure.

Types of Dust
A. *Active dust*

    These are fibrogenic dust and they cause lung fibrosis. They include asbestos, silica, coal and silicate dust (Talc, mica, kaolin and china clay).

B. *Inactive dust*

    Non-fibrogenic dust: These are inert and therefore do not cause lung fibrosis e.g. ferric oxide, siderosis, ferric and silver.

C. *Dust of doubtful activity*

    Aluminium, graphite, tungsten, etc.

D. *Inorganic dust causing chemical pneumonitis*

    These include beryllium, manganese, cadmium, ZnO (metal fumes), etc.

E. *Organic dusts*
    a. Bagasse (sugar cane dust lung, Bagassosis)
    b. Cotton dust (Byssinosis)
    c. Wheat dust (farmer's lung)
    d. Paprika – splitting (parprika – splitter's lung)
    e. Mushroom – mushroom workers lung etc.

F. *Carcinogenic Dust*

    These include arsenic, radioactive dust e.g. uranium, asbestos, thorium, chromate, retort – house gas work, etc.

G. *Gases*

They cause chemical pneumonitis.

They include nitrous fumes, nitrogen dioxide (silofiller's lung), sulphuric fumes, nickel carbonyl fumes, ammonium fumes, kerosene/petroleum product fumes, etc.

Determinants of the type and extent of reaction to dust exposure

1. Nature of inhaled dust
2. Duration of exposure
3. Concentration of particles
4. Individual/host susceptibility
5. Size of inhaled dust

Silicosis

Definition

This results from exposure to silica or silicon dioxide leading to diffuse air-space disease, which is frequently of progressive nature even after termination of the exposure. Pulmonary fibrosis results following several years of exposure and it may continue even after termination of exposure.

Occupations affected

Tunnelling, mining (gold, granite etc), quarrying, sand blasting, ceramic industry, pottery and foundry workers are affected.

Radiological Features

A. **Simple silicosis**

1. Multiple nodular shadows of 2 – 5 mm in diameter seen initially in the middle and upper lung zones.
2. The lesion may progress to involve all the zones but it is more in the upper and middle zones.
3. There is relative sparing of lower zones
4. CT scan demonstrates predilection for the posterior aspect of the lung in both middle and upper zones.
5. There is observance of well-defined uniform densities of about 2 – 5 mm in diameter.
6. Increased density of hilar shadows due to lesion in these areas superimposed on hilar shadows is noted.
7. Multiple linear shadows
8. Septal lines due to thickening of the interlobar and interlobular septa as the lymphatics in these regions try to remove the dust.

CT Scan

What could be observed on CT scan studies include:

1. 3 – 10 mm sized nodules in diameter.
2. Thickened interlobar and interlobular septa
3. Thickened linear and curvilinear densities due to peribronchiolar fibrosis
4. Ground-glass appearance signifying fibrosis with oedema
5. Fibrotic bands within the lung parenchyma
6. Pleural-based nodular densities of varied sizes
7. Bronchiectasis (Traction type)
8. Honey-comb appearance.

B. **Complicated Silicosis**

These are seen radiologically as outlined below:

1. *Confluent homogenous non-segmental shadows*, occurring particularly in the upper lobes. This is refered to as progressive massive fibrosis (PMF).

2. Bigger shadows and opacities which have appeared (PMF) migrate towards the hilar region from the periphery laterally.

3. *Progressive massive fibrosis* is bilateral and symmetrical upper lobe shadows with bat-wing/angel-wing appearance associated with raised ESR and reduced prognosis. PMF is more common in coal worker's pneumoconiosis.

4. Areas of peripheral emphysema are created by the medially migrating shadows. Lesions are seen in plain film but are earlier detected on CT scan.

5. Massive shadows of PMF may cavitate due to ischaemic necrosis.

6. Features of pulmonary arterial hypertension and cor pulmonale develop due to extensive fibrosis.

7. Hilar lymphadenopathy is common.

8. *Egg-shell* or diffuse calcification of enlarged lymph nodes are demonstrated with plain film or CT scan.

9. Features of tuberculosis which frequently complicates PMF or complicated silicosis are seen, but cavity may be due to necrosis of massive fibrosis and not necessarily TB.

10. *Caplan's syndrome:* This is silicosis with multiple rheumathoid lung nodules. Features of rheumathoid arthritis elsewhere in the body can be detected. Caplan's syndrome is more common with coal workers pneumoconiosis.

Complication of Silicosis

Infection: Recorded complications from infections include bronchopneumonia, chronic bronchitis, and pulmonary tuberculosis. Sudden progression of symptoms suggests TB.

Cardiovascular complications: Cor pulmonale, cardiac failure, polycythaemia

Caplan syndrome: Necrobiotic pulmonary nodules of rheumathoid arthritis with pneumoconiosis. They may cavitate.

Amyloidosis: This is extracellular hyaline substance which encroaches on cells and produce cell atrophy. Primary amyloidosis involves the skin, tongue, heart and nerves. Secondary amyloidosis involves the liver, spleen, suprarenals and the kidneys. It causes renal failure in the kidneys.

Asbestosis

This is defined as chronic diffuse progressive pulmonary interstitial fibrosis caused by industrial exposure to asbestos.

Occupations involved

Asbestos mining, asbestos milling, asbestos processing (insulation workers, gasket builders, making of brake lining, asbestos roofing material or ceiling), workers in asbestos construction/demolition work, ship building, manufacture of textiles, living near asbestos work place and living with exposed worker.

Types of asbestos that cause disease

1. Chrysotile (white asbestos): It is the commonest type, relatively benign and found in Canada.

2. Crocidolite (blue asbestos): The most pathogenic (due to very fine fibres, size), it is found in South Africa, Australia.

3. Amosite (Brown asbestos). It is the second most pathogenic.
4. Anthophyllite: It is relatively benign. It is found in North America and Finland.
5. Tremolite: It is relatively benign
6. Actinolite: It is relatively benign

Features

Inhaled fibres are 8 – 32 mm long and 0.25 mm thick and they reach the alveoli, penetrate the pleura and often reach the diaphragm. The gravitation of the fibres to the bases is why the changes are more common in the bases or lower zones than in the middle and upper zones. The fibre cause physical and chemical irritation leading to autoimmune reaction. About 20–30 years of exposure is often required to cause symptoms of asbestosis and/or lung cancer. Cigarette smoking increases the risk of lung cancer by 10 times. Asbestosis increases the risk of lung cancer by five times. Asbestosis and cigarette smoking combined increases the risk of lung cancer by 50 – 90 times.

Radiological Features
A. Pleural changes
  a. Pleural plaques
   1. Thickened dense pleura < 1 cm thick. They are hyalinised collagenous tissue in parietal pleura.
   2. They occur in middle zones and over the diaphragm bilaterally.
   3. Pleural plaques are the most frequent manifestation of previous exposure.
   4. Small plaques are best demonstrated by oblique film, fluoroscopy, ultrasound scan and HRCT.
   5. Plaques do not often calcify but when they do, they present a bizarre appearance.

  b. **Pleural calcification**
   These appear as:
   1. Dense calcification parallel to the lateral chest wall
   2. Dense calcification lines parallel to the diaphragm bilaterally with clear costophrenic angles are characteristic.
   3. Calcification may be seen parallel to the mediastinum and pericardium occasionally.
   4. Thick leaf-like calcification with in-rolled edges
   5. 'Holly-leaf' appearance is seen in advanced cases

  c. **Pleural effusion**
   This is seen in up to 20% of the cases and it occurs early in the disease. It presents as:
   1. Small persistent effusions. They are benign and consist of sterile serous or haemorrhagic exudates.
   2. Large effusions may be bilateral and recurrent and often signify malignancy.
   3. Pleural plaques and calcification may be associated with effusion.

  d. **Pleural thickening**
   This is seen as:
   1. Thickening of visceral and parietal pleura, which may be diffuse. Parietal thickening is more often detected.
   2. Thickened interlobar septa

3. Focal thickening of diaphragm
4. Obliteration of costophrenic angles (rare)
5. Shaggy heart appearance. This denotes bilateral process.

B. Lung Parenchymal changes
1. It is first detected by HRCT. HRCT detects abnormality in up to 25% of patients with asbestosis whose chest radiographs are shown to be normal.
2. Earliest signs are fine reticular, nodular or reticulo-nodular pattern confined to the lower zones.
3. Shaggy heart appearance: Coarse reticulonodular, reticular or nodular appearance with loss of clarity of diaphragm and cardiac margins and cardiac shadow.
4. Involvement of the whole lung but this is more of the lower zones.
5. Areas of emphysema develop but is more in the bases.
6. Pulmonary fibrosis, starting peripherally develops and is earliest detected by HRCT.
7. Parenchymal bands extending inwards from the pleural surface.
8. Distorted lung architecture
9. Sub-pleural linear densities and opacities/septal lines
10. Interstitial fibrosis simulating idiopathic pulmonary fibrosis and presence of pleural dispease suggests asbestosis
11. Honey-comb appearance.

C. Asbestos pseudotumour
It appears as a round pleura or infolding with segmental or subsegmental atelectasis. It is more common in the posterolateral aspect of the lower lobe and may be bilateral.
1. Focal sub-pleural mass abutting on the region of thickened pleura.
2. Little progression but decrease in size may be apparent.
3. Adjacent lung shows volume loss since the lesion is basically an atelectasis.

High resolution computed tomography (HRCT)
1. Wedge-shaped or round density within the lung.
2. Lesion is contiguous with area of pleural thickening or pleural calcification.
3. *Spiculated appearance or crow's feet appearance*: Multiple linear bands radiating from the mass in the lung parenchyma.
4. *Comet-tail or vacuum cleaner sign*: This is bronchovascular marking originating from the subpleural nodular mass and extending towards the ipsilateral hilum.
5. Air-bronchogram effect or Swiss cheese appearance.

D. Asbestos-related carcinoma
Predisposing factors
1. Accumulated dose of asbestos fibres
2. Co-existing smoking
3. Pre-existing interstitial disease
4. Occupational exposure to known carcinogen
Latent period: 20 – 30 years
Location: 1. Lung bases; 2. In any location when associated with smoking.
Cancer types:

1. *Lung cancer*
   a. Bronchoalveolar cell carcinoma (the most common).
   b. Bronchogenic carcinoma (adenocarcinoma (peripheral), squamous cell carcinoma (medial).
2. *Gastrointestinal tract carcinomas*: Oropharynx, oesophagus, stomach, large bowel, peritoneum.
3. *Mesothelioma*
4. *Renal tract carcinoma*

Coal Worker's Pneumoconiosis

Inhalation of coal dust, a non-fibrogenic particle, leads to their deposition in the lungs causing opacities surrounded by emphysema.

Exposed occupation: Coal Miners.

Agents. a. *Coal* which is a type of carbon. It is inert and non-fibrogenic. b. *Coal and silica*. Silica is fibrogenic

Types: 1. Simple coal worker's pneumoconiosis.
   2. Complicated coal worker's pneumoconiosis
      i. Associated with prolonged exposure
      ii. Complicated by (a) infection (b) autoimmune reaction.

Radiological features

A. Simple coal workers pneumoconiosis (>10 years of exposure)
   1. Middle zone, faint, small, indistinct nodules of about 1 – 5 mm in diameter.
   2. Spread of nodules throughout the lungs but more numerous in middle zones.
   3. Opacities do not progress after cessation of exposure.
   4. Nodules correlate with amount of collagen *not* the amount of coal dust
   5. Poor correlation between symptoms, physiological findings and radiological features.

B. **Complicated coal workers' pneumoconiosis (Progressive massive fibrosis (PMF))**
   1. Appearance of larger opacities, of about 1 cm in diameter
   2. Conglomerates of confluent, round or oval homogenous opacities forming non-segmental shadows and fibrosis (PMF)
   3. Lesions seen in middle and upper lobes are bilateral
   4. The round and oval shadows (PMF) migrate towards the hila
   5. Peripheral area of emphysema or bullae. These are created when the opacities of PMF migrate toward the hila
   6. Calcification: The nodular opacities may fibrose and calcify
   7. Cavitation: The area of massive fibrosis may cavitate by necrosis
   8. Confluent non-segmental opacities (PMF) which progress even after cessation of exposure while simple coal worker's pneumoconiosis does not after cessation of exposure.

C. **Caplan's Syndrome**

In this syndrome, there is a combination of rheumatoid nodules and coal worker's pneumoconiosis. Its features are:

1. Multiple oval, well-defined pulmonary nodules 1 – 5 cm in diameter.

2. Lesions appear in crops with simultaneous appearance of cutaneous rheumatoid nodules. These are necrobiotic nodules and should not be misdiagnosed as metastasis
3. Nodules may remain unchanged, calcify, cavitate or regress.

Complications
Chronic obstructive bronchiolitis, cor pulmonale and focal emphysema.

Berylliosis
This is defined as chronic granulomatous disorder resulting from delayed hypersensitivity reaction sequel to exposure to acid salts from beryllium oxide extract.
Occupation that is exposed: Fluorescent lamp factory workers
Types   1. Acute Berylliosis. 2. Chronic Berylliosis

Acute berylliosis
It is defined as acute non-cardiogenic pulmonary oedema caused by beryllium oxide extract chemical pneumonitis

Chronic berylliosis
It requires 5 – 15 years of exposure to occur. It is a widespread systemic disease involving the lungs, spleen, lymph nodes, liver, heart, skeletal muscles and kidneys.
Radiological features
1. Widespread fine nodular non-cavitating granulomas.
2. Irregular opacities in the middle zones sparing the bases and upper zones.
3. Bilateral symmetrical hilar and mediastinal lymphadenopathy (similar to sarcoidosis).
4. Upper lobe emphysema
5. Pulmonary interstitial fibrosis

On HRCT, the findings are:
1. Pneumothorax
2. Bronchial wall thickening
3. Septal lines
4. Ground glass appearance
5. Pleural irregularities

Pneumoconiosis due to inactive dust
These do not cause fibrosis but produce chest x-ray changes by accumulating in the lung and they are usually symptomless.

Siderosis
The disease results from the inhalation of inert iron oxide dust.
Occupation exposed: Arc welding, foundry workers, burning steel, grinders, fettlers, polishers (jewellery).

Radiological features
i.   Reticulonodular opacities in the lungs
ii. Lesions regress when exposure ceases

iii. Absence of secondary fibrosis
iv. Absence of lymphadenopathy
   When mixed with silica (silicosiderosis)
v. Small round opacities are seen
vi. Fibrosis may occur resembling silicosis

Stannosis

Stannosis results from the inhalation of tin oxide dust which causes the disease.
Radiological features are:
i. Multiple, very small and very dense well-defined opacities of 0.5 – 1 mm diameter with miliary appearance.
ii. The opacities are distributed throughout the lung in miliary pattern
iii. There are dense septal lines when particles collect in the interlobular lymphatics.
iv. The opacities have very high density (denser than calcium) because of the very high atomic number of tin.

Barytosis

It results from inhalation of particulate barium sulphate dust.
The radiological features are as follows:
1. Bilateral, very dense nodular opacities in the lungs.
2. Shadows regress after ceasation of exposure.
3. Normal pulmonary function is maintained and it is asymptomatic.
4. The shadows are similar to calcified nodules but denser than calcium/bone
5. There is absence of lymphadenopathy
6. There is also absence of cor pulmonale

Talcosis

This results from prolonged inhalation of magnesium silicate dust, which contains tremolite, anthophyllite and silicate (Amphibole fibres). Exposed occupation are workers in paper, plastic, paint, ceramic, rubber, drug tableting and cosmetic industries.
Radiaological features
a. Features of silicosis (Talcosilicosis)
   1. Round small and large opacities
   2. Pulmonary fibrosis which does not regress after ceasation of exposure
   3. Features of progressive massive fibrosis of silicosis
   4. Features of end-stage sarcoidosis

b. Features of Asbestosis (Talcoasbestosis)
   1. Massive and bizarre pleural plaques
   2. Calcification of pleura
   3. Encasement of the lung by pleural calcification

c. Features in those that inject tables intravenously (drug abusers).

Magnesium trisilicate is used as fillers and lubricants in the preparation of tablets intended for oral use. However, among drug abusers these tablets may be grounded, dissolved and injected intravenously.

The talc accumulates in the pulmonary circulation and the deposits may then cause numerous small foreign body reactions in the form of granulomas. With persistent use, the nodules can coalesce to form larger masses.

Hyperdense micronodules of less than 1 mm in diameter are seen with CT particularly in the lower lobes. These nodules are *birefrigent to polarized light* and are within giant cells in areas of pulmonary fibrosis when examined histologically. Ground glass appearance may be seen as well as conglomerate masses.

Extrinsic Allergic Alveolitis (Hypersensitivity Pneumonitis)

This is an allergic inflammatory granulomatous reaction in the lungs characterised by inappropriate host response to inhaled dust containing organic allergens or proteins that are frequently related to the patient's occupation or addicter's hobby (table 2.21).

Causes

It is caused by occupational or habitual exposure to organic dust of < 5 – 10 mm particle size that acts as allergen (table 2.21).

Mechanism

Antigenic particles reaching previously sensitized lungs cause hypersensitivity reaction. The presence of host antibodies, which are meant to neutralize the antigen, may, by their combination with the antigen, cause damage to the tissue and elicit reactions, which are progressive and causing disease.

Types of reactions involved:

Type III hypersensitivity reaction

Type IV hypersensitivity reaction

Exposed occupations: Various types of farming, animal farming and husbandry, bird farming and other occupations as shown in the table below (table 2.21).

Radiological features

These depend on the length of exposure and the balance between progressive lesion and development of fibrosis.

Acute extrinsic allergic alveolitis (AEAA)

1. Chest x-ray may be normal in up to 50% of the cases at the initial stages
2. Patchy or nodular opacities.
3. Diffuse alveolar consolidation due to pulmonary oedema
4. Fine nodular opacity
5. Generalised ground glass appearance
6. Lymphadenopathy develops in recurrent cases

CT scan

1. Patchy opacities
2. Ground glass appearance even in those with normal radiographs
3. Varied-size round opacities depicting granulomas
4. Diffuse confluent dense pulmonary consolidations

Chronic extrinsic allergic alveolitis

Fibrosis: Reticular/nodular/reticulonodular shadows which progress to coarse linear shadows of fibrosis
Mid and upper lobe affectation. Lesions are seen in middle and upper zones
Loss of volume. Severe contraction in the middle and upper zones due to cicatrization atelectasis
Pleural effusion rare

Table 2.21: Hypersensitivity pneumonitis, related occupations and implicated infective agents or antigens[1-6]

Disease	Occupation/source	Organism involved
Farmer's lung	Wheat workers, grain farmer or millers (mouldy hay).	*Micropolyspora faeni, Thermoactinomyces vulgaris* or *Aspergillus, actinomycetes*
Bird-fancier's or Bird-breeder's lung	Bird fancier, poultry worker, bird hobbyist, bird pet-store workers	Feathers, droplets containing bird serum or protein
Mushroom grower's lung	Mushroom worker's lung (exposure to compost)	Fungal spores containing *Micropolyspora faeni, Thermoactinomyces vulgaris Thermophilic actinomyces*
Bagassosis	Sugar cane workers	Bagasse, mouldy sugar cane residue contaminated with *Micropolyspora faeni, Thermoactinomyces sacchari/vulgaris.*
Malt worker's disease/	Malt worker or farmer	Malt dust containing *Aspergillus clavatus*
Marple worker's disease	Saw millers or wood workers	Mouldy marple bark containing *Cryptostroma corticale*
Byssinosis	Cotton workers or farmers	Cotton dust
Suberosis	Cork workers	Mouldy cork dust containing *Penicillium glabrum (frequentans), aspergilus species*
Sequiosis	Saw millers or wood workers	Mouldy red wood dust containing *Thermophylic actinomycetes*
Pandoram pneumonitis	Centrally air-conditioned, large buildings, humidified or heated large buildings	Forced air or air-conditioned equipments containing *Thermophylic actinomycetes*
Japanese summer disease	Worker or persons exposed to Tatamic rats	*Trichosporum asahii*
Isocyanate penumonitis	Painters lung (paint spray, plastics workers)	*Isocyanates*
Hot tub lung	Hot tub users	*Microbacterium avium complex*

Honey-comb appearance
Bronchiectasis and cyst formation
CT scan
Honey-comb appearance
Focal air-trapping
Emphysema formation
Co-existence of subacute changes/acute changes due to on-going process.

Treatment
1. Remove from the exposure
2. Reduce contact to minimum by using masks, filters, industrial hygiene, reposting staff to safer environment.
3. Change/alter air-conditioning system
4. Steroid is not useful

Differential diagnosis of upper lobe fibrosis
1. Cryptogenic fibrosing alveolitis
2. TB
3. Bronchopulmonary aspergillosis
4. Ankylosing spondylitis
5. Histoplasmosis.

Silo-Filler's disease
This is an occupational lung disease that results from inhalation of nitrogen dioxide (NO_2) gas from fresh silage usually filled in the last quarter of the year. Toxic gases such as nitrogen dioxide penetrate the lung and alveoli and may manifest with several respiratory illnesses such as pulmonary oedema, hyalinised alveolar membranes and a form of acute respiratory distress syndrome. In some parts of the world when long vacation is taken during the end of the year, fresh silage may be by the New Year in which case, the disease will be by the first quarter of the year.

(Adam & Dixon, 2008; Dahnert, 2011; Sutton, 2003, Palmer & Reeder, 2001).

References
1. Akira M. High-resolution CT in the evaluation of occupational and environmental disease. Radiol Clin North Am 2002; 40:43-59.
2. Kim KI, Kim CW, Lee MK, Lee KS, Park CK, Choi SJ, Kim JG. Imaging of occupational lung disease. Radiographics 2001; 21:1371-91.
3. Shida H, Chiyotani K, Honma K, Hosoda Y, Nobechi T, Morikubo H, Wiot JF. Radiologic and pathologic characteristics of mixed dust pneumoconiosis. Radiographics 1996;16:483-98.
4. Brown K, Mund DF, Aberle DR, Batra P, Young DA. Intrathoracic calcifications: radiographic features and differential diagnoses. Radiographics 1994;14:1247-61.
5. Gotway MB, Golden JA, Warnock M, Koth LL, Webb R, Reddy GP, Balmes JR. Hard metal interstitial lung disease: high-resolution computed tomography appearance. J Thorac Imaging 2002;17:314-8.
6. Kim JS, Lynch DA. Imaging of non-malignant occupational lung disease. J Thorac Imaging 2002; 17:238-60.

2.3   DIFFERENTIAL DIAGNOSIS OF AN ELEVATED RIGHT HEMIDIAPHRAGM

Definition
Diaphragm
The diaphragm is a thin, flat fibro-muscular structure and organ of respiration, which forms the convex floor of the thoracic cage, separating the thorax from the abdomen. It has sternal, costal and vertebral origins and forms a central tendon in the centre.

The diaphragm has two domes or hemidiaphragms. The right dome or hemidiaphragm is usually higher than the left due to the heart depressing the left side and not the liver pushing up the right side. The diaphragm is 2 – 3 mm thick.

The combined wall of the stomach and diaphragm, when measured on the left, and made clear by gastric air bubble, is 5 – 8 mm thick. The hemidiaphragms may lie at the same level in a small percentage of people. In about 3% of people, the left hemidiaphragm is higher than the right.

Unilateral elevation of right hemi-diaphragm
The right hemidiaphragm is elevated if the vertical height between the dome of the right and left hemidiaphragm is greater than 3 cm.

Causes of Elevated Right hemidiaphragm (unilateral)
Normal Variants (congenital)
Diaphragmatic hump, dromedary hump and eventration.

Pulmonary lesions
Lower lobe collapse, pulmonary hypoplasia, lower lobar pneumonia, pulmonary embolism and pneumonectomy.

Pleural lesions
Pleural thickening, pleurisy and subpulmonic effusion

Subdiaphragmatic lesions
Chilaiditi's syndrome (interposed gas-distended bowel), right subphrenic abscess, abdominal mass/hepatic mass, hepatomegaly, hydatid cyst/disease and hepatic abscess (amoebic, pyogenic, hydatid cyst) and hepatic metastasis.

Paralysis of diaphragm (Phrenic nerve paralysis)
Surgery or trauma involving right hemithorax, idiopathic, radiotherapy (fibrosis), diabetes mellitus (neuropathy), neoplastic diseases (lung tumours, mediastinal tumours, lymphomas, metastatic lymphadenopathy), infections: tuberculous lymphadenopathy and Herpes zoster

Bone lesions
Scoliosis, concave to the right and rib fractures (with diaphragmatic splinting)

Diaphragmatic hernias
Hiatus hernia, Morgagni hernia, Bochdalek hernia and rupture of diaphragm with herniation

Diaphragmatic tumours
Lipomas, neurofibromas, cysts and fibromas, sarcomas.

Radiological investigative modalities
1. Plain film
2. Ultrasound
3. Conventional tomography
4. CT scan
5. MRI
6. Radionuclide studies
7. Angiography

Discussion

Congenital diaphgamatic lesions
Diaphragmatic hump
There is no diaphragmatic defect but there is incomplete formation of diaphragmatic muscle, leaving the membranous part to be larger than usual. These are found in the anterior part of the diaphragm and more often right-sided. It is actually a mild form of eventration. In PA view of the chest, hump gives the diaphragm a double lobulated appearance or a double contour. It also appears as a round mass in the right cardiophrenic angle whose inferior limit is continuous with the diaphragm.

On lateral view, the round mass overlies the cardiac shadow.
Ultrasound scan of the right hypochondrium will show a normal liver without any mass effect and no metastatic lesion or cystic mass. CT scan is not necessary but if done, the lung and the liver are shown to be perfectly normal.

Dromedary diaphragm
This is a more severe form of diaphragmatic hump. A more, well-defined round double mass with inferior limit continuous with the diaphragm is seen. The double contour appearance is better defined. The mass is seen in the cardiophrenic angle and the differential diagnoses, which are the same as of diaphragmatic hump, are cardiac fat pad, pericardial cyst, lipoma, Morgagni hernia, middle lobe collapse, hepatic masses/metastasis and hydatid cyst. It overlies the heart in the lateral view. The ultrasound and CT features are as in diaphragmatic hump.

Eventration
The diaphragmatic muscle is thin, weak with reduced movement. There may be paradoxical or absent movement on fluoroscopy. The membranous part is virtually the entire diaphragm. Eventration is rare on the right compared to the left. There is mediastinal displacement to the contralateral side. It is associated with gastric volvulus if found on the left. The differential diagnoses are diaphragmatic paralysis (this does not present with mediastinal displacement), absence of diaphragm (extremely rare), rupture of diaphragm (history of trauma) and gastric volvulus (barium meal/swallow will confirm this).

Pulmonary Lesion
Right lower lobe collapse
The right hemidiaphragm is elevated with increased opacity of the right lower lobe on frontal view. There is downward displacement of the minor fissure and the oblique fissure is not visible until the collapse is almost complete. When completely collapsed, it may flatten and merge with the elevated hemidiaphragm towards the mediastinum appearing like a hump. Frontal and lateral views as well as assessment of orientation of the fissures will lead to the diagnosis. There may be air bronchogram if the air is not completely absorbed.

Right pulmonary hypoplasia
Small lung with triangular thoracic configuration and skeletal dysplasia are seen. Obstructive uropathy or renal aplasia is often associated with it. It is frequently a fatal disease. Ultrasound (echocardiography) will show if there is intracardiac lesion/pathology. Cardiac catheterization and pulmonary angiography will confirm the diagnosis and differentiate it from many other condition.

Right lower lobe pneumonia
There is right lower lobe shadowing obscuring the diaphragmatic margin. There is air bronchogram. The opacity is limited by the minor fissures anteriorly in oblique film and the right cardiac margin is visible. There will be complete clearing with sensitive antibiotics therapy.

Right pulmonary embolism
Blockage of pulmonary artery leads to the lack of perfusion of the lung and to absence of aeration. There is a reduction in the lung volume which appears as elevated hemidiaghram. Mild pleural effusion may follow lung infarction. It is common on the right. Isotope lung scanning will help identify the sub-acute cases where perfusion defect is seen even with normal ventilation. In chronic cases, there is dilated central pulmonary artery with peripheral pruning and in lung scan there is widespread perfusion defect with normal ventilation.

Right pneumonectomy
The hemidiaphragm is elevated because of the volume loss. There is often scoliosis and mediastinal shift to the ipsilateral side. Rib lesion or sternal lesion or defects or surgical clips due to previous surgery may be obvious. The presence of Lucite ball or cellophane often packed to reduce volume loss may be appreciated. Complete obliteration of hemithorax is seen after about 2– 3 months.

Pleural Lesions
Pleural thickening
Previous pleurisy can present as pleural thickening. Localised pleural thickening extending upwards to oblique or minor fissures may produce appearance of tenting of diaphragm or pulmonary scaring from previous infection or infarction. Pleural fibrosis and fibrothorax may follow trauma, thoracotomy, pleural effusion or empyema. There is reduced ventilation with decreased volume of hemithorax and elevated hemidiaphragm.

Right pleurisy
Associated pain and reactive fluid will cause guarding of the diaphragm and lack of adequate ventilation and diaphragmatic elevation. Thus poor inspiratory effort from pain of the pleurisy will eventually lead to that hemidiaphragm being elevated relative to the contralateral hmithorax.

Right subpulmonic effusion

Fluid accumulation may occur between the diaphragm and the under surface of the lung. The diaphragm is elevated and its apex is more laterally situated with associated blunting of costophrenic angle.

Diaphragmatic Lesions
Bochdalek hernia

A congenital diaphragmatic defect arising posterolaterally usually on the left in over 90% of the cases but it can also be observed on the right. It occurs through a defect in the pleuroperitoneal membrane (pleuroperitoneal canal). It is a cause of neonatal respiratory distress and may simulate cystic adenomatous malformation of the lung. The diaphragm is elevated. The hernia may contain omentum, bowel, spleen, part of the liver, kidney, pancreas, small bowel and rarely stomach. There is bowel gas-shadow in the chest with contralateral mediastinal shift and ipsilateral hypoplastic lung. Barium swallow, meal or enema will confirm the diagnosis. CT scan and MRI of the chest can confirm the diagnosis without the need for contrast injection. If a solid organ like the liver is herniated into it, then ultrasound scan will effectively comfirm the lesion by showing a defect in the diaphragm through which the liver herniated into the chest.

Morgagni Hernias

Morgangni hernias are right-sided and located anteriorly in majority of the cases. A Morgagni hernia often appears as a homogenous shadow in the right cardiophrenic angle. It may contain fat, omentum, bowel (colon) or liver. Rarely the heart may herniate to the abdominal cavity through the defect. It is caused by a defect in the development of diaphragm between the septum transversum and the right and left costal origins of the diaphragm. Barium swallow or meal or rarely barium enema may show the tenting of the bowel to the hernia site.

Ruptured diaphragm

It is often left-sided and there may be herniation of the stomach with volvulus. However, it may occur on the right where it may simulate eventration. If there is rupture without herniation the appearance is that of elevated hemidiaphragm with irregular outline or non-visualisation of contour, or obscured outline. The causes of diaphragmatic rupture are trauma, surgery and they are occasionally idiopathic. There may be mushroom mass of herniated liver in the right hemithorax with or without basal lobar consolidation and haemothorax. Lower rib fracture adjacent to the diaphragm may be seen. CT scan will show abrupt and sharp discontinuity of hemidiaphragm. There may also be features suggestive of absent diaphragm because the diaphragm could not be seen. Ultrasound will show the tear or where there is lack of continuity in the diaphragm and may show both pleural fluid and haemoperitoneum.

Diaphragmatic tumours

Tumours of the diaphragm are rare and they include lipomas, sarcomas, fibromas, neurofibromas and cysts. They appear as lobulated, smooth, round masses. When they have wide base, they completely appear as elevated hemidiaphragm or diaphragmatic humps. However, if the base is less wide they appear as liver metastasis, pulmonary metastasis or hernias. Pleural effusion is seen especially in sarcomas. CT scan and MRI will clearly show the masses as diaphragmatic masses.

Lesions below the Diaphragm
Chilaiditis syndrome

This is interposition of gas-distended bowel loop, usually the colon, between the liver and diaphragm. The diaphragm is elevated and there is obvious haustral pattern of the colon. This condition is common, transient and the haustral markings confirm that the gas is not free.

Right Subphrenic abscess

The hemidiaphragm is elevated with associated reduced movement. Occasionally, paradoxical movement is noted on fluoroscopy. Abdominal gas shadow is found below the diaphragm when there is infection with gas–forming organisms and this is best appreciated with horizontal beam. There is also depression of the liver edge. Reactive pleural effusion is common. These are found in patients with recent surgery or sepsis. Ultrasound scan will show the abscess as hypoechoic area with multiple internal echoes. The liver edge and diaphragmatic edge will be shown. CT scan is also diagnostic and both CT and ultrasound scan can be used to guide abscess drainage. Differential diagnosis is post-operative gas seen up to 10 days after the surgery. Any large intra-abdominal mass or massive ascites will cause elevated diaphragm but this is often bilateral. However, occasionally it can be unilateral if the mass is more on the right. Examples of such masses are renal or adrenal masses.

Hepatomegaly

Enlarged liver, and when gross, will cause elevated hemidiaphragm. Ultrasound scan and CT scan will clearly demonstrate that the lesion is hepatomegaly. Other signs of enlarged right lobe of the liver are depressed hepatic flexure and duodenum, depressed right kidney (occasionally), bulging of the right lateral properitoneal fat line and occasionally splaying of the right lower ribs.

Infection and Infestations
Hydatid cyst

This is a cystic lesion of *Echinoccocus granulosus* in the liver. It appears as oval, round, well-circumscribed mass of homogenous density. Calcification may rarely occur. A wavy band of detachment of germinal layer (endocyst) produces *"floating membrane" or "water-lily sign"* on plain film or CT. Undulating membrane which is the end product from separation of the endocyst from the pericyst is seen at ultrasound scan and if the patient's position is changed while scanning this gives a *"snowstorm"* pattern or appearance. Radionuclide liver scan detects it more than plain film. They are often unilocular and may be mistaken for elevated hemidiaphragm. They are sub-capsular and if longstanding may contain bright nodules on the inner lining of their walls. Fluid-level may be seen following rupture of hydatid cyst into the pleural cavity and this gives a *"meniscus sign"* on plain film or CT scan. *"Racemose"* or *"wheel spoke"* or *"cartwheel"* appearance on CT scan is produced by multiple cysts and echogenic areas that are enclosed together within a capsule. *"Rosette sign"* in CT scan is created by high attenuating fluid surrounding the daughter cyst within the mother cyst occupying almost the entire volume of mother cyst and looking like septa. Low signal intensity rim of the parasitic membrane and pericyst on T2-weighted image is known as *"Rim sign'* and is characteristic. *"Snake sign"* on MR imaging represents collapsed parasitic membranes secondary to damage or degeneration of a hydatid cyst. Liver cyst can also elevate the hemidiaphragm.

Amoebic liver abscess

This is caused by *Entamoeba histolytica*. It is a protozoan found in the tropics and subtropics. A large hepatic amoebic abscess may by its size on the liver cause hepatomegaly and right diaphragmatic elevation. It may also erode through the diaphragm and cause diaphragmatic elevation. It also causes pleural effusion, lung cavitation and lower lobe consolidation. Sonography will show a well-defined hypoechoic liver abscess and pleural effusion as the cause of elevated hemidiaphragm. Males are more frequently affected and the patients are usually of younger age and more sick than those with pyogenic abscess.

Pyogenic hepatic abscess

They are usualy solitary with no sex predilection but are often found in middle aged patients. It is hypoechoic or hyperechoic on USS with well-defined and sometimes irregular capsule. Gas within it causes high intensity echoes with linerar echoes or shadowns with reverberation artefacts or "*comet sign*". The abscess in CT is low attenuating and the capsule rarely enhances.

Lesions causing Phrenic Nerve Paralysis
Diabetic neuropathy

Nerve paralysis due to diabetic neuropathy will cause elevated hemidiaphragm. There is no mediastinal displacement (this is seen in eventration). Paradoxical or absent movement is seen on fluoroscopy. History and basic examination of blood sugar will confirm the diagnosis. When one side is more affected, unilateral elevation of the hemidiaphragm may occur. History of diabetes mellitus is essential for accurate diagnosis in many cases.

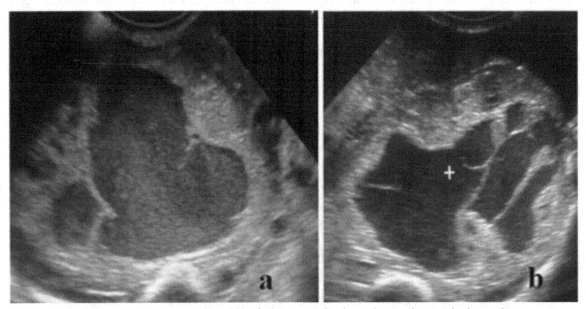

Figure 2.31: Sonograms (a and b) of a large amoebic liver abscess that resulted in right diaphragmatic elevation. In (a), there is a large hypoechoic area within the liver with well-defined edges. In (b), multiple internal septations are noted within the abscess cavity.

Neoplastic tumour (causing paralysis of phrenic nerve)

Lung carcinoma, mediastinal tumours, lymphomas, metastatic lymphadenopathy are some of the tumours that could invade the phrenic nerve and causes its paralysis. They may also erode into the phrenic nerve or destroying the nerve. The appearances are as in diabetic neuropathy for the diaphragm. Chest x-ray, CT scan and MRI may show the tumour masses and biopsy will confirm the diagnosis.

Infection (TB lymphadenopathy/Herpes zoster)

Herpes zoster affects the nerve root and the supplied dermatome. The features are those of phrenic nerve paralysis. TB lymphadenopathy may compress the nerve and have similar appearance as neoplastic tumours. However, there may be features of tuberculosis like fibrocystic changes, cavitary components, upper lobe fibrosis and nodular infiltrates. *Myasthenia gravis* may also affect the phrenic nerve and cause its paralysis. CT and MRI may show anterior mediastinal tumour. Or the tumour may be completely absent. Biochemical tests for this disease using neostigmine may establish the diagnosis.

Various other Lesions
Metastasis

Nodular, peripheral and sub-capsular metastatic disease within the lung or pleura or diaphragm or the liver may cause elevated hemidiaphragm. In sonography, they are often multiple, well-defined and there may be evidence of primary site in the abdomen. History also may be able to identify primary tumour mass and that pain originates from the site of existing mitotic disease. Often, when the primary site is not identified, biopsy is needed for histological diagnosis. CT and MRI will also be helpful in identifying multiple liver masses, lymphadenopathy and other organs of origin of the primary.

Scoliosis

This is lateral curvature of the spine. Scoliosis of the dorsal spine has accompanying diaphragmatic elevation on the concave side of the curvature.

Rib fractures

The appearance of haemothorax, haemopneumothorax or intrapulmonary haemorrhage associated with rib fracture may obscure the outline of the hemidiaphragm and simulate elevated hemidiaphragm. Pain and guarding associated with rib fracture, especially if the rib fractures are multiple, may cause splinting of the diaphragm and lack of excursion on respiration and therefore elevated hemidiaphragm. Oblique view of the chest, CT scan and MRI will clearly, individually or complimentary to each other, lead to the diagnosis.

Post-radiotherapy fibrosis (Radiation lung injury)

The elevated hemidiaphragm is seen months or years after the injury. The changes are seen, usually when over 6000 Rad is used. There is elevated hemidiaphragm because of the volume loss. This occurs mostly when the radiotherapy is for breast cancer since only one side is then treated. Mediastinal radiotherapy for lymphoma and lung carcinoma is often bilateral. The pulmonary fibrosis has a sharp linear vertical margin between the fibrotic area and the normal lung corresponding to the geometric shape of the radiotherapy portal. There may be consolidation with or without air-bronchogram effect, and pleural effusion. History is often helpful and together with the shape may be confirmatory.

Surgery and Trauma

Thoracotomy, chest/cardiac surgery and trauma may injure the phrenic nerve and cause paralysis. History, presence of surgical clip for thoracotomy and evidence of previous rib fracture may help in the diagnosis.

Other types of infections

Fungal abscess (histoplasmosis and candidiasis of the liver), schistosomiasis, viral infection, cat-scratch disease and bacilliary angiomatosis (peliosis hepatitis) caused by *Bartonella henselae* in immunocompromised patients, are some of the other infections that can cause elevated hemidiaphragm. Ancilliary investigations and histology of specimen are invaluable to their accurate diagnsosis.

Causes of Unilateral Elevated Left Hemidiaphragm

All of the above, pancreatitis, splenomegaly and prominent gastric air bubble

Causes of Bilateral Elevated Hemidiaphragm
Technical

Poor inspiratory effort, supine view, expiratory view and post-operative radiography (due to chest pain).

Subdiaphragmatic lesions

Ascites, obesity, bowel distension, pregnancy and large intra-abdominal mass.

Reduced lung compliance

Lymphangitis carcinomatosa, systemic lupus erythematosus (SLE), fibrosing alveolitis, radiation lung injury for mediastinal lesion and bilateral chest injury.

Pulmonary lesion

Bilateral atelectasis and bilateral partial pulmonary hypoplasia.

Neuromuscular lesions

Diabetic neuropathy, myasthenia gravis and myotropic lateral sclerosis

(Adam & Dixon, 2008; Dahnert, 2011; Sutton, 2003; Swischuk, 2004; Palmer & Reeder, 2001).

References

1. Shin SW, Do YS, Choo SW, Lieu WC, Cho SK, Park KB, Yoo BC, Kang EH, Choo IW. Diaphragmatic weakness after transcatheter arterial chemoembolization of inferior phrenic artery for treatment of hepatocellular carcinoma. Radiology 2006; 241:581-8.
2. Ghamande S, Ramsey R, Rhodes JF, Stoller JK. Right hemidiaphragmatic elevation with a right-to-left interatrial shunt through a patent foramen ovale: a case report and literature review. Chest 2001;120: 2094-6.
3. Chen F, Nakai M, Aoyama A, Isowa N, Chihara K. Diaphragmatic elevation of a patient with chronic obstructive pulmonary disease after left upper lobectomy. Interact Cardiovasc Thorac Surg 2003;2:688-91.

2.4   RADIOLOGICAL FINDINGS IN PULMONARY TUBERCULOSIS

Definition
Pulmonary tuberculosis is the disease caused by infection with *Mycobacterium tuberculosis* that affects the lungs. Robert Koch first isolated mycobacterium tuberculosis in 1882 even though the disease, tuberculosis (TB), had been with man, afflicting him since antiquity.

Other *Mycobacterium non-tuberculous organisms are also involved*
These causes the infection called *atypical tuberculosis*, which manifests clinically as disease in 5% of cases of pulmonary (tuberculosis) infections. Such atypical mycobacterium includes *Mycobacterium Avium – Intracellulare, Mycobacterium kansasii, Mycobacterium fortiuiform, Mycobacterium xenopi, Mycobacterium battei.* They cause more cavitary thin-walled lesions and are less likely to spread. They also cause less fibrosis and are less sensitive to antituberculous drugs. They may also cause infection that co-exists with mycobacterium tuberculosis.

Mode of infection
By inhalation: The particles measuring 1–5 μm in size can be kept airborne by normal air currents for prolonged periods, resulting in dispersion throughout a room or building.

Mode of transmission
Droplets – inhalation with critical dose of viable organism.

Susceptible group
Infants, children, pubertal adolescence, elderly, alcoholics (socially deprived) immunocompromised especially AIDS, diabetes, measles, post-gastrectomy patients, patients on steroid therapy, pregnancy, silicosis, sarcoidosis, poor nutrition and malignant diseases, workers in pathology departments (pipetting) are also susceptible.

Immunity
These confer immunity and render hypersensitivity reaction to tuberculoprotein (tuberculin test). 1. Previous subclinical infection. 2. Bacille Calmette-Guérin (BCG) vaccination. In about 5% of infected persons, immunity is inadequate and clinically active disease develops within 1 year of infection resulting in primary tuberculosis; and in another 5% of the infected population, endogenous reactivation of latent infection (which was not initially active) occur remote from time of initial infection resulting in post-primary tuberculosis.

Progress of infection
1. Primary tuberculosis: The patient was not previously sensitized.
2. Post-primary tuberculosis: The patient was previously sensitized and with reactivation of latent initially dormant infection.

Risk of progression of disease in persons that are co-infected with HIV
Simultaneous co-infection of HIV and *M. tuberculosis* is the strongest known risk factor for both immediate (primary) and delayed progression from infection (post primary) to active tuberculosis. This risk of progression to disease for co-infected persons is 5%–10% per year compared with a 5%–10% lifetime risk for persons who tested HIV-negative.

Epidemiology[1-3]

- Over ninety percent (90%) of all the cases and 95% of the deaths from pulmonary tuberculosis occur in developing countries.
- Of the over 3 million cases of TB notified to the WHO in 1995, over 75% were from Asia, Sub-Saharan Africa and Island regions.
- Prevalence rate is as follows: Southeast Asia (rate is over, 230 per 100,000) and sub-Saharan Africa (rate is over, 190 per 100,000).
- In poor underdeveloped countries about 80% of involve persons or more are in their productive years (15–59 years of age).

PRIMARY TUBERCULOSIS

Usually in children, but increasingly found in adults.

Symptoms and signs

1. Asymptomatic or subclinical >90%.
2. Symptomatic 5 – 10%

Clinical symptoms

Fever, chest pain, cough, malaise, night sweats, haemoptysis, difficulty with breathing (due to chest pain), erythema nodosum, weight loss, loss of appetite, failure to thrive.

Site of predilection

Organisms multiply and settle in the alveolus of any part of the lung. Nevertheless, commonly in subpleural site of:

1. Apico-posterior segment of upper lobe
2. Middle lobes
3. Well-ventilated lower lobe.

Reason for affectation of the lung and the prevalent sites

1. Low or poor lymphatic distribution and drainage of the lung
2. High oxygen tension or saturation of the lung (the organism is air-seeking).

Radiological Features

Lobar consolidation (The Ghon focus)

The area of the peripheral lung adjacent to the subpleural area where the organism settles may become consolidated. Increased opacity with air-bronchogram is seen. This may not take any shape or it may appear as lobar pneumonia (unresponsive to pyogenic antibiotics). Consolidation may appear as well-defined round nodules. Healed lobar consolidations may leave a scar in the lung as thin linear fibrotic strands. The appearances are summarised below:

i. Pulmonary parenchymal involvement in primary pulmonary TB most commonly appears as an area of homogeneous consolidation with air-bronchogram effect.
ii. Patchy, linear, nodular, and mass-like forms may occur.
iii. Consolidation typically occurs in a segmental or lobar distribution; multifocal involvement is identified radiographically in 12%–24% and found at autopsy in 16% of the affected population.
iv. Right-sided predominance in the distribution of Ghons foci (consolidation) and Ranke complexes is agreed to reflect the greater statistical chance of an airborne infection involving the right lung due to its short length and more steep orientation.

v. Finding of normal chest films and consolidation confined to the lower lung zones are other atypical radiographic patterns that are well-documented to be associated with endobronchial TB.

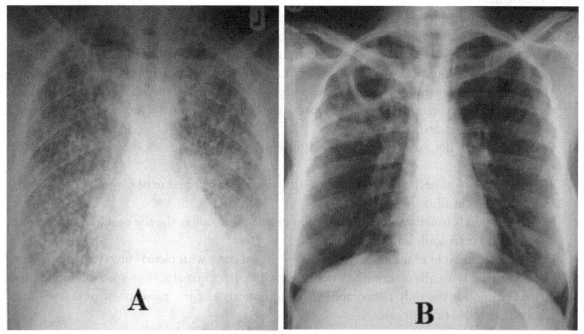

Figure 2.41: Chest radiographs in pulmonary tuberculosis showing multiple pin-head size opacities due to miliary tuberculosis (A); and a tuberculous cavity with surrounding fibrocystic changes (satellite lesions) in the right upper lung zones (B).

Enlarged lymph nodes

Lymphadenopathy is the *radiologic hallmark of primary* TB.

i. Enlarged lymph nodes occur in 83%–96% of paediatric cases but the prevalence decreases with increasing age.

ii. Massive hilar lymphadenopathy is seen in over 60% of children and is more common on the right side.

iii. Right paratracheal lymphadenopathy are more commonly involved, followed by the enlargement of hilar stations although any combination of groups of lymph node enlargement can occur, including bilateral hilar or isolated mediastinal lymphadenopathy. The spread of the infection from draining lymphatics of area of Ghons focus to the lymph nodes is what results in lymphadenopathy (1 and 2 are referred to as primary complex).

iv. Healed primary tuberculous lesion may calcify, although viable organisms will still be present within it.

v. Contrast material–enhanced CT scans, show mediastinal tuberculous lymphadenitis, especially when nodal size exceeds 2 cm in diameter. The lymph nodes may have a characteristic appearance consisting of central areas of low attenuation associated with peripheral rim enhancement and obliteration of surrounding perinodal fat.

Mediastinal lymphadenopathy (This is seen more in adults).

Pleural effusion

The subpleural infection may cause serous effusion to develop or it may rupture into pleura causing effusion. If patient has a history of trauma, it may be confused with haemothorax.

i.   Pleural effusions typically develop 3–6 months in primary TB after infection and results from a hypersensitivity response to a small amount of tuberculoprotein released into the pleural space.

ii.   There is paucity of organisms in pleural fluid and positive cultures are obtained only in 20%–40% of cases where as a single closed needle biopsy of the pleura substantially increases the diagnostic yield to approximately 65%–75%.

iii.   Pleural effusion is not a common manifestation of primary TB in infants and young children (<2 years of age)

iv.   The prevalence of pleural effusion increases with age and is reported to be 6%–11% in children, and 29%–38% in adults.

v.   Pleural effusion is usually observed to develop on the same side as the site of initial tuberculous infection and is typically unilateral.

vi.   Bilateral affectation of effusions occurs in 12%–18% of cases with pleural involvement.

vii.   Even though it is usually observed in association with parenchymal and/or nodal abnormalities, pleural effusion is the only radiographic finding indicative of the presence of primary TB in approximately 5% of adult cases.

Bronchopneumonia

Erosion of caseous nodes into the airway may ensue. Bronchopulmonary or bronchogenic spread of infections with small multiple nodular changes may lead to bronchopneumonia. This is caused by weak response and further spread. Small multiple cavitations may occur.

Pneumothorax

Rupture of small, multiple cavities in a disease with weak reactive immunity, renders the features in-between primary and post primary tuberculosis. Pneumothorax develops if the cavity ruptures into the pleural space.

Miliary tuberculosis

Radiographically, this appears as multiple pin head-sized opacities of soft tissue density measuring 1 – 2 mm in diameter and scattered almost evenly throughout the lung fields (figure 2.41 A).

It can occur in both primary and post primary tuberculosis. Erosion of caseous nodes into the pulmonary vessels leads to haematogenous spread, releasing a large number of viable bacilli that embolize to capillary beds in multiple organs. The lung is the most commonly involved organ. The sputum contains acid-fast bacilli in the minority of cases, and therefore bronchoscopy with transbronchial biopsy is often necessary for the accurate diagnosis apart from chest radiography and CT scan.

Multiple organ involvement is the rule and prognosis is poor without treatment but there is rapid complete clearing with appropriate, sensitive antituberculous drug with excellent prognosis.

Atelectasis

Lung collapse may occur and results from:

i.   Endobronchial tuberculosis with caseous nodules compromising the calibre of the airway.

ii. Atelectasis can also occur from complete occlusion of the airway by external compressive effect of enlarged lymph nodes. Obstructive atelectasis and over inflation resulting primarily from compression by adjacent enlarged nodes have been reported to occur in 9%–30% and 1%–5% of children with primary TB, respectively. Distribution is typically right-sided with obstruction occurring at the level of the lobar bronchus or bronchus intermedius.

iii. Extrinsic airway obstruction is observed much less frequently in the adult population because of their larger-calibre airways and lower prevalence of lymphadenopathy. Involvement of the airway by endobronchial TB in adults with primary disease may manifest radiologically as atelectasis and endoluminal or peribronchial masses simulating neoplastic disease.

Tuberculoma

Granuloma that develops from primary tuberculosis may form a solitary, well-defined pulmonary nodule of 0.5 – 5 cm in diameter. It commonly calcifies but very rarely cavitates. It may have lobulated margin.

Destroyed lung syndrome

The enlarged lymph nodes in primary tuberculosis may compress the bronchus and cause bronchial obstruction. Infection of distal obstructed segment of the bronchus by pyogenic and tuberculous bacteria may lead to continuous series of changes leading to fibrosis, cystic changes, lung collapse and eventually destruction of the lung. In plain radiograph, the heart (mediastinum) is completely shifted to the hemithorax with the collapsed lung. Opacity, cystic changes and air-trapping are seen in the affected lung. The contralateral lung is often normal. Destroyed lung syndrome is more common in the left side because the left main bronchus is longer than the right and therefore more prone to compression by enlarged lymph nodes.

Air-trapping with hyperinflation

This may be caused by extrinsic compression of bronchi by lymphadenopathy or by endobronchial TB. Both of them can compress the airway leading to air trapping and hyperinflation (ball-valve effect).

POST-PRIMARY TUBERCULOSIS

This occurs as a result of:
1. Re-infection leading to reactivation of latent disease acquired in childhood (most common).
2. Re-activation of initial focus acquired in childhood after a latent period as a result of depressed immunity without re-infection.
3. Continuation of initial primary infection progressing without intervening latent period (rare)
4. Initial infection in individuals vaccinated with BCG, which because it still confers some immunity produces post-primary tuberculosis.

Pathology

Caseous necrosis with formation of multiple nodular opacities by the caseated necrotic materials, which spread downwards to middle and lower lobes. Areas of necrosis and areas where necrotic nodules have spread may have inflammatory exudation leading to pneumonia. Necrotised area form cavity. Fibrosis is attempt of the lung at healing.

Site

Right lobe of the lung is more affected than the left. Apical posterior segment of upper lobe is more commonly involved, followed by superior segment of lower lobe. Mixed location can occur.

Age

Adolescents and young adult. Adult population of predisposed group with primary tuberculosis.

Radiological Features

Hilar and Medistinal lymphadenopathy

Hilar and mediastinal lymph enlargement are uncommon manifestations of post-primary TB and occur in only approximately 5% of cases.

Lung consolidation/lobar pneumonia

i.   In the early stages, this can appear as ill-defined area of increased opacity often associated with nodular and linear components and is observed radiating outward from the hilum or in the periphery of the lung.

ii.   Later it appears most commonly as heterogeneous opacities or in the form of lobar pneumonia or may be partly nodular, and ill-defined. This is due to local exudatory inflammation.

iii. As the disease progresses, other opacities develop that may coalesce, and are, sometimes, seen in association with distortion of adjacent bronchovascular and mediastinal structures consistent with pulmonary fibrosis.

Multiple nodular opacities

The necrotic caseated material appears as multiple nodular opacities in the lung. These solid caseating materials are in the terminal or respiratory bronchioles.

Pulmonary fibrosis and cystic changes

Lung fibrosis shows as thickened strands in the lung. It also shows as reduction in the lung volume, marked by elevation of right minor fissure, upwards pull of the hilum and sometime ipsilateral shift of the mediastinum.

Cystic changes: This appears as area of extremely small cavities or holes in the lungs where caseous materials have been extruded from.

Fibrocystic changes: The appearances of fibrosis and cystic changes give *fibrocystic changes*. These are intermixture or co-existence of multiple oval cystic areas and multiple linear fibrotic strands. They are diagnostic of TB in the presence of positive sputum smear.

Increased drainage markings towards ipsilateral hilum

Any pulmonary opacity with multiple minute nodular opacities usually in linear beaded rows towards the hilum is significant of tuberculosis.

Cavitation

This can be thin-wall (early stages) or thick-walled in late stages. Cavitation is the hallmark of post-primary tuberculosis. It is due to caseous necrosis of the lung with formation of a space or "*hollow*" where the necrotic material was extruded from. It occurs in about half of all adult post-primary tuberculosis (figure 2.41 B).

Tuberculous cavity

A tuberculous cavity can be described as a space or hole in the lung where semisolid caseous materials was extruded from due to tuberculous caseation. It is the hallmark of post-primary tuberculosis. A tuberculous cavity has the following features.

i.   *Wall thickness:* It can be thick-walled or thin-walled, smooth or irregular/nodular. Thick-wall means increased activity.
ii. *Number of cavity:* It can be single or multiple occurring in 40%–45% of cases of post primary TB.
iii. *Wall lining:* Tuberculous cavities are lined by granulation tissue.
iv. *Satellite lesion:* Tuberculous cavities may be associated with satellite cavity or fibrotic changes, calcification, tuberculoses nodule or area of consolidation elsewhere in the lung but usually close to the cavity.
v.   *Location:* Upper lobe predominance and often bilateral but worse on one side.
vi. *Rasmussen aneurysm:* A cavity may be traversed by remnant bronchial or terminal part of pulmonary artery. Secondary inflammatory necrosis of the incompletely obliterated vessel wall causes it to dilate. If it ruptures, it can lead to life-threatening haemoptysis.
vii. *Air-fluid level:* Air-fluid levels are reported to occur in 9%–21% of tuberculous cavities often indicates active infection.
viii. *Fungus colonization:* Residual tuberculous cavity may be colonized by *Aspergillus* species. The fungus ball or aspergilloma consists of a cluster of intertwined hyphae matted together with a variable amount of mucus and cellular debris and trapped air between the hyphae.

Pulmonary atelectasis

This is cicatrisation type. There is volume loss due to fibrosis.

Pleural thickening/ Apical cap

This may be seen in the apex where it accompanies the fibrosis of apical tuberculosis that is healing. Elsewhere it may be due to healed empyema or pleural effusion. This may be difficult to differentiate from Pancoast tumour or small pleural effusion. It is often due to thickened apex from fibrosis, or thickened extra-pleural fat or pleura in the superior sulcus.

Endobronchial TB

This involvement occurs in approximately 2%–4% of persons with pulmonary TB. The main, upper, and lower lobe bronchi account for three-quarters of the involved sites. Upper lobe predominant-parenchymal opacities, segmental or lobar atelectasis are radiographically apparent. Endobronchial TB typically manifests as irregular or smooth circumferential bronchial narrowing associated with mural thickening on CT scan.

Pneumothorax

This may be seen as the first sign of TB. It follows rupture of subpleural cavitary lesion with escape of air into the pleural space. When massive it results in tension pneumothorax.

Pleural effusion

This is area of exudative pleural fluid collection due to subpleural and pleural infection.

i.   Pleural effusions are less commonly a manifestation of post primary tuberculosis even though a large number of organisms are spilled into the pleural space from rupture of a cavity or adjacent parenchymal focus and pleural aspirate are usually positive for acid fast bacilli.

ii.   Tuberculous pleural effusion, although usually regarded as a manifestation of primary disease, may occur in association with post primary disease in up to 19% of detected cases.

iii. Pleural effusion is observed radiographically in 16%–18% of persons with post primary TB and is typically unilateral in distribution.

iv.   *Air-fluid level, when shown within the pleural cavity,* indicates the presence of a bronchopleural fistula.

v.   *Split pleura sign.* Smooth thickening of visceral and parietal pleural surfaces separated by a variable amount of fluid demonstrated in contrast-enhanced CT evaluation of post-primary tuberculous is called *split pleura sign.*

vi.   Pleural effusions may progress to form empyemas, pleural thickening in healed stage or pleural calcification after long time of healing.

vii. Loculated pleural effusions that are stable in size for years or persistent fluid within a calcified fibrothorax detected by CT typically means active disease and chronic tuberculous empyema.

Pleural empyema

Pleural effusion in patients with post primary TB is true empyema, and therefore, acid-fast smears and mycobacterial cultures of the pleural aspirates are usually positive. Detection of persistent fluid within a calcified fibrothorax at CT should raise concern for active disease and chronic tuberculous empyema. Tuberculous effusions are typically loculated and may be stable in size for many years.

Tuberculoma

Tuberculoma is defined as a localised tuberculous granuloma appearing as round or oval, sharply marginated lesions and usually measuring between 0.5–4.0 cm in diameter. In 3%–6% of cases of post primary disease, tuberculomas are the predominant parenchymal manifestation. Tuberculomas are typically solitary but may be multiple, have regular or irregular (lobulated) margins, and often demonstrate calcification as well as proximity to adjacent small *satellite* nodules. Cavitation is rare but it often calcifies.

Bronchopneumonia

Patchy, nodular areas of consolidation with multiple lobar bronchial spread. This is due to bronchogenic spread of disease, occurring when an area of caseous necrosis liquefies and communicates with the bronchial tree. It is seen in radiographs of approximately 20% of cases of post primary TB and manifests as multiple, ill-defined, 5- to 10-mm nodules distributed in a segmental or lobar distribution, distant from the site of cavity formation and typically involving the lower (dependent) lung zones

Miliary tuberculosis

Fibrosis or other lesion of primary tuberculosis is rarely seen in military TB due to primary TB but common in military TB due to post-primary TB. Military TB is haematogenous spread of infections that have ruptured into a bronchial or pulmonary artery. It is seen in both primary (see above) and post-primary tuberculosis (figure 2.41 A).

Characteristic radiographic findings of miliary Tuberculosis

i. *Number:* They are innumerable, multiple and widespread, round or oval small nodules.

ii. *Size:* The nodules are of various sizes of 1–4 mm in diameter.

iii. *Uniformity in size and distribution:* The nodules tend to be uniform in size and distribution as they represent the release of simultaneous sloughs via the pulmonary artery circulation.

iv. *Calcification:* The pulmonary nodules are not calcified (miliary TB does not have time to calcify).

v. *Diffuse spread:* They are scattered throughout both lungs but more at the bases, (the lung being a cone is thicker at the bases and with more blood flow here).

vi. *Mild basal predominance:* There is mild basilar predominance due to increased volume of lung tissue at the bases and increased basal blood supply.

vii. *Satellite lesion:* There are associated radiographic findings that may suggest the diagnosis (satellite lesion) of TB and are present in up to 30% of affected persons and include consolidation, cavitations, calcified lymph nodes, fibrosis and lymphadenopathy.

viii. *Normal lung at early stages:* There are normal radiographic findings in the early stages of those with miliary disease; these are well-recognized and occur in 25%–40% of persons at initial presentation.

ix. This is the *window period* when there is time lag between the pathology and the appearance of the nodules radiographically. Typical miliary lesions may not be visible until 3–6 weeks after haematogenous dissemination.

x. *Diffuse alveolar pattern:* This is rarely observed in patients with miliary TB-associated adult respiratory distress syndrome·

xi. *Early demonstration by CT:* CT scan can demonstrate miliary disease before it becomes radiographically apparent.

xii. *Septal thickening on CT:* Using high resolution, thin-section CT, a mixture of both sharply and ill-defined, 1–4-mm nodules are seen in a diffuse, random distribution often associated with intra- and interlobular septal thickening are seen.

xiii. *Seen in both primary and post-primary TB:* Miliary opacities in tuberculosis can be seen in a background of both primary and post-primary tuberculosis.

Tuberculous lymphadenitis of the neck

Multiple round masses may appear in both sides of the neck laterally and palpable clinically. Some of them may calcify and identifiable radiologically. They represent lymphadenopathy caused by TB.

Destroyed lung syndrome

This can occur also in post-primary tuberculosis. (See primary tuberculosis).

Bronchiectasis

This may be as a complication of healed tuberculosis or may be due to current infection, which waxes and wanes.

Complications of Tuberculosis

Empyema thoracis

Abscess formation due to infected pleural effusion, which may need surgery for removal. This may form bronchopleural fistula, osteitis of adjacent rib, pleurocutaneous fistula and asymmetrical thoracic cage due to thoracoplasty to treat lesion.

Bronchiectasis

The upper lobes are involved and are identifiable in 71%–86% of persons with prior disease on thin-section CT scans. An ectatic bronchus may be colonized by *Aspergillus* species and form the fungus ball.

Miliary tuberculosis

This may disseminate to distant organs and cause extra-pulmonary tuberculosis affecting particularly the lymph nodes, liver, spleen, kidneys, adrenals, prostate, seminal vesicles, epididymis, Fallopian tube, endometrium, meninges, brain, skeleton, eye, intestines, omentum, pericardium and the spinal cord.

Pseudoaneurysm of pulmonary artery

Rasmussen aneurysm is a pseudo-aneurysm of a pulmonary artery usually caused by erosion of the vessel from an adjacent tuberculous cavity. It may form months to years after formation of the cavity. It is uncommon. Haemoptysis is the usual presenting symptom, it may occasionally be massive (>300 ml / 24 hours) and life threatening.

Broncholithiasis

This is characterized by calcified peribronchial nodes that either erode into or cause marked distortion of an adjacent bronchus. Radiologic findings show calcified peribronchial nodes, segmental or lobar atelectasis, obstructive pneumonitis, branching opacities in a "V" or "Y" configuration (obstructive bronchocele), and rarely, focal hyperinflation. The observed presenting symptoms include cough, haemoptysis, wheezing, or signs of recurrent pneumonia. Even though any bronchus may be involved, a right-sided predominance is observed.

Aspergilloma

Fungal colonization of residual cavity appears as a roughly spherical nodule or mass separated by a crescent-shaped area of decreased opacity from the adjacent cavity wall (whorl-like). At CT it characteristically appear as a mobile intra-cavitary nodule or mass that is usually surrounded by air but it may completely fill the cavity and may also gravitate to dependent part on prone and supine CT images.

Other complications are destroyed lung syndrome and fibrosing mediastinitis

(Adam & Dixon, 2008; Dahnert, 2011; Sutton, 1998 and 2003, Palmer & Reeder 2001).

References

1. Leung AN. Pulmonary Tuberculosis: The Essentials. Radiology 1999;210:307-322
2. Jeong YJ, Lee KS. Pulmonary Tuberculosis: Up-to-Date Imaging and Management. Am J Roentgenol 2008; 191: 834 - 844.
3. Dogru D, Ozcelik U, Gocmen A, Merino JM. Pediatric Primary Pulmonary Tuberculosis. Chest 2002; 121: 1722 - 1722.
4. Khan MA, Kovnat DM, Bachus H, Whitcomb ME, Snider GL. Clinical and roentgenographic spectrum of pulmonary tuberculosis in the adult. Am J Med 1977; 62:31-38.
5. Makanjuola D, Adeyemo AO. Lower lungfield tuberculosis in a rural African population. West Afr J Med 1991;10:412-9.

6. Elegbe IA, Salawu L, Adeyemo AO. Pulmonary tuberculosis in Nigeria. J R Soc Health 1986;106:69-71.
7. Makanjuola D. Fluid levels in pulmonary tuberculosis cavities in a rural population of Nigeria. AJR Am J Roentgenol 1983;141:519-20
8. Ahidjo A, Hammangabdo A, Anka MK. The chest radiographic appearance and frequency distribution of cavities in pulmonary tuberculosis among adults in northeastern, Nigeria. Afr J Med Med Sci 2005;34:281-4.
9. Erinle SA. An appraisal of the radiological features of pulmonary tuberculosis in Ilorin. Niger Postgrad Med J 2003;10:264-9.
10. Ahidjo A, Anka MK, Yusuph H. Radiograghic evaluation of lymphadenopathy in pulmonary tuberculosis in Northeastern, Nigeria. Niger J Med 2006;15:68-71.

2.5 ROLES OF RADIOLOGY IN THE DIAGNOSIS AND MANAGEMENT OF A PATIENT WITH BLUNT CHEST TRAUMA

Definition
Blunt chest trauma is defined as a non-penetrating chest injury without an open wound in the skin.

Causes
Fall from height, assault (blows, use of blunt instruments), blasts from bombs, or other explosive or exploding structures, road traffic injury and trauma to other parts of the body may have chest injury component.

Role of radiology
1. To make diagnosis of the injury
2. To diagnose any possible complication
3. To monitor progress for improvement/complication
4. Interventional study – ultrasound-, CT-, MR-guided drainage, embolisation of bleeding vessel.
5. To check other associated injury – head injury, fracture of other parts of the body, ruptured abdominal viscus.

Radiologic Techniques
Plain films
PA, High kV, Lateral, Supine AP (severely injured patient), Lateral decubitus, computed radiography (wide latitude of detector, reduces need for repeats, maintains consistent quality between examinations, reporting from remote location by experts possible).

Ultrasound
Conventional, echocardiography, Doppler, transoesophageal sonography, and ultrasound-guided interventional studies are possible.

CT scan
It defines fracture better and both interventional studies and CT guided biopsy can be undertaken.

MR Imaging
It has multiplanar capability, better soft tissue details and interventional studies can also be undertaken.

Radionuclide studies
This is capable of showing fracture even where other methods fail especially at the healing stages.

Other views
- Plain skull x – ray PA, Lateral, CT scan of skull, MRI of body/skull
- Abdominal Ultrasonography, Transfontanel ultrasonography
- Plain x-ray examination of limbs for fractures of other parts of the body.

Injury to the Thoracic Cage

Rib fractures: This may be single, multiple, unilateral or bilateral.

a.   Haematoma with extrapleural mass may suggest rib fracture.

b.   Fracture of 1 – 3 ribs is associated with severe intrathoracic injury.

c.   Fracture of 3 – 6 ribs may involve injury to the abdominal organs.

Flail chest: Several ribs adjacent to each other fracture in more than one segment.

Fracture of sternum: It is seen in lateral view or CT scan.

Fracture of clavicle

1.   Injury to brachial plexus, subclavian artery may occur.

2.   If fractured segment is posteriorly displaced, injury to trachea, oesophagus, superior mediastinum, nerves and great vessels may occur.

Fracture of thoracic spine: Single or multiple vertebral fractures with or without pain, spinal haematoma/shadow.

Injury to the Pleura

Pneumothorax: Lucency in pleural space devoid of long markings following rib fracture or pneumomediastinum or lung laceration.

Haemothorax: It presents as different grades of opacity of a haemithorax. This is caused by laceration of intercostal or pleural vessels. It may follow rib fracture.

Hydropneumothorax: Air-fluid level seen, the fluid being blood. Best shown by horizontal beam view.

Pleural effusion: Lung contusion/laceration, osteomyelitis of ribs, pneumonia following lung injury may later present with pleural effusion.

Empyema thoracis: This occurs many weeks or moths after the trauma and is more common if there is unrecognised infected open wound.

Injury to the Lung

Contusion: Severe trauma to the lung may lead to haemorrhage into the alveoli and interstitial space. Sudden appearance of patchy non-segmental consolidation, which starts to improve in 2 days and clears in 3 – 4 days, is diagnostic.

Laceration: Traumatic thin-walled cystic spaces. This may be obscured in acute stages by consolidation or lung contusion. The cystic space may appear as round opacity if it is filled with blood. Fluid level may develop if only partially filled with blood. They may be multiple and resolution may take a few months.

Torsion: Twist of the lung around hilum through 180° seen in blunt trauma commonly in children. Opaque haemithorax may be seen if unrelieved and gangrenous.

Lung collapse: Decreased respiratory movements. Mucus or haematoma blocking a major bronchus may cause lung collapse.

Compensatory hyperinflation: This occurs because of lung collapse of one part or the entire contralateral lung field.

Pulmonary oedema: Features of adult respiratory distress syndrome with widespread consolidation as a result of massive injury, fat embolism, or bone marrow embolism released during the trauma.

Fat embolism: Embolism of lung with lung collapse as a result of fat deposits from bone marrow entering the systemic circulation. Multiple round opacities in the lungs are seen. *The presence of fat globules in urine or sputum confirms the diagnosis.* Ventilation/perfusion study may be useful in early assessment of the lesion for diagnosis.

Injury to the Trachea/Bronchi

Rupture or laceration of the trachea may present as mediastinal emphysema / pneumothorax. Injury occurs often at / around the carina.

Injury to the Mediastinum
Pneumomediastinum

Air between tissue planes of the mediastinal structures.

Gas shadows may extend up the neck.

Mediastinal pleura may be displaced laterally.

The causes are oesophageal perforation, ruptured trachea/bronchi, from pneumoperitoneum or penetrating injury.

Pneumopericardium

"Continuous diaphragm sign" may be produced by pneumomediastinum or pneumopericardium as air collects within (pneumopericardium) or below the pericardium (pneumomediastinum) making the central part of diaphragm visible.

Mediastinal haemorrhage

This causes widening of mediastinum bilaterally or a localised bulge due to local haematoma. Aortic rupture, and dissecting aortic aneurysm or other vessels may bleed into mediastinum.

Traumatic aortic transaction/Ruptured Aorta

The isthmus, site of ligamentum arterosum is the commonest affected site. Findings in plain chest radiography include mediastinal widenning, mediastinum to chest ratio of greater than 0.25 or a mediastinal width greater than 8 cm signifies large mediastinal haematoma due the condition. Deviated of the oseophagus to the right of the transverse process of the fourth thoracic vertebra; apical extrapleural cap and a left haemothorax are some of the features that may be demonstrated. There is a right-side and anteroinferior push or shift of the left main stem bronchus. There is also compression or deviation of the trachea to the right. Fractures of the first two ribs or sixth cervical to the eight thoracic vertebrae mean that transaction is very likely and should be actively excluded. Left apical cap, right lateral displacement of superior vena cava, opacification of medial border of left lung, obscured aorto-pulmonary window, and widened right with left paraspinal stripe are among other signs of aortic transaction. Saccular aortic arch aneurysm may develop with time. Angiography (aortography) is the definitive diagnostic modality but CT scan, MRI and transoesophageal echocardiography are also highly sensitive.

Cardiac Rupture

Myocardial contusion, infarction and in severe cases cardiac rupture may occur. Rhythm disturbances, cardiac tamponade, pericardial haematoma, ventricular aneurysm and septal defects may occur. Echocardiography from the chest or transoesophageal route is highly sensitive. However, echoplanar MR imaging (EPI) and dynamic spatial reconstructed CT imaging techniques are excellent diagnostic tools.

Oesophageal Rupture (Rare in blunt trauma alone).
Pneumothorax, pneumomediastinum or hydropneumomediastinum (often left-sided) may occur. Barium swallow studies using water-soluble low-osmolar contrast medium is preferred to confirm diagnosis instead of barium.
Chylothorax: Thoracic duct damage may occur leading to chylothorax.

Injury to the Diaphragm
Laceration: This may lead to reduced excursion or movement.
Ruptured diaphragm: More common on the left. Herniation of stomach, omentum, bowel or kidneys and spleen may be immediate or delayed.
The appearance shows increased opacity of the affected haemithorax with obscured diaphragmatic margins.
Ultrasound will demonstrate pleural effusion/haemothorax, ascites/haemoperitoneum, herniated organs in the chest and may show point of rupture of the diaphragm.
Barium studies will confirm the herniation of stomach, small or large intestine.

Injury to the Subcutaneous Soft Tissue
Haematoma: Subcutaneous soft tissue haematoma in any part of the chest will be demonstrated by ultrasound scan, CT scan or MRI.
Subcutaneous emphysema: Air from pneumomediastinum may dissect through the neck and cause subcutaneous emphysema. The neck may be swollen by subcutaneous air and respiratory embarrassment may occur. Gas may also extend extra-pleurally over the diaphragm. It may also extend over the chest wall.
Herniation of the lung: Grossly displaced rib fracture may lead to herniation of the lung to the exterior. This is best shown by tangential view.

Acute respiratory distress syndrome (ARDS)
This can occur in massive initial injury and consists of extensive bilateral air space opacities. It is earliest seen with 2 days of the injury and it is very vital that the diagnosis is recognised so the appropriate treatment is started to keep the patient alive. Intensive care unit (ICU) is the best place to keep such patients.

Osteomyelitis
This may follow fracture. Osteomyelitis may develop after some time has elapsed if the rib fracture is infected.

Other Injuries Elsewhere
Skull: Plain x-ray and CT scan of the skull may show or exclude fractures, subdural/epidural/intracerebral haemorrhage/haematoma.
Limbs: Fracture of the upper/lower limbs may be shown by x-ray of affected part.
Abdomen: Ultrasonography will quickly check for normality/abnormality of intra-abdominal organs. Ultrasonography will also confirm viability of foetus in case of pregnant patient.
Interventional study
Ultrasound-/CT-guided drainage of haemorrhage/haematoma using wide-bore catheters/needles.

(Adam & Dixon, 2008; Dahnert, 2011; Sutton, 2003; Swischuk, 2004).

References

1. Van Hise ML, Primack SL, Israel RS, Müller NL. CT in blunt chest trauma: indications and limitations. Radiographics 1998; 18:1071-84.
2. Kaewlai R, Avery LL, Asrani AV, Novelline RA. Multidetector CT of blunt thoracic trauma. Radiographics 2008; 28:1555-70.
3. Zinck SE, Primack SL. Radiographic and CT findings in blunt chest trauma. J Thorac Imaging 2000; 15:87-96.
4. Kuhlman JE, Pozniak MA, Collins J, Knisely BL. Radiographic and CT findings of blunt chest trauma: aortic injuries and looking beyond them. Radiographics 1998; 18:1085-11068.
5. Iochum S, Ludig T, Walter F, Sebbag H, Grosdidier G, Blum AG. Imaging of diaphragmatic injury: a diagnostic challenge? Radiographics 2002; 22 Spec No:S103-16.
6. Alkadhi H, Wildermuth S, Desbiolles L, Schertler T, Crook D, Marincek B, Boehm T. Vascular emergencies of the thorax after blunt and iatrogenic trauma: multi-detector row CT and three-dimensional imaging. Radiographics 2004; 24:1239-55.
7. Methodius-Ngwodo WC, Burkett AB, Kochupura PV, Wellons ED, Fuhrman G, Rosenthal D. The role of CT angiography in the diagnosis of blunt traumatic thoracic aortic disruption and unsuspected carotid artery injury. Am Surg 2008;74:580-6.
8. Umerah BC. Radiology of trauma. In: Umerah BC (Ed), (1989). Medical practice and the law in Nigeria. Longman, Ikeja, Nigeria. 88-94.

2.6   RADIOLOGICAL FINDINGS IN ENDOMYOCARDIAL FIBROSIS

Definition

Endomyocardial fibrosis (EMF) is a progressive cardiac disease in which there is a swelling of the endocardial connective tissue and accumulation of acid mucopolysaccharides in the endocardium followed by scarring and fibrosis.

Pattern of involvement

It affects one or both ventricles primarily and other cardiac chambers to a lesser extent. It is primarily and specifically a cardiac disease, never accompanied by lesion in other parts of the body.

Geographical distribution

1. It is endemic in the tropics, especially Africa.
2. It is more common in West and East Africa.
3. It commonly affects lower socioeconomic groups due to poor nutrition, although it affects well-nourished Caucasian immigrants to Africa as well.

Causes

The aetiology is unknown

Filariasis has been implicated.

Hypersensitivity and immunological damage are also implicated

Viral involvement has been questioned.

Pathology

There is the laying down of fibrous tissue on the inner aspect of the ventricle (endocardium) starting from and more severe in the apex and spreading to involve the inlet valves. Ventricular capacity is reduced to about one-third (⅓). Fusion of the cardiac walls can occur. The disease is dominantly on one side but both sides and atria are affected in up to half of the cases. The heart is usually enlarged but not increased in weight. High protein-content effusion often accompanies the changes. Lesions do not occur elsewhere in EMF except as complications. Valvular incompetence leads to heart failure. Pulmonary embolism occurs and to lesser extent embolus formation in systemic circulation. Rheumatic heart disease may accompany it. Intra cardiac calcifications also occur especially of the ventricular apex.

Clinical features

Acute febrile illness, malaise and anorexia. Fever continues until heart failure develops and most of the EMF are chance findings at autopsy.

Radiological Features

Left-sided EMF

The disease may show dominance of one side or the other but it is rarely truly unilateral and radiographic findings will depend on the stage in which the disease is observed or when the patient presented.

Plain films
1. Routine plain chest radiograph will show cardiomegaly, which is non-specific.
2. Evidence of mitral valvular disease like mitral valvular calcification may be observed.
3. Small aorta with enlarged infundibulum may be noted.
4. There could be enlarged pulmonary bay/conus with flattened or bulging left cardiac border.
5. There could be left atrial enlargement evidenced by double density behind the heart. Left atrial enlargement is only mild to moderate and not as large as in rheumatic mitral incompetence or right-sided EMF.
6. Enlarged and pulsating main pulmonary arteries that do not extend peripherally.
7. Pulmonary oedema appearing like cotton wool opacities or bat's-wing pattern opacities. Visible septal lines are not common.
8. Intra-cardiac calcification of left ventricular apex occurs infrequently but when seen is characteristic.
9. Differentiation of EMF and rheumatic mitral valve disease using only plain films is not possible.
10. There could be features of cardiac failure and most patients present at this stage.

Ultrasound
1. The heart is often normal in size and shows good systolic function with good contraction and emptying.
2. There is difficulty in filling the ventricles
3. Features of mitral incompetence with regurgitation and stenosis often co-exist.
4. If mitral regurgitation is severe, the heart size may increase.
5. Doppler ultrasound shows impaired compliance.
6. Pericardial effusion is confirmed
7. Partial obliteration or amputation of the cavity at left ventricular apex with a ring of calcification around it.
8. Short axis dimension of the ventricle more than the long axis dimension due to apical obliteration.
9. Mitral valve crescent due to fibrosis of mitral valve cusp.
10. Dilatation of the left and right atria
Abdominal sonography will show ascites, which may be massive.

Angiocardiography (Findings are characteristic)
1. Small and irregular left ventricle
2. Filling-defect or amputation and smoothing-off of the apices of the left ventricle
3. Almost constant volume of the left ventricle with little change between systole and diastole.
4. Near-impossibility in identifying the mitral valve cusps.
5. Demonstration of mitral incompetence is easy but in a few cases, it may be difficult to identify.

MR Imaging
1. Apical hyperenhancement shown by Myocardial delayed enhancement (MDE-MR) cardiovascular magnetic resonance (CMR) is highly suggestive of endomyocardial fibrosis.
2. Hypoenhancing areas correspond to areas of calcification and/or thrombi formation.

CT Scan
1. Myocardial delayed enhancement computed tomography (MDE-CT) shows left ventricular apical obliteration with areas of MDE associated to calcified areas.
2. Using MDE-CT, hyperenhancement images demonstrate fibrosis and calcification areas.

3. Hypoenhancement areas could also suggest thrombi.
   Massive apical subendocardial calcification may be shown by MDCT calcium score images, Sometimes the density of calcification can be denser than the patient's spine and if this in the left ventricular apex, the diagnosis is certain

Right Sided EMF
Plain films
1. Routine chest radiograph will show marked (non-specific) cardiac enlargement with smooth and globular outline. It is quite difficult to decide whether the cardiomegaly is due to pericardial effusion, generalised cardiac enlargement or specific enlargement of the right atrium.
2. Calcification at apex of right ventricle or at the base of pulmonary conus. This is best demonstrated using high-speed Bucky film.
3. Striking and marked oligaemia of the lung fields which appear clear with no evidence of pulmonary oedema.
4. There may be pericardial effusion.

Fluoroscopy
1. Minimal cardiac pulsation and cannot differentiate pericardial effusion from myocardiopathy.
2. It will demonstrate intracardiac cardiac calcification at the cardiac apex.
3. There will be cardiac hypokinesia demonstrated.
4. The globular shape of the heart is shown.

Ultrasound (Echocardiography)
1. It will show presence or absence of pericardial effusion.
2. Weak movement of cardiac muscles.
3. Tricuspid valvular incompetence shown by regurgitation, stenosis, or both.
4. Echogenic substance within the atrium or ventricle may be shown due to thrombus. This may embolize.

Angiocardiography
1. Normal outflow portion but contracted and restricted inflow tract.
2. Distended but continuous functioning outflow tract may occasionally be observed.
3. Filling-defect within the atrium and/or ventricle due to thrombus formation. This is rarely symptomatic except when it embolizes.
4. Dilated right atrium.
5. Stasis of contrast material within the right atrium because of decrease in size of right ventricle and tricuspid incompetence. Contrast may persist within right atrium for up to 12 seconds.
6. Obliteration of cardiac apex which is often progressive.
7. Dilatation of veins of the neck due to incompetence of these and azygos veins.
8. Reflux filling of perivertebral venous plexuses may occur.

MR Imaging
1. Apical hyperenhancement shown by Myocardial delayed enhancement (MDE-MR) cardiovascular magnetic resonance (CMR) is highly suggestive of endomyocardial fibrosis.
2. Hpoenhancing areas correspond to areas of calcification and/or thrombi formation.

CT Scan
1. Myocardial delayed enhancement computed tomography (MDE-CT) shows right ventricular apical obliteration with areas of MDE associated to calcified areas.
2. Using MDE-CT, hyperenhancement images demonstrate fibrosis and calcification areas.
3. Hypoenhancement areas could also suggest thrombi.
4. Massive apical subendocardical calcification may be shown by MDCT calcium score images.

Differential diagnoses
1. Pericardial effusion.
2. Cardiac failure from other causes
3. Mitral stenosis/incompetence from other causes.
4. Rheumatic heart disease.

(Adam & Dixon, 2008; Dahnert, 2011; Sutton, 2003; Swischuk, 2004; Palmer & Reeder, 2001).

References
1. Falase AO, Kolawole TM, Lagundoye SB. Endomyocardial fibrosis. Problems in differential diagnosis. Br Heart J 1976;38:369-74.
2. Cockshott WP, Sarić S, Ikeme AC. Radiological findings in endomyocardial fibrosis. Circulation 1967;35:913-22.
3. Sliwa K, Mocumbi AO. Forgotten cardiovascular diseases in Africa. Clin Res Cardiol 2010;99:65-74
4. O'Hanlon R, Pennell DJ. Cardiovascular magnetic resonance in the evaluation of hypertrophic and infiltrative cardiomyopathies. Heart Fail Clin 2009;5:369-87.
5. Bukhman G, Ziegler J, Parry E. Endomyocardial fibrosis: still a mystery after 60 years. PLoS Negl Trop Dis 2008;2:e97.
6. Paydar A, Ordovas KG, Reddy GP. Magnetic resonance imaging for endomyocardial fibrosis. Pediatr Cardiol 2008;29:1004-5.
7. Senra T, Shiozaki AA, Salemi VM, Rochitte CE. Delayed enhancement by multidetector computed tomography in endomyocardial fibrosis. Eur Heart J 2008;29:347.
8. Namboodiri KK, Bohora S. Images in cardiology. Clenched fist appearance in endomyocardial fibrosis. Heart 2006;92:720.
9. Goo HW, Han NJ, Lim TH. Endomyocardial fibrosis mimicking right ventricular tumor. AJR Am J Roentgenol 2001;177:205-6.

CHAPTER 3

GASTROINTESTINAL
TRACT AND ABDOMEN

3.1   RADIOLOGY OF HAEMATEMESIS

Definition
Haematemesis is defined as vomiting of blood. The blood loss in haematemesis is derived from acute upper gastro-intestinal (GI) haemorrhage. Upper GI bleeding is defined as haemorrhage occurring proximal to the duodenal–jejunal flexure, which means proximal to the ligament of Treitz. In haematemesis, blood from such haemorrhage is passed out retrogradely usually initiate by the force of vomiting.

Causes of haematemesis
Oesophageal lesion
This is caused by bleeding from:
Oesophageal varices, oesophageal erosion/oesophagitis, Mallory-Weiss tear, oesophageal laceration/perforation by foreign body, oesophageal carcinoma, Iatrogenic, via endoscopes, nasogastric tube injury, biopsies, Hiatus hernia, aorto–oesophageal fistula, oesophageal polyp/adenoma and oesophageal diverticulum

Stomach or gastric lesions
It can be from bleeding:
Gastric ulcer, gastritis/gastric erosion, gastric carcinoma, gastric lymphoma, gastric varices, gastric adenoma, gastric polyp, aorto–gastric fistula and gastric diverticulum.

Duodenal lesions
It can be from bleeding:
Duodenal ulcer, ampullary tumours, duodenitis/duodenal erosion, biliary system/haemobilia, duodenal diverticulum, Aorto–duodenal fistula, duodenal varices, duodenal polyp and duodenal adenoma.

Systemic lesions
Bleeding disorders/blood dyscrasias, disseminated intravascular coagulation with bleeding, viral haemorrhagic fever, haemorrhagic disease of the newborn, vomiting of swallowed blood by the newborn, septicaemia and schistosomiasis

Vascular anomalies (developmental lesions).
These could be bleeding from:
Arteriovenous anomalies/masses, haemangioma, haemorrhagic telangiectasia (Osler-Weber-Rendu Syndrome), pseudoxanthoma elasticum and Ehlers-Danlos syndrome.

Rupture of surrounding organs
These could be bleeding from rupture or leaking:
Aortic aneurysm into oesophagus, rupture of prosthetic graft into oesophagus, stomach or duodenum, rupture of gastrectomy suture and anastomotic bleed.

Contribution of causes of upper gastrointestinal bleeding
1. Peptic ulceration 70 – 80%
2. Erosions 10 – 15%
3. Varices 3 – 5%

Table 3.11: Radiological investigative modalities

Angiography – Arteriography, venography

Endoscopic Ultrasonography

Barium swallow/meal

Radionuclide studies – ^{99m}Tc sulphur colloid

Ultrasound – conventional, colour Doppler

CT scan – contrast, non-contrast, helical CT, CT Angiography

MRI – contrast and non-contrast (intravenous and oral), MRA

Transjugular intrahepatic porto-systemic shunt (TIPS)

Plain chest X-ray

Plain abdominal X-ray (Erect and supine)

Plain film of the neck (AP/lateral)

Pre-radiological management
1. Take a quick accurate history and physical examination to establish
    1. Chronic conditions like peptic ulcer disease, gastric ulcer, cirrhosis of the liver, schistosomiasis, carcinoma anywhere in the body.
    2. Haemorrhagic disease like haemophilia, sickle cell disease, platelet deficiency disease, other clothing factors deficiency
    3. Infections (viral haemorrhagic fever and septicaemia)
    4. Establish whether haematemesis or haemoptysis
    5. Recent swallowing of foreign body, impaction, fish bone impaction, artificial denture impaction
    6. Establish whether recent endoscopy/endoscopic procedure or biopsy was undertaken.
2. Stabilize the patient, correct hypovolaemia by replacing fluid and electrolyte quickly to avoid hypotension which can cause myocardial infarction in the elderly.
    Do full blood count and check clotting time, group and cross-match 5 or more units of fresh, whole blood. Transfuse if necessary. Bring patient out of shock state. Hypovolaemic shock causes

acute renal failure with high mortality. Inform surgeons, physicians and anaesthetists. Get the theatre ready.

Investigations and Radiological Findings
Endoscopy

Even though not a radiological procedure, it is the first line of investigation to establish diagnosis. It can diagnose varices, oesophageal/gastric erosions, masses, foreign bodies, rupture of peptic/ gastric ulcer, and gastric mass lesions.

The advantages of endoscopy are that it can:

1. Identify the bleeding site even when this is different from the patient's established chronic conditions.

    For instance, a patient with oesophageal varices may be bleeding from gastric erosion from aspirin ingestion and not from the varices. A patient with peptic ulcer disease may be bleeding from Mallory – Weiss tear instead of the peptic ulcer disease.
2. Be used to stop bleeding by application of diathermy or balloon tamponade or laser.
3. It can visualise all the other structures outside and not just the bleeding site so that a more wholesome treatment is planned.
4. Endoscopy can be used to remove foreign body and if tumour is discovered, biopsy can be undertaken at the same time (table 3.11).

Arteriography

This is positive contrast examination of the arterial supply of the duodenum, stomach and oesophagus using selective and highly selective Seldinger's technique through catheterization of the femoral artery. Arteriography will promptly show the site of the bleeding, the bleeding vessel and there may be multiple bleeding points. The greatest advantage of arteriography is the possibility of carrying out interventional procedures simultaneously. This is done by injection of sclerosants, gelfoams, vasoconstrictive agents (vasopressin and glucagon) to block the bleeding artery and stop the bleeding or to reduce blood supply to vascular bleeding tumour. It is the first modality after endoscopy. Angiography requires bleeding rate of about 0.5 ml per minute for detection and it can detect over 63% of bleeding sites.

Endoscopic ultrasonography

High frequency radial electronic driven ultrasound transducers mounted on a fibre-optic endoscope form an endoscopic ultrasound device. This is widely available in developed countries and is used to carry out quick survey of the oesophagus and stomach. Knowledge of normal anatomy of upper GIT is essential for accurate assessment. The probe is applied to the wall of the GIT or via water-filled balloon and the endoscope withdrawn. Strictures need prior dilatation before the passage of the endoscopic ultrasound transducer. Carcinomas are excellently diagnosed as well as haemangiomas within the muscle coat. Endoscopic ultrasound will show collaterals from varices in perioesophageal and perigastric locations but the submucosal oesophageal varices are not shown. Endoscopic sonography is also used as follow up after sclerosant injection and also for assessment for the risk of re-bleeding which is high.

Barium meal/swallow

This is inferior to both endoscopy and arteriography in demonstrating upper GIT bleeding. Barium studies should not be done before arteriography as residual contrast may obscure diagnosis with arteriography. Barium swallow using thick viscous barium will show varices as multiple worm-like, beaded or serpiginous filling defects which change position in different films. Valsalva's or Mullers manoeuvres will show varices better.

Radionuclide studies

This shows even the smallest intestinal bleeding. The site is not always specified. Technetium 99m sulphur colloid or Tc – 99m pertechnetate or Tc-99m-labelled RBC (with invitro labelling preferred) is used. Tc – 99m sulphur colloid detects bleeding rate of [3] 0.05 ml / minute and more sensitive than angiogram but image degraded by respiratory and bowel motions. Tc-99m-labelled red blood cell (RBC) is more than 90% sensitive for blood loss above 50 ml per 24 hours.

CT scanning

This can show gastric carcinomas, lymphomas, metastatic masses of the adrenal, liver, transcoelomic spread of Kruckenbeurg's tumour of the ovaries. CT scanning can also show aortic aneurysm and aorto – duodenal fistulas. This occurs from pressure necrosis of 3rd part of duodenum where it crosses over or lies above aortic aneurysm or where there is infection of top end of prosthetic graft. This will also show thickened oesophageal, gastric or duodenal wall with hypodense non-contrast are due to bleeding displacing the contrast medium within the bowel.

MR imaging

This will show the features as demonstrated by CT scan. However, it can reveal vascular anatomy like aneurysms, collateral circulations and fistulas without the use of contrast medium. It can also differentiate flowing from stagnant blood. It has no ionizing radiations and can image in different planes. Cost still limits its use particularly in the developing countries. Radiolucent foreign body in the neck can be visualised.

Transjugular intrahepatic portosystemic shunt (TIPS)

This is used to quickly undertake intervention for shunting of high pressure portal blood to the low pressure systemic circulation. The portal blood is decompressed through percutaneously established shunt with expandable metallic stent between the hepatic and portal veins within the liver. The size of the stent is at least 10 mm wall stent. Mean portal venous blood velocity is aimed to be increased from 18 cm/s to 55 cm/s and mean portal pressure decreased from 37 mmHg to 22 mmHg.

Plain chest radiograph

This will show air under the hemidiaphragm in perforated peptic ulcer disease or gastric ulcer. Metastatic lesions are seen as pleural effusion, osseous osteolytic or sclerotic changes, plate-like atelectasis, lymphangitis carcinomatosa, solitary or multiple pulmonary nodules. Widening of the mediastinum due to bleeding within the mediastinum may be seen and there may also be bleeding outside the oesophageal wall due to iatrogenic perforation or biopsy. Hydrothorax, pneumomediastinum and pneumothorax may be seen. Osseous metastatic lesions can be seen in the bones in the case of carcinomas.

Plain radiograph of the neck

This will show any radio-opaque foreign body in the neck.
It will also show retropharyngeal abscess if this has developed as a result of endoscopy or biopsy. Subcutaneous emphysema, pneumomediastinum may also be seen.

Differential diagnosis

Peptic ulceration

This is common in the duodenum occurring about two to three times more than in the stomach and about seven or more times more common in males than females. Over 90% of ulcers are at the bulbar region. Giant ulcers are more than 2 cm in diameter and may resemble diverticula or deformities of duodenal cap. On double-contrast barium study, duodenal ulcer craters appear as sharply defined pockets of barium collections. This may sometimes show area of surrounding oedema or mucosal fold radiating to the ulcer crater. The mucosal fold will be irregular if the ulcer is penetrating. Chronic duodenal ulcer may show deformity of involved parts as well as pockets of barium collection in ulcer craters in barium meal studies (figure 3.11). Erosion or penetration of the ulcer may lead to intraperitoneal bleeding, haematemesis or melaena. In unsuspected perforation, barium meal studies will show extraluminal flakes of barium within the peritoneal cavity (figure 3.12). Active bleeding ulcer can be detected by angiography if the bleeding is at a rate of 0.5 ml / min.

Gastric ulcer

Benign gastric ulcers are commonest in lesser curvature. *Geriatric ulcers* are commonest in dependent part of greater curvature and are more than 3 cm in diameter, often caused by aspirin and non-steroidal anti-inflammatory drugs. On barium meal study, benign ulcer has ulcer crater with radiating mucosal folds when seen in profile, protrudes outside the expected line of the stomach wall. A halo defect which is a wide lucent band encircles the ulcer signifying oedema. Ulcer on nondependent side are seen as ring shadows when seen en face. Malignant ulcer are more common at the apex of a protruding tumour mass within the outline of the stomach. Margins of malignant ulcers have surrounding, rolled shouldered edges. These ulcers are also diagnosable using endoscopy. Erosion, penetration or perforation leads to bleeding and haematemesis. On barium study, ulcer crater that is bleeding may contain a central filling-defect produced by blood clot.

Erosive gastritis

These are small mucosal erosions or ulcerations which do not penetrate the muscularis mucosa that are seen on barium meal study as small shallow pools of barium and measuring 1-2 mm in diameter. These erosions, also called *aphthous ulcers* are often bordered by a translucent halo of oedema when they are called *varioloform* or *complete erosions*. In the absence of the halo they are called *incomplete erosions* and may in that case appear as short linear or serpentine lines or blot of barium collections. They often lie on rugal folds, giving the folds a scalloped margin. Endoscopy is best for diagnosis of gastric erosions particularly, the single or incomplete erosions. Aspirin, indomethacin and phenylbutazone are recognized causes. Haematemesis may result from severe erosive gastritis. Infusion of vasopressin and embolisation of supplying arteries are used for control of the bleeding.

Erosive duodenitis

This rarely causes haematemesis. There is the development of gastric metaplasia of the duodenal cap, which becomes colonized by Helicobacter Pylori, and may result from antral gastritis associated with *Helicobacter* Pylori. The duodenal cap is mainly affected and there may be co-existing duodenal ulcer. On barium meal studies, it shows as coarsening of duodenal folds. On double contrast barium meal, it shows as spots of barium collection, with or without a radiolucent halo. A combination of coarsening of duodenal folds and complete erosions gives the duodenal cap a 'cobblestone' appearance on double contrast barium meal studies. Crohn's disease and AIDS are other conditions that can cause duodenitis.

Caustic oesophagitis/erosion

The early stages show mucosal sloughing, coagulative necrosis and ulceration with haematemesis. Fistulation and rarely perforation may later result. Household agent and those used in some particular occupations are frequently drunk accidentally or in attempted suicide. The implicated caustic agents are alkali such as sodium bicarbonate, lye, iodine and bleach. The commonly ingested acid includes hydrochloric acid (HCl) and sulphuric acid (H_2SO_4). There is narrowing of the oesophagus with fibrosis in late stages. History is often diagnostic but upper gastrointestinal series may show long-length narrowing with preserved mucosal pattern.

Drug-induced oesophagitis/erosion

Several drugs can cause oesophageal erosion, ulcer, inflammation and in late states benign stricture. These drugs may be trapped in areas of constrictions of the oesophagus or may be refluxed back to the oesophagus even in dissolved state. The implicated drugs are aspirin, indomethacin, quinidine, tetracycline, doxycycline, butazolydone and phenylbutazone.

Erosive changes from these drugs are the cause of the haematemesis and such erosion may appear as aphthoid ulcers on barium swallow. History is essential but conditions that cause dysphagia such are cardiomegaly, oesophageal diverticulum and, reflux oesophagitis may predispose to this condition as the drugs may be trapped or refluxed. On barium swallow studies, there may be mucosal irregularities, nodularity with thickened fold due to oesophagitis and the appearance may resemble varices.

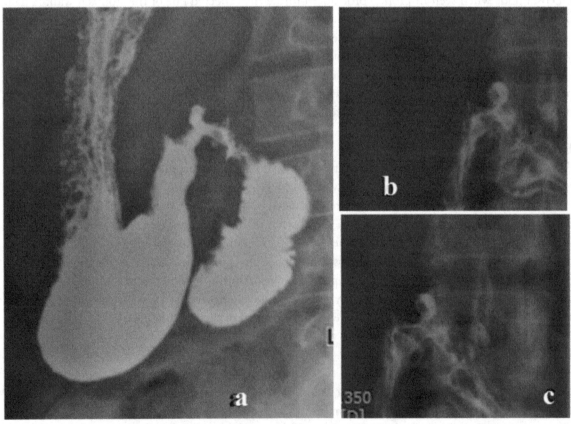

Figure 3.11: Radiographs of images of barium meal examination in a patient with chronic peptic ulcer disease. Note the distortion of the duodenum and multiple ulcer craters (**a**, **b**, and **c**).

Oesophageal Varices

Oesophageal varices are dilated oesophageal submucosal veins. They may run the whole length of the oesophagus or be confined to the upper thoracic oesophagus depending on the type of the shunting. On a chest radiograph there may be a posterior mediastinal mass behind the heart, which is associated with a dilated azygos vein. On barium swallow studies, when seen en face, varices appear as multiple serpiginous translucent filling-defects which changes position in different films. Profile view shows varices as lines of nodular or scalloped filling- defects that changes position in different films. Oesophagitis and varicoid carcinoma of oesophagus may simulated varices and must be differentiated. Arteriography or endoscopy is used to demonstrate bleeding varices as the true cause of the haematemesis.

Gastric varices

Gastric varices are dilated submucosal venous plexus in the fundus of the stomach. Contrast-enhanced CT shows varices as an enhancing thickening of the oesophageal wall. On endoscopy, they produce a lobular or nodular contour on the fundus of the stomach. On barium meal studies, they may be seen as multiple serpiginous filing-defects in the stomach extending to the duodenum, this appearance changes position with different films. Solitary varix may enlarge and produce a smooth submucosal tumour but this is rare. Tear or rupture of the varices is a cause of haematemesis.

Duodenal varices

Varices are encountered occasionally in the duodenal cap and loop. They occur mainly in patients with extrahepatic portal hypertension, but may occur in portal hypertension without evidence of extrahepatic obstruction. It is associated with oesophageal and gastric varices but could, tear and bleed on its own causing haematemesis. The varices may tear, bleed and cause haematemesis. Endoscopy is useful in their diagnosis.

Mallory-Weiss syndrome

This is a tear of mucosa and submucosa of the lower oesophagus with involvement of venous plexus resulting from a sudden increase in intraoesophageal pressure precipitated by violent vomiting or retching. On endoscopy, the mucosal tear is visible occurring above the gastro-oesophageal junction. On double contrast barium study, the tear is seen as a vertical short white line. Haemorrhage or barium may enter the tear and dissect out the mucosa from underling circular muscle coat either circumferentially or vertically producing obstructive, annular, constrictive broad-based filling defect or narrowing the lumen respectively. Catheter embolisation or open surgery is the treatment options.

Dieulafoy's lesion (*exulceratio simplex Dieulafoy*)

This is the occurrence of a large dilated and tortuous arteriole in the wall of the stomach that erodes and bleeds causing massive life-threatening haematemesis. It is a development abnormality of the stomach and causes less than 5% of all gastrointestinal bleeding in adults. It is also called "*calibre-persistent artery*" or "*aneurysm*" of gastric vessels. Dieulafoy's lesion appears as a single large tortuous submucosal arteriole which fails to branch or forms a branch with calibre that is more than 10 times the normal diameter of mucosal capillaries. Minute submucosal defects caused by protrusion of the dilated arterioles into the gastric submucosa may lead to bleeding. It is diagnosed using angiography, endoscopy or endoscopic ultrasound, and sclerotherapy and embolisation can be performed to obliterate it.

Water melon stomach

The antrum of the stomach is invaded by vascular ectasia, which may bleed at any time leading to haematemesis. The condition is diagnosed at endoscopy as the ectatic submucosal vessels are clearly visualized. Thickened folds, which is similar to the submucosal varices that are occasionally seen in barium studies. Such patients may also have portal hypertension.

Aortoenteric fistula

There are two types of aorto-enteric fistula, namely the more common secondary type which results from complication of aortic reconstructive surgery and the primary type that results from complication of atherosclerotic aortic aneurysms. If the fistula is in the upper GIT particularly the third and fourth part of duodenum, it may bleed and lead to haematemesis. Plain films may show pneumoperitoneum and CT scan of abdomen will show intra – and periaortic gas. Sonography may demonstrate aneurysm of the abdominal aorta. Abdominal aortic angiography may demonstrate bleeding from the aneurysm signifying rupture. This is evidenced by extravasations of contrast from the abdominal aorta into a bowel.

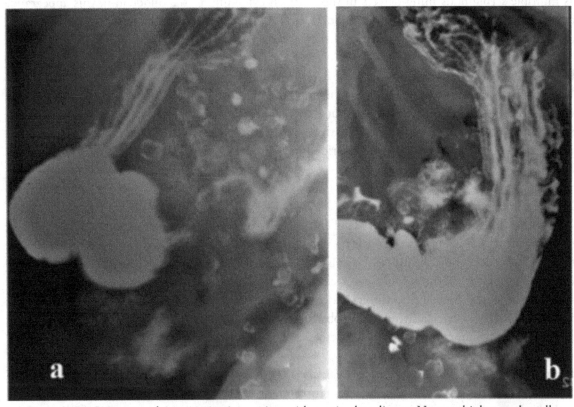

Figure 3.12: Barium meal examination in a patient with peptic ulcer disease. Note multiple round small extraluminal flakes of contrast due to age of contrast through the site of unsuspected perforation (**a** and **b**).

Gastro-duodenal haemangiomas

They can be solitary or multiple and may be found anywhere within the upper GIT and are a source of bleeding that are vomited out as haematemesis. They are made of capillary and cavernous types. The cavernous type may occasionally contain calcified phleboliths, which aids its recognition by plain film or CT scan. They are diagnosed using endoscopy. At barium meal study, they simulate submucosal tumour. Haemangiomas appear as well-defined lesions with a lobular outline and show homogeneously high signal on T2-weighted, which further show rapidly enhancing vessels at their periphery visible in the arterial phase images. The lesions will 'fill in' centripetally to become isointense or slightly hyperintense with the adjacent parenchyma within a period of minutes. CT study reveals a well-defined, lobulated lesion with density similar to that of blood in non-enhanced scan. The pattern of enhancement shows the lesion filling-in centripetally and finally merging with the background parenchyma similar to MR imaging. Their supplying artery can be identified in super selective angiography and embolised to obliterate the haemangioma.

Gastric carcinoma

These are malignant tumour of gastric epithelium that has invaded the muscularis propria. They may be polypoid or fungating and may ulcerate when they have protruded into the gastric lumen. 'Leather bottle' stomach or 'linitis plastica' appearance may occur caused by excessive infiltrating type that grossly narrows the gastric lumen. Calcification may be seen in mucin-producing type. At early stages, ulcerating tumours may resemble benign peptic ulcers, except for its nodularity and the fact that malignant ulcers project into the lumen of the stomach in profile on barium meal studies. CT scan will show the extent of the tumour and its protrusion into the gastric lumen. Biopsy for histology is required for accurate diagnosis. The haematemesis is from bleeding when the tumour erode or ulcerate into blood vessel.

Iatrogenic perforation injury

This results from instrumentation mostly endoscopy procedures, dilatation of stricture, bougie, disruption of suture line following surgical anastomosis, attempted intubation and malposition of nasogastric tubes. The upper cervical and upper thoracic oesophagus are involved in over 80% of cases. The injury is in the form of penetrating intraluminal erosion, laceration or tear of the oesophagus resulting in haematemesis. Plain chest x-ray may show intraluminal gas behind the heart. Subcutaneous emphysema dissecting up the neck, mediastinal emphysema and pneumothorax may be seen in chest radiography. Mediastinal abscess may develop without antibiotics therapy. Gastrografin or other iodine based contrast swallow procedures may show the site of perforation.

Barrett's oesophagus

This is columnar metaplasia of mucosal cells of distal oesophagus which are normally squamous. Ulceration of junction of normal and metaplastic mucosa, circumferential finger-like projections, fine reticular mucosal pattern resembling appearance of areae gastricae and stricture formation are variably demonstrated by barium swallow. Significant erosion of the oesophageal mucosa with involvement of highly vascularised tissues and bleeding leading to haematemesis.

Bezoar and phytobezoars

Bezoars and phytobezoars result from constant accumulation of ingested foreign matter in intestines, which due to their large size and indigestibility fails to exit stomach, or intestines causing gastric outlet obstruction, gastric hypomotility or intestinal obstruction. On plain abdominal radiograph, there may be an intraluminal mass with air-crevices of whorl-like appearance. Barium studies may show an intraluminal mass causing filling-defect, which shows change in position in different films. There are crevices within the mass that are filled with barium or rarely a coiled-spring appearance may be observed. Haematemesis may occur from ulceration, pressure necrosis of bowel mucosa or perforation. These may co-exist with signs of partial or complete intestinal obstruction.

Intussusception

There could be haematemesis in partial jejunogastric intussusception. However, most times, the presentation is asymptomatic. The intussusception tends to involve the efferent loop in 75% of the cases while the afferent loop is involved in about 25% of the cases of acute form of the obstruction. The presentations are signs of high intestinal obstruction, left hypochondriac mass and haematemesis. There is also the chronic intermittent form, which may be self-reducing, and in this, a coiled spring appearance of a gastric filling defect is seen in barium study. Another variety of the obstruction is the gastrojejunal or gastroduodenal mucosal prolapsed which is often asymptomatic but may also present with haematemesis if it causes partial obstruction.

Oesophageal squamous cell carcinomas

This comprises over 50% of oesophageal carcinomas. There is high prevalence in China, Middle East and South Africa due to diet. Other predisposing factors are achalasia cardia, chronic caustic stricture, coeliac disease, irradiation, asbestos exposure, Plummer-Vinson syndrome and *ptylosis palmaris et plantaris*. Short-segment narrowing with shouldering, mucosal destruction, dilatation of proximal segment and apple-core deformity are seen in classical cases in barium swallow.

Adenocarcinoma

About 40% of oesophageal carcinoma is adenocarcinoma occurring at oesophago-gastric junction. On barium swallow, studies will depict intraluminal filling-defect, which may show ulceration. Rigid, thickened, mucosal fold are seen in varicoid form resembling varices but the affected area shows loss of peristalsis unlike varices. CT malignant nodules are usually lager than 1 cm. MRI and CT detect tracheo-oesophageal invasion if trachea is displaced forward. It may produce achalasia-like lesion on barium swallow film. There is an increased risk in scleroderma and other lesions that cause Barrett's oesophagus.

Annular pancreas

This presents with haematemesis in about 10% of the cases. It occurs when abnormal migration of head and the uncinate process of the pancreas causes a ring of normal pancreatic tissue to encircle the duodenum. On plain abdominal radiograph in the neonates, there is double bubble sign signifying dilated stomach and proximal duodenum. The head of pancreas is seen enlarged in sonography. On barium study, there is peculiar narrowing of the second part of duodenum with reverse peristalsis and incompetent pyloric canal. CT scan will demonstrate the pancreatic tissue encircling the descending part of the duodenum. ERCP will show the pancreatic body and tail to have normally located main duct but a small duct originating on anteriorly and passing posteriorly around duodenum and communicating with main pancreatic duct.

Other malignant oesophageal tumours

Spindle-cell carcinoma presents as bulky polypoid mid oesophageal lesions
Leiomyosarcoma occurs in the lower two-third of oesophagus as a posterior mediastinal mass lesion. Strictures develop with classical carcinoma picture of narrowing; irregular mucosal pattern and apple-core deformity on barium swallow examination.
Malignant melanoma is a primary tumour appearing as a bulky, polypoid, intraluminal mass lesion on barium swallow studies.

Neuroendocrine carcinoma of the oesophagus occurs in the elderly males and presents with dysphagia and vomiting. It is often polypoid and ulcerated located mostly in the lower oesophagus and rarely in the middle oesophagus. Immuno-histochemistry shows at least one of the neurocrine antigens.

Neurofibroma

This presents with haematemesis, haematochezia or melaena. The symptoms include intestinal obstruction, nausea, vomiting and abdominal distension. The types of obstructions are intussusception and colonic volvulus. Those that cause haematemesis are located in the jejunum, stomach, duodenum or ileum. On barium meal there may be submucosal filling-defect in the stomach or duodenum. Mural thickening and narrowing may be seen in infiltrating type. Intraluminal multiple eccentric polypoid filling-defects is also noted. When rarely mesenteric fat are seen trapped within entangled network of tissue, the diagnosis is almost certain. Other findings on barium meal include multiple leiomyomas that may have associated ulcerations. Endoscopic biopsy for histology is the final arbiter of the nature of these polyps.

Foreign bodies

Foreign body erosion, impaction and perforation are common in children and results from objects such as coin, metallic button, safety pin, radiolucent plastic toy, cap of bottled drinks, and other metals around where the child plays such as knots and nails. If radiopaque, plain film of the cervical region and chest are adequate for the diagnosis. Endoscopic removal is the preferred treatment. Laceration, erosion and vascular injury are responsible for the haematemesis.

Oesophageal diverticulum

This is seen in the mid oesophagus at level of the carina. It is a traction type with wide neck. It is produced by traction from fibrosis or increased intraluminal pressure. As it widens it descends lateral to the oesophagus and exerts pressure effect with compression. Inflammatory changes may occur in it with ulceration, bleeding and haematemesis. Barium swallow demonstrates the diverticulum.

Oesophageal diverticulosis

These are multiple, flask-shaped oesophageal out-pouching on barium swallow filled with contrast. Abscess, fistulations, and perforation may occur. The oesophagus is thickened and long-length tapered stricture develops. Reflux oesophagitis, inflaming the over 300 glands in the oesophagus is the most common predisposing factor. Carcinoma rarely predisposes to it.

Oesophageal intramural pseudodiverticulosis (EIPD)

There is dilatation of the submucosal oesophageal glands in this disease condition. The exact cause unknown but dysphagia is the major presenting symptom. It is diagnosed radiologically by noting multiple small collections of barium or other positive contrast media in the out-pouched oesophageal glands in barium swallow studies. It is a rare disease but it is more common in adult than children.

Factitious haematemesis

This is a gastrointestinal manifestation of Munchausen's syndrome. Children predominate in the cases and there may be connivance of the mother. The haematemesis is pretended and the patient may undergo extensive and invasive investigations. The patient may secure the blood that he uses to colour the urine red through a self-inflicted external skin wound. The patient may undergo extensive invasive radiological investigations including the use of surgeries before the diagnosis is discovered.

Its early detection is vital in order to avoid unnecessary, invasive and expensive investigations some of which may result in iatrogenic complications.

Modalities to stop the bleeding
1. Bleeding may stop spontaneously without any treatment.
2. Check and correct any clotting disorders
3. Intravenous ranitidine injection in small bleeding.
4. Balloon tamponade in endoscopy
5. Selective infusion of vasopressin via intraluminal arterial catheter at angiography
6. Selective arterial embolisation using embolic materials like gelfoams.
7. Transjugular intrahepatic percutaneous porto-systemic shunt, (TIPS)
8. Surgery. Operation aimed at stopping the bleeding, if the artery is identified it can be ligated. However, gastrectomy may be undertaken in difficult-to-treat cases that are life-threatening.

(Adam & Dixon, 2008; Dahnert, 2011; Sutton, 1998 and 2003, Palmer & Reeder 2001).

References
1. Gralnek IM, Barkun AN, Bardou M. Management of acute bleeding from a peptic ulcer. N Engl J Med 2008; 359:928-37.
2. Cheung FK, Lau JY. Management of massive peptic ulcer bleeding. Gastroenterol Clin North Am 2009;38:231-43.
3. Mylona S, Ntai S, Pomoni M, Kokkinaki A, Lepida N, Thanos L. Aorto-enteric fistula: CT findings. Abdom Imaging 2007;32:393-7.
4. Caldwell SH, Hespenheide EE, Greenwald BD, Northup PG, Patrie JT. Enbucrilate for gastric varices: extended experience in 92 patients. Aliment Pharmacol Ther 2007 ;26:49-59.
5. Ohanaka CE, Ofoegbu RO. The pattern of surgical cancers in Nigeria: the Benin experience. Trop Doct 2002;32:38-9.
6. Vu QD, Menias CO, Bhalla S, Peterson C, Wang LL, Balfe DM. Aortoenteric fistulas: CT features and potential mimics. Radiographics 2009; 29:197-209.
7. Elusoji SO, Tabowei BI. Fatal haematemesis due to impacted foreign body in the oesophagus. J Pak Med Assoc 1993;43:39-40.
8. Olokoba AB, Olokoba LB, Jimoh AA. Upper gastrointestinal tract bleeding in Ilorin, Nigeria--a report of 30 cases. Niger J Clin Pract 2009;12:240-4.

3.2 RADIOLOGY OF DYSPHAGIA

Definition
Dysphagia can be defined as difficulty in swallowing. Often times there is associated pain during swallowing (odynophagia).

Causes/Differential diagnosis
Lesions within the mouth
Stomatitis, glossitis, tonsillitis and lymphoma of Tonsil.

Lesions within the pharynx
Retropharyngeal abscess, pharyngitis, pharyngeal adenoma, pharyngeal lymphoma, adenoid hyperplasia, Eagle's syndrome, tuberculous lymphadenopathy and, laryngeal/pharyngeal carcinoma.

Lesions of the oesophagus
Extrinsic compressive lesion of the oesophagus
Osteophyte (from cervical vertebrae), enlarged cricopharyngeal muscle (*cricopharyngeal achalasia*), goitre, large parathyroid tumour, right-sided aortic arch and descending aorta, enlarged left atrium, enlarged left ventricle, aberrant right subclavian artery, coarctation of aorta, unfolded atheromatous descending aorta, aneurysm of descending aorta, pericardial effusion, mediastinal lymphadenopathy, mediastinal tumours, bronchogenic carcinoma and metastasis

Lymphoma/oesophageal lymphoma
Intrinsic lesion of oesophagus
Achalasia, oesophageal web, Zenker's diverticulum, caustic oesophageal stricture, caustic acid stricture, drug-induced stricture, benign stricture, radiation stricture, peptic stricture, reflux oesophagitis /stricture, long indwelling nasogastric tube causing stricture, Zollinger-Ellison syndrome (lower oesophageal reflux stricture), Barrett's oesophagus, oesophageal diverticulum, oesophageal diverticulosis, Chagas disease (Trypanosomiasis) and oesophageal rings

Malignant stricture of oesophagus
Squamous cell carcinomas, adenocarcinoma, spindle-cell carcinoma, leiomyosarcoma and malignant melanoma

Oesophagitis
Candidiasis/monoliasis, tuberculosis, cytomegalovirus (AIDS, giant ulcers), Herpes simplex infection, drug-induced, caustic erosion, radiation-induced, peptic disease and HIV/AIDS and immunocompromised

Foreign body
Coin (Metallic money), drink covers (coca cola, beer and other soft drink covers), dentures (artificial dentures), drugs (big-sized tablets swallowed at bed time may be impacted especially potassium chloride and quinidine), meat/fish bones, meat/fish/food bolus, screws and knots used in mechanical appliances and seeds (beans, corn).

Systemic lesion
Scleroderma, dematomyositis and presbyoesophagus

Central nervous system lesions
Myasthenia gravis, bulbar / pseudobulbar palsy, neuritis such as diphtheria (upper one-third affected), Parkinson's disease (upper third of oesophagus affected), diabetic autonomic neuropathy, ischaemic stroke, brain stem infarction, truncal bilateral vagotomy, poliomyelitis and syringomyelia.

Psychiatric lesion
Globus hystericus

Iatrogenic lesions
Perforation of oesophagus during endoscopy, perforation of oesophagus by surgical clips, metallic stents in aortic/bronchial surgery, fracture/knotting of endoscopic tips, catheters, balloons and dilators with dislodgement and injury to oesophagus.

Causes of dysphagia in the neonate
Congenital lesions:
Choanal atresia (choanography is diagnostic), cleft palate, macroglossia, glossoptosis, oesophageal atresia, vascular rings, congenital heart disease, aberrant right subclavian artery, right-sided aortic arch, aberrant left pulmonary artery (rare) and neuromuscular defects.

Delayed neuromuscular maturity due to:
Prematurity, mental subnormality, delayed development/developmental milestones and muscles dystrophy.

Discussion

Lesions within the Mouth
Stomatitis and Glossitis: These two are diagnosed clinically.
Tonsilitis: Lateral view of the nasopharynx may show tonsilar enlargement. This appears as a soft tissue mass with lobulated margin in the area of the tonsil. It can also appear as widening of the prevertebral soft tissue.
Lymphoma of tonsil: This is often larger than the enlargement of inflamed tonsil.

Lesions within the Pharynx
Pharyngitis
This is often caused by moniliasis or other infections that can occur post-surgery. The diagnosis is clinical by pharyngoscopy.

Pharyngeal adenoma and Pharyngeal lymphoma/sarcoma
These can present as intrinsic filling-defect within the pharyngeal lumen in pharyngography. CT and MRI will clearly demonstrate the well demarcation of the masses as well as their intraluminal location. Histology is necessary for definitive diagnosis.

Adenoid hyperplasia

Lobulated, enlarged soft tissue mass in the area of adenoid is shown on lateral radiograph of nasopharynx or pharyngography.

Retropharyngeal abscess

It appears as an enlarged retropharyngeal soft tissue with gas and mottled opacities found within the soft tissue. Osteomyelitis of adjacent cervical vertebrae or foreign body like fish bone may be identified within the soft tissue.

Eagle's syndrome (ES)

The syndrome occurs when an elongated or hypertrophied styloid process or calcified stylohyoid ligament causes recurrent throat pain, neck pain or foreign body sensation, dysphagia, or facial pain. These symptoms arise from compression of neurovascular structures by the hypertrophied styloid process. The neck or throat pain could radiate to the ipsilateral ear. It is diagnosed by physical examination and confirmed radiologically. The causes of the styloid process elongation or hypertrophy include congenital anatomical variation, aging and trauma. The treatment is surgical by shortening of the styloid process or removal of the impinging part of the calcified stylohyoid ligament through an intraoral or external approach.

Tuberculous lymphadenopathy

This appears as extrinsic compressive lesion on a barium-filled oesophagus. It may resemble carcinoma in appearance if a caseous necrotic lesion ulcerates from outside to the lumen of the pharynx.

Laryngeal/pharyngeal carcinoma

It presents as a compressive mass lesion with invasion, infiltration and destruction of adjacent structures and bones. Compression may necessitate tracheostomy and gastrectomy for breathing and for feeding of the patient.

Extrinsic Compressive Lesion of the Oesophagus
Osteophytes

These are from the cervical vertebrae. They produce impressions on the posterior aspect of barium–filled oesophagus on lateral view. These impressions are often multiple and serrated or undulated. The causes are osteoarthritis, rheumatoid arthritis and ankylosing spondylitis.

Enlarged cricopharyngeal muscle
Cricopharyngeal achalasia

This is caused by failure of the cricopharyngeus to relax. A smooth oblique or transverse impression on the posterior aspect of barium-filled oesophagus is seen on lateral view of barium swallow film. This is the third most common cause of dysphagia in some studies. *Vigorous contraction* to propagate primary and secondary peristaltic waves beyond this part may lead to appearance of *vigorous achalasia*, which is development of non-propulsive tertiary contraction waves seen on barium swallow films.

Goitre

Enlarged thyroid gland especially retrosternal goitre may be gross but unnoticed. This may displace the upper oesophagus and trachea to one side. It also produces smooth narrowing of the oesophagus causing dysphagia.

Large parathyroid tumour
Parathyroid tumours, often carcinomas, large enough to indent the oesophagus do so on the lateral side and cause impressions or irregular indentations (demonstrable on barium filled oesophagus) with dysphagia.

Right-sided aortic arch and descending aorta
A right-sided aortic arch can cause dysphagia and is noted in barium swallow study. The left aortic arch impression is absent on barium swallow study.

Forestier disease
In this condition, there is ossification of the anterior spinal longitudinal ligament (ALL) in at least three adjacent vertebrae, and diffuse spinal enthesopathy. It is a systemic disorder and the patient presents with dysphagia, respiratory distress and hoarseness of voice. Plain film and CT scan are usually adequate for the imaging diagnosis. Excision of the osteophyte or bony exostosis is the surgical treatment.

Enlarged left Atrium
This produces anterior impression on barium-filled lower oesophagus. There is posterior displacement of oesophagus and to the right. This is best seen in lateral view. There is obstruction to passage of food bolus and tablets (potassium chloride) (ulceration and stricture may develop if tablets or food bolus are trapped for long time). This is seen in cardiac failure, mitral valvular disease (aneurysm and regurgitation) and left atrial myxoma.

Enlarged left ventricle
There is an anterior larger impression on the oesophagus and at a level lower than the impression of left atrium. The oesophagus is displaced posteriorly and to the right. Cardiac failure and left ventricular aneurysm are the usual causes. Dilated cardiomyopathy also contributes to the causes.

Aberrant right subclavian artery
Arises from aortic arch distal to the origin of left subclavian artery. Passes upwards and to the right behind the oesophagus. Shows smooth oblique indentation on posterior wall of barium-filled oesophagus.

Coarctation of aorta
A reversed-3 impression is seen on left side of oesophagus on barium swallow study. This is caused by pre-stenotic and post-stenotic dilated descending aorta causing extrinsic impression on the barium-filled oesophagus.

Unfolded atheromatous descending aorta
This has a tortuous course. It displaces lower third of oesophagus anteriorly to one side. Transmitted pulsation of oesophagus is seen on fluoroscopy. Distal oesophageal narrowing by extrinsic impression on erect and supine position is relieved by turning the patient prone in barium swallow examination.

Aneurysm of descending aorta
Localised dilatation of descending aorta will cause localised displacement which may be marked. It is seen in hypertension, syphilis, trauma, diabetes mellitus (inflammatory aneurysm), Marfan's syndrome, Ehlers–Danlos syndrome, previous aortic injury (degenerative atherosclerosis) and Takayasu disease. Aortic aneurysm is the most common cause of mediastinal mass of vascular origin and 10% of mediastinal masses are of vascular origin.

Pericardial effusion

This causes cardiomegaly with water bottle or palm wine keg configuration and pencilled-out cardiac margins with oligaemic lung fields on plain chest x-ray. Echocardiography will show the pericardial fluid as anechoic area encircling the heart. Myocardial infarction, uraemia, tuberculosis, metastasis, purulent infection, cardiac failure, hypoproteinaemia are some of the causes.

Mediastinal lymphadenopathy

Middle third of the oesophagus is affected. It occurs mostly from primary malignant lesions, infections (tuberculosis) and metastases. Lymphoma involves the sub-carinal lymph nodes. Metastases are usually from carcinoma of bronchus or breast. Extrinsic compressive lesion is seen at early stages. Invasion of the oesophagus may occur if tumour encircles the oesophagus or ulcerates. Chest x-ray will show hilar enlargement and CT scan will confirm the masses.

Mediastinal tumours

Middle and posterior mediastinal masses indent the oesophagus. Most of the lesions frequently encountered include abscesses, haematomas, and mediastinal cysts (bronchogenic cyst). CT scan will confirm the nature of the mass seen on plain chest x-ray.

Bronchogenic carcinoma

This causes direct invasion of the oesophagus with typical shouldering, mucosal destruction and apple core deformity of oesophagus as seen in primary carcinoma of oesophagus. Collapse, mediastinal shift and lung fibrosis associated with bronchogenic carcinoma can also cause dysphagia.

Metastasis

This is rare. However, the primary lesions are most frequently from breast and bronchus. Established cases may come to resemble changes of primary carcinoma. Appearances seen on barium meal may be difficult to exclude from achalasia. Pancreatic metastasis from tail of pancreas to the oesophagus produces achalasia-like lesions. Muscle coat is infiltrated by carcinoma together with mucosa and muscularis propria whereas in achalasia cardia, infiltration is limited to mucosa and muscularis propria. Metastases from malignant melanoma produce broad-based submucous nodule and polypoid lesion with stricture, which may simulate benign or malignant lesion.

Lymphoma

This is rare. It is usually the Hodgkin's type. It appears as diffuse nodularity throughout the length of the oesophagus. It resembles carcinoma but the long length of affectation is in favour of lymphoma. Lymphomas may simulate achalasia cardia by infiltration of the submucosa of distal oesophagus. Invasion and compression of mid-oesophagus may occur with lymphomatous mediastinal nodes.

Intrinsic Lesion of Oesophagus
Achalasia

Achalasia cardia is narrowing of oesophagus usually the distal third, caused by degeneration of neuronal fibres of Auerbach's plexus with failure of propagation of primary and secondary peristaltic waves beyond the point of narrowing. Proximal oesophagus dilates with stasis of food and fluid, air–oesophagogram, right vertical paravertebral mass with air- fluid levels are seen. Scanty or absent gastric air bubble is seen. Distal third of oesophagus has rat-tail narrowing on barium studies (figure 3.21). Fibrotic changes in the lung due to repeated aspiration pneumonia may be seen in chest radiograph.

Oesophageal web

Constriction of oesophagus by 1 – 2 mm thick mucosal infolding. Oesophagus balloons proximal to the web. Seen in association with epidermolysis bullosa, bullous pemphigoid, reflux oesophagitis, Plummer–Vinson's syndrome and aging. Passage of endoscope often destroys a web. Rarely balloon dilatation may be necessary.

Zenker's diverticulum

Pulsion diverticulum of posterior pharyngeal pouch. This develops at the site of Killian's dehiscence. This is a site of weakness of posterior pharyngeal wall between oblique and horizontal fibres of inferior constrictor muscles.

Diverticulum displaces the oesophagus forward and causes dysphagia. A posterior diverticulum is noted in upper third of oesophagus in lateral view of barium swallow study.

Caustic oesophageal stricture

There is narrowing of the oesophagus with fibrosis. The early stage shows mucosal sloughing, coagulative necrosis, ulceration, fistulation and rarely perforation. The causative agents are household materials often used daily at home. Children and adult may drink it accidentally. Attempted suicide may be the cause of the swallow. The implicated caustic alkali includes sodium bicarbonate (caustic soda), lye (sodium hydroxide), iodine and bleaches (sodium hypochlorite). Long length narrowing with preserved mucosal pattern is seen.

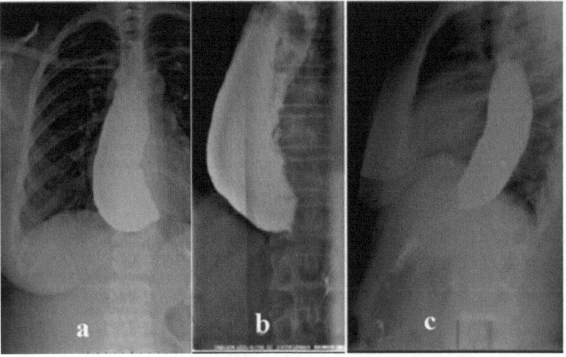

Figure 3.21: Radiographs of images of barium swallow study of a patient with dysphagia due to achalasia, AP view (a), oblique (b) and lateral (c) views. Note the grossly dilated oesophagus with severe rat-tail narrowing at the distal third and scanty bowel gas in the stomach.

Caustic acid Stricture

Similar to alkali ingestion. However, it causes less severe damage. There is also long length stricture with preserved mucosal pattern. Hydrochloric acid (HCl) and sulphuric acid (H_2SO_4) are commonly ingested. This is common among battery chargers and their families.

Drug-induced stricture

Several drugs can cause oesophageal erosion, ulcer, inflammation and in late stages benign stricture. These drugs may be trapped in areas of constrictions of the oesophagus or may be refluxed back to the oesophagus even in dissolved state. The implicated drugs are aspirin, indomethacin, quinidine, tetracycline, doxycycline, butazolydone etc. There may be mucosal irregularities due to oesophagitis or long-length narrowing due to benign stricture.

Radiation stricture

This can cause oesophageal inflammation, erosion, ulceration and stricture. Usually 3000 – 4500 Rad is required. Stricture develops 6-8 months after irradiation. Often diseases of adjacent organs like bronchogenic and breast carcinomas are what actually the irradiations were for. Obliterative endoarteritis, oesophagitis and strictures develop. Similar changes are seen with the use of adriamycin and actinomycin D, or these may potentiate the effect of irradiation.

Peptic stricture

Oesophageal stricture may develop from peptic ulcer disease. This is most likely if the ulcer is above a co-existing hiatus hernia. Short-segment strictures with tapered margins and smooth lumen are seen. The proximal part may be dilated giving a rat-tail appearance. The mucosal pattern is preserved so it is essentially a benign stricture.

Reflux oesophagitis/stricture

Rat-tail appearance of lower oesophageal stricture from reflux of acid and peptic content is observed. There is often co-existing hiatus hernia. Reflux often occurs if the lower oesophageal pressure is less than 15 mmHg. Occasionally it can occur intermittently with normal lower oesophageal pressure. The reflux oesophagitis appearance on endoscopy is oedema of mucosa, loss of vessel pattern and blurring of squamo-columnar junction. Mucosal nodularity appears in double contrast barium swallow. Thickened mucosal fold of >3 mm seen on film of collapsed oesophagus is seen.

Felinization of oesophagus is seen as transverse ridges of contracted muscularis mucosa (as seen in cat oesophagus). Appearances similar to varices, ulcers and out-pouching may progressively occur. In many studies, oesophageal reflux is the commonest cause of dysphagia.

Long in-dwelling nasogastric tube causing stricture

This predisposes to oesophageal reflux of gastric peptic content. Three days of catheter has caused severe stricture in some patients. Severe long length stricture with preserved mucosal pattern appearance in the barium swallow is seen in late stages.

Zollinger-Ellison syndrome (stricture)

Gastric contents with very low pH seen in this condition often reflux to the lower oesophagus and damage the mucosa. Long-length benign stricture or rat-tail appearance of lower oesophagus is seen in barium swallow.

Barrett's oesophagus

This is columnar metaplasia of mucosal cells of distal oesophagus which are normally squamous. Ulceration of junction of normal/metaplastic mucosa, circumferential finger-like projections, fine reticular mucosal pattern resembling appearance of areae gastriae and stricture formation may occur and are demonstrated by barium swallow.

Oesophageal diverticulum

This is observed in the mid oesophagus at the level of the carina. It is a traction type with wide neck. It is produced by traction from fibrosis or increased intraluminal pressure. As it widens it descends lateral to the oesophagus and exerts pressure effect with compression. Inflammatory changes may occur in it with ulceration, bleeding may occur. Barium swallow demonstrates this.

Oesophageal diverticulosis

These are multiple, flask-shaped oesophageal out-pouching on barium swallow filled with contrast. Abscess, fistulations, and perforation may occur. The oesophagus is thickened and long-length tapered stricture develops. Reflux oesophagitis, inflaming the over 300 glands in the oesophagus is the most common predisposing factor. Carcinoma rarely predisposes to it.

Oesophageal intramural pseudodiverticulosis (EIPD)

This is a disease condition in which there is dilatation of the submucosal oesophageal glands. The exact cause is unknown but dysphagia is the major presenting symptom. It is diagnosed radiologically by noting multiple small collections of barium or other positive contrast media in the out-pouched oesophageal glands in barium swallow studies. It is a rare disease but more common in adult than in children.

Chagas disease (Trypanosomiasis)

This causes secondary degeneration of neuronal fibres of myenteric (Auerbach's) plexus. The strictures and pathology seen are as in achalasia.

Ventricular aneurysm and ventricular dilatation are also seen on plain film and echocardiography and are due to myocarditis. Megacolon is seen on barium enema. *Trypanosoma cruzi* transmitted by the *reduvid* bug is the causative organism. The disease is endemic in Central and South America. The bug lives in thatched roof of houses and cracks in walls of buildings.

Oesophageal rings

Schatzki's ring located at lower oesophagus causes annular narrowing of the lower oesophagus. This produces obstruction and dysphagia when the lumen is narrowed to less than 13 mm in diameter. If not significantly narrowed however, it may be asymptomatic. Inflammation and fibrosis contribute to narrow it to the critical level for symptoms to develop. It is associated with hiatus hernia. Distended oesophagus is necessary for proper demonstration in barium swallow examination.

Malignant Oesophageal Stricture

Squamous cell carcinomas

This comprises 60% of oesophageal carcinomas. Alcohol and smoking are synergistic risk factors. There is high prevalence in China, Middle East and South Africa due to diet. Other predisposing factors are achalasia cardia (which leads to chronic mucosal irritation), chronic caustic stricture, coeliac disease, irradiation, asbestos exposure, Plummer-Vinson syndrome and *ptylosis palmaris et plantaris*. Short-segment narrowing with shouldering, mucosal destruction, dilatation of proximal segment and apple-core deformity are seen in classical cases in barium swallow.

Adenocarcinoma
About 40% of oesophageal carcinoma is adenocarcinoma. It occurs at oesophago-gastric junction. Nodules larger than 1cm on CT are malignant. MRI and CT detect tracheo-oesophageal invasion if trachea is displaced forward. It may produce achalasia-like lesion on barium swallow film. There is an increased risk in scleroderma and other lesions that cause Barrett's oesophagus.

Spindle-cell carcinoma
It presents as bulky polypoid mid oesophageal lesions. It is seen in the elderly with history of smoking and alcohol consumption

Leiomyosarcoma
It occurs in the lower two-third of oesophagus as a posterior mediastinal mass lesion. Strictures develop with classical carcinoma picture of narrowing, irregular mucosal pattern and apple-core deformity on barium swallow examination.

Malignant melanoma
It is a primary tumour. It appears as a bulky, polypoid, intraluminal mass lesion.

Neuroendocrine carcinoma of the oesophagus
It occurs in the elderly males and presents with dysphagia and vomiting. The tumour is often polypoid and ulcerated when seen with endoscope and the location is mostly lower oesophagus but may be seen in the middle oesophagus. Three cell types has been described including small cell carcinoma, adenocarcinoma and squamous cell carcinoma and immunohistochemically each one shows at least one of the neurocrine antigens.

Oesophagitis-Causing Conditions
Candidiasis
It is seen in immunocompromised patients, achalasia due to stasis of food. There is mucosal plaques on barium study. Erythema seen in endoscopy and plaques give the long mucosal folds nodular appearance similar to varices. Upper third of oesophagus is usually involved unlike varices that affect distal third.

Tuberculosis
It may present as deep ulcers, fistulas, scarring and strictures. Caseating tuberculous nodes compressing and eroding into the oesophagus is the cause.

Cytomegalovirus (AIDS, giant ulcers)
It appears as granular mucosal pattern with diffuse involvement. Marginal ulceration can occur. Perforation, fistulation and long-segment stricture are rare complications.

Herpes
It occurs in the immunocompromised and present as mid-oesophageal ulceration.

Drug-induced oesophagitis
The usual drugs that causes this are potassium chloride, quinidine, doxycycline, tetracycline, aspirin, ferrous sulphate, indomethacin, phenylbutazone, ascorbic acid, clindamycin, etc.

Caustic erosion
It is observed as ulceration, mucosal sloughing and healing by fibrosis. There is a history of ingestion of caustic soda solution.

Radiation-induced oesophagitis
There is mucosal irregularity with ulceration and aperistalsis of the oesophagus is observed after 6 months. History of recent radiation therapy for lesion of the chest or head and neck is usually obtained. In many studies, radiation-induced dysphasia is the second most common cause of dysphagia.

Peptic disease
This is reflux of high acid gastric contents into the oesophagus due to lax lower oesophageal sphincter, hiatus hernia, and is caused by long-indwelling nasogastric tube, etc.

HIV/AIDS and immunocompromised state
HIV virus may produce oesophageal ulcer on itself. AIDS and immunocompromised status lead to multiple opportunistic infections including candidiasis, Herpes simplex, cytomegalovirus infection, tuberculosis and actinomycosis. Mild to severe oesophagitis with ulceration, perforation, fistulation and stricture formation may be produced by these opportunistic infections.

Eosinophilic oesophagitis (EO)
This is a chronic condition in which there is immune reaction most likely directed to foods but in some occasions also to aeroallergens or inhaled irritants. There is immune or antigen-mediated oesophageal disease resulting in dysphagia due to stricture. Eosinophil-predominant oesophageal inflammation results with fifteen or more eosinophils per high-powered field of blood/tissue film, now generally accepted as a basic cut-off level of infiltration. This, together with other clinical data such as oesophageal pH and impedance studies, can help discriminate this condition from other possible causes of such symptoms such as gastro-oesophageal reflux disease. Removal of the type of food that the patient is reacting to is an essential part of the treatment.

Foreign Body/Swallowed Impacted Substances
Foreign body
Plain radiograph may show radio-opaque foreign body in the oesophagus.
Radiolucent lesion may be shown by endoscopy which may also be used to remove the foreign body if it can enter the endoscope. Materials often swallowed include:
1. Coin (Metallic money).
2. Bottled drink covers (coca cola, beer and other soft drink covers).
3. Dentures (artificial dentures).
4. Drugs (Big or large-tablet drugs swallowed at bed time may be impacted in the oesophagus). The drug most commonly involved are potassium chloride (slow-K) and quinidine.
5. Meat or fish bones.
6. Meat, fish or food bolus.

7. Screws and knots used in mechanical appliances.
8. Seeds, beans, corn.

Systemic Lesion
Scleroderma
This occurs in the lower two-thirds of the oesophagus. It causes *Barrett's oesophagus* and *air oesophagogram*. Small bowel hypomotility with delayed transit, bowel dilatation and coiled spring small bowel is shown in barium follow-through.
Aperistalsis of distal two-third of the oesophagus on fluoroscopy is shown. Dilated featureless, distal two-third of oesophagus is also shown in barium swallow. Degeneration of muscularis mucosa causes air to enter the bowel wall causing *pneumatosis cystoides intestinalis.* Wide-necked pseudosacculations in small and large bowels are seen. Basal pulmonary fibrosis due to aspiration pneumonia occurs. Nephrocalcinosis, hypertension and renal failure due to vasculitis develop. CREST syndrome may occur.

Dermatomyositis
This disease affects the lower two-thirds of the oesophagus and there are associated skin lesions. Polymyositis, amyopathic dermatomyositis and inclusion body myositis also causes dysphagia. Biopsy for histology will be required to differentiate the heterogenous group of conditions classified as inflammatory myositis.

Oesophageal lichen planus
This is a rare inflammatory mucocutaneous disease affecting the skin and and mucous membranes, including oral and genital mucosa. Oesophageal mucosa is rarely involved and this causes significant dysphagia and oesophageal strictures and stenosis. Oesophageal lichen planus presents with a spectrum ranging from lichenoid tissue reactions of skin, mucous membrane or other body tissues to systemic manifestations. Dysphagia may lead to significant weight-loss, malnutrition syndrome and chronic respiratory distress resulting from recurrent aspiration pneumonia. Co-existence of muco-cutaneous lesions and characteristic endoscopic and histological findings are essential in accurate diagnosis of this rather under-reported condition. Treatment includes the use of systemic cyclosporine A, vitamins and nutrition supplements. It is more common in adult females.
Others are *presbyoesophagus, oesophageal Crohn's disease* and *ulcerative colitis.*

Central Nervous System Lesions
Myasthenia gravis
It affects the upper one-third (upper 4 cm of oesophagus), and presents with paralysis of oesophagus and phrenic nerve with lack of diaphragmatic movement on the affected side. Mediastinal mass is identified with CT or MR imaging in most cases.

Wallenberg's Syndrome
In this condition, dysphagia occurs after lateral medullary infarction (LMI). The dysphagia in Wallenberg's syndrome is dynamically characterized by a failure in initiating or triggering of the pharyngeal phase of swallowing movements, reduced movement output, and lack of coordination of swallowing motion. Thus, there is swallowing pattern abnormality. The diagnosis is based on the absence of upper oesophageal sphincter (UES) opening of the unaffected side of the medullae with failure of bolus passage through the intact side of the upper oesophageal sphincter UES, occurring

at least once during the videofluorographic evaluation of each individual. The treatment includes rehabilitation through respiratory treatment, food adaptation, postural changes, and oral care. In severe cases, botulinum toxin injection or surgery to prevent aspiration and adequate nutrition are essential part of the management.

Brain stem infarction

There is impaired relaxation of lower oesophagus similar to achalasia due to destruction of dorsal nucleus of vagus nerve.

Syringomyelia

This is cystic- or fluid-degenerative appearance within the spinal cord with wasting of muscles supplied by nerves originating from the affected area. If the syringomyelia is from the cervical region, upper limb and upper third of oesophagus are affected by paralysis. Dysphagia may then occur.

Parkinson's disease

There is degeneration of the nuclei in the brain stem that controls deglutition. The upper third of the oesophagus is affected. Sialorrhea caused by retention of saliva may be an initial presentation and is indicative of subclinical dysphagia. Frank dysphagia may occur and is caused by muscle rigidity. Barium swallow will show signs of brain induced swallowing difficulty. History and physical examination of the patient will be very beneficial.

Rabies

The patient has a history of exposure to wild animal or a dog bite. Vomiting, paresthesias of upper limbs, fever, seizures, dysphagia and autonomic dysfunction are some of the complaints. Rarely this disease can be transmitted through solid organ donation in a patient with long incubation period for rabies.

Diabetic autonomic neuropathy

A variable length of the oesophagus is involved.

Poliomyelitis: There is paralysis of proximal third of oesophagus contributed by striated muscles.

Truncal bilateral vagotomy: There is impaired relaxation of lower oesophagus similar to achalasia.

Bulbar/Pseudobulbar palsy/amyotrophic lateral sclerosis: Upper one-third of oesophagus affected.

Neuritis (Diphtheria): Upper one-third affected

Tumour of the vagus nerve (schwannoma).

Myotonic dystrophy

Distal oesophageal spasm

Psychiatric Conditions
Globus hystericus

This is an anxiety condition in which there is a false feeling and complaint of lump in the throat and that this is causing restriction of swallowing. It occurs in generalized anxiety disorder, panic disorder, agoraphobia and obsessive compulsive disorder. Most importantly, the people are usually physically normal without any abnormality detected radiologically or using other methods. As the anxiety disorder improves, this complaint may reduce or disappear.

Iatrogenic Lesions
Perforation of the oesophagus
Perforation of oesophagus during endoscopy with the development of oedema, swelling, inflammation, tenderness and dysphagia.

Perforation of oesophagus by surgical clips, metallic stents in aortic/bronchial surgery.

Fracture of tips or knotted tips of endoscopic tips, catheters, balloons, dilators with dislodgement and injury to oesophagus.

Causes of Dysphagia in the Neonate
Congenital conditions
These include choanal atresia (choanography is diagnostic), cleft palate, macroglossia, glossoptosis and oesophageal atresia (barium swallow with water-soluble contrast medium is diagnostic) and oesophageal webs.

Vascular rings
These include aberrant right subclavian artery, right-sided aortic arch, double aortic arch and aberrant left pulmonary artery (rare).

Neuromuscular defects
This includes delayed neuromuscular maturity due to prematurity, Down's syndrome, mental subnormality, gastroesophageal reflux diseases and delayed development or developmental milestones.

Congenital heart diseases
Infants with complex congenital heart malformations show signs and symptoms of dysphagia and even after open heart surgeries they keep on showing signs of dysphagia and may have aspiration pneumonitis. Videofluoroscopic studies is required for accurate diagnosis of exact causes of the dysphagia.

(Adam & Dixon, 2008; Dahnert, 2011; Sutton, 1998 and 2003, Swischuk, 2004; Palmer & Reeder 2001).

References
1. Umerah BC, Mukherjee BK, Ibekwe O. Cervical spondylosis and dysphagia. J Laryngol Otol 1981;95:1179-83.
2. Canon CL, Morgan DE, Einstein DM, Herts BR, Hawn MT, Johnson LF. Surgical approach to gastroesophageal reflux disease: what the radiologist needs to know. Radiographics. 2005;25:1485-99.
3. Odita JC, Omene JA, Okolo AA. Gastro-oesophageal reflux in Nigerian newborn infants. Trop Geogr Med 1984;36:169-73.
4. Ofoegbu RO. Incidence, pattern, and African variations of common benign disorders of the esophagus. Experience from Nigeria. Am J Surg 1982;144:273-6,
5. Okoye IJ, Imo AO, Okwulehie V. Radiologic management of impacted coin in the oesophagus--a case report. Niger J Clin Pract 2005;8:56-9.
6. Eze KC, Awosanya GOG. Retropharyngeal abscess sequel to swallowed meat bone. West African Journal of Radiology 2006; 13:18-21.

7. Luedtke P, Levine MS, Rubesin SE, Weinstein DS, Laufer I. Radiologic diagnosis of benign esophageal strictures: a pattern approach. Radiographics 2003; 23:897-909.

8. Bello IS, Arogundade FA, Sanusi AA, Adesunkanmi AR, Ndububa DA. Gastro-oesophageal reflux disease: a review of clinical features, investigations and recent trends in management. Niger J Med 2004;13(3):220-6.

9. Adegboye VO, Brimmo AI, Adebo OA, Ogunseyinde OO, Obajimi MO. The place of clinical features and standard chest radiography in evaluation of mediastinal masses. West Afr J Med 2003;22(2):156-60.

10. Ofoegbu RO. Benign peptic strictures of the oesophagus in the absence of hiatus hernia. Experiences from Nigeria. J R Coll Surg Edinb 1984;29(1):18-21.

3.3 RADIOLOGY OF PORTAL HYPERTENSION

Definition
Portal hypertension is said to occur when the portal venous pressure rises above 12 mmHg despite formation of portal collateral channels or vessels. Normal portal venous pressure is 10 mmHg or less. In pre-sinusoidal portal hypertension, the portal venous pressure may be normal.

Pathophysiology
Increased intrahepatic resistance with inadequate collateral channel formation (collateral vessels are present but unable to fully compensate for the degree of resistance). In this condition, the portal flow becomes slow, stagnant or even reversed.

Decreased hepatic perfusion from any cause can lead to increased splanchnic vasodilatation and increased cardiac output to conserve the hepatic function. Portal venous flow is greatly increased above 15 ml/kg/min. This exceeds the normal hepatic blood flow of 500 – 900 ml/minute of which two-thirds is contributed by portal blood flow.

Cause of Portal Hypertension

Increased Portal Resistance
Prehepatic increased portal resistance
1. *Portal vein thrombosis*
   Portal phlebitis, oral contraceptive, pancreatitis, neoplastic invasion, neonatal omphalitis/umbilical sepsis (from EBT) and coagulopathy (clotting disorder, bleeding diathesis, polycythaemia)
2. *Portal vein compression*
   Lymphadenopathy, pancreatic pseudocyst, trauma/haematoma, portal phlebosclerosis and tumour (carcinoma, lymphoma, metastasis)
3. *Splenomegaly*
   Hypersplenism and tropical splenomegaly syndrome

Intrahepatic obstruction (of portal venules)
a. *Presinusoidal (hepatic function relatively unimpaired)*
   Schistosomiasis, chronic malaria, idiopathic non-cirrhotic fibrosis, primary biliary cirrhosis, reticuloendotheliosis/lymphoma (Hodgkin's), myelofibrosis / myeloproliferative disorder/ leukaemia, alpha-1-antitrypsin deficiency, toxic fibrosis (copper, arsenic, polyvinyl chloride), Felty's syndrome, sarcoidosis of liver, Wilsons disease, and cystic fibrosis
b. *Sinusoidal*
   Sickle cell disease and Hepatitis
c. *Post Sinusoidal*
   Cirrhosis (commonest cause) and veno-occlusive disease of the liver (Jamaican bush tea).

Post-hepatic increased portal resistance
Budd–Chiari syndrome (hepatic vein obstruction), constrictive pericarditis, cardiac failure (tricuspid incompetence) and inferior vena caval obstruction.

Dynamic Portal Hypertension
i.   Congenital arterio-venous fistula
ii. Traumatic arterio-portal fistula
iii. Neoplastic arterio-portal fistula

Radiological Investigative Modalities
1. Plain films
    Chest, PA, lateral; Abdomen, skull, extremities
2. Conventional tomography
3. Ultrasound scan (3.5 MHz, 7.5 MHz transducers)
    Transabdominal, transrectal, endoscopic
4. Colour Doppler ultrasonography/Duplex Doppler Scanning
5. Intra-arterial Doppler scan through 5 F catheter into superior mesenteric artery.
6. Echocardiography
7. Endoscopy
8. Barium studies (barium swallow, barium meal, and enema)
9. Computed Tomography/Helical CT
10. Magnetic Resonance Imaging, MR Angiography
11. Angiography (Arteriorgraphy and venography)
    i.   Percutaneous splenic puncture
    ii.   Operative mesenteric phlebography
    iii. Arterio-portography
    iv.   Transhepatic portal phlebography
    v.   Hepatic vein catheterization
    vi.   Superior mesenteric arteriography
    vii. Splenic arteriography
    viii. Direct portography
12. Radionuclide studies
13. Interventional techniques
    i.   Endoscopic sclerotherapy
    ii. Endoscopic balloon tamponade
    iii. Ultrasound- / CT-guided liver biopsy
14. Transjugular / transfemoral catheter procedures
    i.   Balloon dilatation to re-establish hepatic vein patency
    ii. Clot thrombolysis via transhepatic approach
    iii. Dilatation of stenosis, surgical porto-caval shunt with balloon catheter via inferior vena cava.
    iv. Embolization of splenic artery (for hypersplenism)
    v.   Transjugular intrahepatic porto-systemic shunt (TIPS).

Radiological Findings
Plain films (plain radiography)
Hepatosplenomegaly: Dense opacity of the liver and spleen in the right and left hypochondrium respectively is shown in portal vein thrombosis, cardiac failure, schistosomiasis, etc.
Enlarged azygos vein: Opacity, of soft tissue density in the right tracheobronchial angle superiorly, measuring above 1 cm in diameter. This alters in shape during Valsalva manoeuvre or change in

posture. It is caused by dilated azygos vein due to inferior vena caval obstruction, portal hypertension, superior vena caval obstruction or congenital azygos continuation of the inferior vena cava.

Paraspinal varices: Enlarged paraspinal vessels are seen in portal vein thrombosis and may cause defects in the vertebral bodies.

Mediastinal widening: This occurs from varices, lymphoma, haemorrhage, lymphadenopathy.

Vertebral collapse/destruction: This may be as a result of carcinoma, metastasis, leukaemia, lymphoma, sickle cell anaemia which caused the portal hypertension

Cholelithiasis: This may occur as a result of sickle cell anaemia.

Sclerotic changes in the bone: These may be seen as a result of osteoblastic metastasis, sickle cell bone infarction or myelofibrosis. It may give a clue as to the cause of portal hypertension.

Very dense shadow of liver in Wilson's disease.

Features of cardiac failure: Cardiomegaly, upper lobe blood diversion, pulmonary oedema, pleural effusion

Changes in the chest due to cystic fibrosis:
Consolidation, fibrocystic changes, pneumothorax, peribronchial thickening, peripheral nodular thickening, hilar lymphadenopathy and signs of air trapping

Calcification of pericardium: This is seen in chronic constrictive pericarditis. It occurs in the anterior and lateral parts of the heart particulay seen along the margins of the left lateral margin of the heart.

Calcified spleen or autosplenectomy in sickle cell disease.

Takayama's syndrome: Miliary opacities in the chest are shown in early stages of schistosoma infection of the chest.

Features of tricuspid incompetence: Enlargement of right atrium, bulging of cardiac shadow to the right with inferior vena cava entering inferiorly.

Ultrasound Scan

Hepatomegaly: The liver's supero-inferior diameter will measure above 15 cm. This is seen in cardiac failure and schistosomiasis, portal vein thrombosis, sickle cell disease.

Splenomegaly: Hypersplenism and TSS are among the lesions. The largest spleen is seen in these conditions.

Cirrhosis: The liver will appear shrunken and echogenic in late stages with evidence of ascites (transsonic free fluid within the peritoneal cavity). It is enlarged in early stages. Nodular surfaces with shrunken right lobe and signs of portal hypertension develops at late stages.

Lymphadenopathy: Enlarged para-aortic, para-hepatic and lumbar lymph nodes will be detected by ultrasound in reticulosis or lymphadenopathy.

Hepatitis: There is hypoechoic liver with evidence of hepatomegaly.

Pancreatic pseudocyst: A large hypoechoic area consisting of the cyst is observed posterior to the stomach and displacing the stomach anteriorly on lateral view.

Enlarged hypoechoic pancreas measuring above 2.5 cm in diameter at the head is seen in acute pancreatitis.

Gamna–Gandy siderotic nodules: Areas of trabecular / perifollicular haemorrhages within the liver. They appear as multiple small hyperechoic spots on US.

Recanalised paraumbilical vein: These are visualised as hypoechoic channels at the ligamentum teres and measuring equal to or more than 2 mm in diameter on Ultrasound. They exhibits hepatofugal flow on Doppler studies.

Increased diameter of portal vein above 13 mm

Collateral vessels are seen in the lower oesophagus and the cardia of stomach

Collateral channels in splenic hilum

Splenic vein enlargement: There is enlargement of splenic vein.

Non-visualisation of extrahepatic portal vein with collaterals in and around the gall bladder, duodenum and pancreas, with evidence of solid material (thombus) within the portal vein is seen in portal vein thrombosis.

Tumours of pancreas, liver, kidney, spleen and neuroblastoma causing obstruction of portal vein will be identified.

Thickened lesser omentum.

Metastasis: Multiple oval hypoechoic areas in the liver, spleen, kidney, pancreas and with ascites may be shown in metastasis.

Echocardiography

Constrictive pericarditis: Echogenic areas at the margins of the heart with distal acoustic shadowing impairment of cardiac chamber filling, thickening and rigidity of the pericardium involving mostly the right side of the heart.

Cardiac failure in tricuspid incompetence: Incompetent tricuspid valve identified by incomplete closure. It is often due to rheumatic fever or may be functional. The liver is engorged and pulsatile with raised jugular venous pressure. The right atrium is enlarged. The tricuspid valve is thickened.

Doppler Ultrasonography

Loss of respiratory change in portal venous flow with continuous featureless flow.

Loss of flow in portal vein during expiration

Marked reduction in mean portal vein velocity to about 7 – 12 cm/second (Normal = 12 – 30 cm/second)

Hepatofugal flow (Reversal of portal venous flow direction).

High resistive index in dilated hepatic artery > 0.78.

Development of collateral channels in the splenic hilum, renal hilum, lower oesophagus, cardia of stomach and gall bladder and anterior abdominal wall (caput medusae).

Echogenic material within the portal vein lumen (thrombus) with enlargement of thrombosed area in portal vein thrombosis.

Lack of flow in post-prandial colour Doppler studies due to blockage of the vein by the thrombus.

Doppler scan with decrease in hepatic artery resistive index is also seen in portal vein thrombosis.

Cirrhosis: There is portalization of hepatic waveform (the hepatic waveform simulates that of portal vein); oscillation of hepatic vein waveform (oscillation of hepatic vein is dampened similar to that of portal vein).

Budd-Chiari syndrome: There is absence or reversal of flow in the inferior vena cava with loss of variation in hepatic vein pulsation with heartbeat.

Endoscopy

Dilated submucosal oesophageal veins are directly identified.

Site of bleeding oesophageal varices can be directly sisualised and identified.

Lesions such as gastric tumours, pancreatic pseudocysts can be directly identified.

Barium Swallow and Meal

Multiple thickened, coarse sinuous, interrupted mucosal folds (earliest sign).

Multiple serpiginous filling-defects that change position on different films are seen on oblique view of barium swallow studies.

Smooth-lobulated worm-like filling defects are seen in the upper stomach in gastric varices.

Hypotonic Duodenography

Widened C–loop of duodenum is seen with Frostberg's reversed–3 signs and is noted in carcinoma of pancreatic head and in acute pancreatitis.

Computed Tomography Scan

The following ffeatures can be demonstrated.

Thickened oesophageal wall with multiple lobulated contour due to varices.

Right- and left-sided oesophageal soft tissue mass in the outer wall due to paraoesophageal varices.

Nodulated or scalloped oesophageal outline or masses within the lumen due to oesophageal varices.

Marked contrast enhancement of masses in contrast CT scan studies due to varices.

Low-density centre in the portal vein (thrombus) with circumferential enhancement are shown with contrast CT in portal vein thrombosis.

The aortic density is higher than portal vein density on contrast CT studies in portal vein thrombosis

Enhancement of enlarged caudate lobe with failure to identify hepatic vein in Budd-Chiari syndrome.

CT/spiral CT with small amount of contrast will show dilated vein in the head and neck and upper limbs in superior vena caval obstruction.

Magnetic Resonance Imaging

Porto-systemic collateral channels identified without the use of contrast injection.

Dilated portal vein > 15 mm in diameter

Flow void in portal vein

Dilated oesophageal/gastric vein with flow void.

Features of the causes of portal hypertension identified

Abnormal signal intensity within the portal vein in portal vein thrombosis.

Angiography

Coeliac arteriography: This may demonstrate angiomas or arteriovenous malformation, which is a rare cause of upper GIT bleeding because of dynamic portal hypertension.

Percutaneous Splenic Puncture

High value of intra-splenic pressure with reflux of blood at considerable speed.

Enlarged/dilated portal vein >15 mm in diameter

Gastric/oesophageal varices demonstrated by dilated collateral channels in these areas.

Failure of visualisation of portal vein (may very rarely be normal).

Distortion of intrahepatic vascular pattern

Demonstration of numerous collateral channels.

Operative Mesenteric Phlebography

This is done during laparotomy to prove the patency of the portal veins where the findings by other techniques are inconclusive.

Arterioportography

Super selective catheterization and injection into splenic, common hepatic, left hepatic or superior mesenteric artery.

Dilated portal vein: Portal vein is shown at various phases of the arteriography as dilated above 15 mm in diameter.

Hepatofugal flow into portal vein by injection into hepatic artery.

Oesophageal and gastric varices are shown by injection into the short gastric artery.

Collateral flow into superior mesenteric veins can be shown by injecting into the superior mesenteric artery.

Transhepatic-portal Phlebography

The major indications are severe cirrhosis in patients in whom surgery is contraindicated.

Selective catheterization and obliteration by embolization can be done to the varices.

Venous sampling for assay from the pancreatic drainage veins into splenic or inferior mesenteric veins can be obtained for hormone-producing pancreatic tumours.

Interventional Procedures

Endoscopic sclerotherapy: Injection of sclerosants to obliterate the various veins in the lower oesophagus and gastric cardia can be done using endoscopy.

Endoscopic balloon tamponade: Bleeding oesophageal varices can be compressed and the bleeding stopped by balloon tamponade under endoscopic control.

Ultrasound- /CT-guided biopsy: This is done for histology of liver, spleen, pancreas and lymph node to establish diagnosis/cause of tumour mass or bleeding.

Transfemoral / transjugular catheter procedure

Balloon dilatation can be done to re-establish hepatic vein patency which drains into inferior vena cava.

Clot thrombolysis in hepatic vein or portal vein is done via transhepatic approach.

Dilatation of stenosing surgical porto-caval shunts with balloon catheters via inferior vena cava is feasible.

Embolization of splenic artery

This is done for hypersplenism as its treatment or to reduce blood supply before surgery. The procedure is complicated by infection and abscess formation.

Transjugular Intrahepatic Porto-systemic Shunt (TIPS)

Expansible metallic stent inserted percutaneously is used to establish connection between hepatic vein and portal vein within the liver.

Features observed on Doppler ultrasound scan after TIPS include:

Decompression of portal vein with reduced portal venous pressure to about 22 mmHg from pre-TIPS value of about 37 mmHg.

Re-establishment of high velocity flow in portal vein of 50 – 250 cm/second from pre – TIPS value of 10 – 30 cm/second.

Re-establishment of cardiac beat and respiratory movement variation of hepatic and portal veins.

The velocity in hepatic artery is increased from pre – TIPS value of 77 cm/second to about 119 cm/second.

Reversal of flow: There is reversal of hepatofugal flow to flow towards the liver. Shunt obstruction is a complication and may occur in less than 40% of cases after ten years following shunt operation

(Adam & Dixon, 2008; Dahnert, 2011; Sutton, 2003; Swischuk, 2004; Palmer & Reeder, 2001).

References

1. Liu CH, Hsu SJ, Liang CC, Tsai FC, Lin JW, Liu CJ, Yang PM, Lai MY, Chen PJ, Chen JH, Kao JH, Chen DS. Esophageal varices: noninvasive diagnosis with duplex Doppler US in patients with compensated cirrhosis. Radiology 2008;248:132-9.

2. Kishimoto R, Chen M, Ogawa H, Wakabayashi MN, Kogutt MS. Esophageal varices: evaluation with transabdominal US. Radiology 1998;206:647-50.

3. Pilette C, Oberti F, Aubé C, Rousselet MC, Bedossa P, Gallois Y, Rifflet H, Calès P. Non-invasive diagnosis of esophageal varices in chronic liver diseases. J Hepatol 1999;31:867-73.

4. Piscaglia F, Donati G, Serra C, Muratori R, Solmi L, Gaiani S, Gramantieri L, Bolondi L. Value of splanchnic Doppler ultrasound in the diagnosis of portal hypertension. Ultrasound Med Biol 2001;27:893-9.

5. Piscaglia F, Valgimigli M, Serra C, Donati G, Gramantieri L, Bolondi L. Duplex Doppler findings in splenic arteriovenous fistula. J Clin Ultrasound 1998;26:103-5.

6. de Franchis R; Baveno V Faculty. Revising consensus in portal hypertension: report of the Baveno V consensus workshop on methodology of diagnosis and therapy in portal hypertension. J Hepatol 2010 ;53:762-8.

7. Qamar AA, Grace ND, Groszmann RJ, Garcia-Tsao G, Bosch J, Burroughs AK, Ripoll C, Maurer R, Planas R, Escorsell A, Garcia-Pagan JC, Patch D, Matloff DS, Makuch R, Rendon G; Portal Hypertension Collaborative Group. Incidence, prevalence, and clinical significance of abnormal hematologic indices in compensated cirrhosis. Clin Gastroenterol Hepatol 2009 ;7:689-95.

8. Grace ND, Groszmann RJ, Garcia-Tsao G, Burroughs AK, Pagliaro L, Makuch RW, Bosch J, Stiegmann GV, Henderson JM, de Franchis R, Wagner JL, Conn HO, Rodes J. Portal hypertension and variceal bleeding: an AASLD single topic symposium. Hepatology 1998; 28:868-80.

3.4   RADIOLOGICAL FEATURES OF INTESTINAL OBSTRUCTION

Definition
Intestinal obstruction is defined as impedance, blockage, constraint or barrier to the bowel lumen or the normal pathway of progression of food and gas from the stomach to the anal opening. The normal peristaltic wave cannot pass distal to the obstacle, leading to dilatation of bowel proximally and expulsion of bowel content distally with collapse.

Classification
Dynamic or mechanical obstruction: This is caused by intrinsic or extrinsic bowel mass, constriction or bowel twist or herniation.
Adynamic obstruction or paralytic ileus: Partial or complete paralysis of bowel due to electrolyte imbalance with bowel dilatation, or defects in the neural supply to the bowel walls.

Causes of intestinal obstruction
Strangulated external hernia is the commonest cause in developing countries.
Bands and adhesion from previous surgeries are the commonest cause in Europe and other high-income countries (tabes 3.41 and 3.42).

Table 3.41: Common causes of dynamic intestinal obstruction in adults

Volvulus	Appendicitis
Intussusception	Infection/Inflammations
Strictures	Aortic aneurysm
Neoplasm	Mesenteric artery syndrome
Meckel's diverticulum	Haematoma of bowel wall
Meconium ileus	Chronic duodenal ulcer
Vascular insufficiency	Perforated cholecystitis
Enteric duplication	Gastric volvulus
Foreign bodies	Bezoars / trichobezoars
Parasitic – Ascariasis	Corrosive gastritis/colitis
Blood dyscrasias	Endometriosis
Blunt trauma	Pelvic abscess/diverticulitis
Faecal impaction	Mesenteritis/adenitis

Radiological investigative modalities
1. Plain film: Chest x-ray: PA, lateral and lateral decubitus
   Plain abdominal radiography: Erect, supine and left lateral decubitus, lateral Radiography of spine, pelvis, skull
2. Ultrasound scan, Doppler ultrasound scan
4. CT scan and Spiral CT with angiography
6. MRI, MR angiography
7. Barium studies: Swallow and meal, barium follow through, small bowel enema and barium enema

8. Angiography (Arteriography and phlebography)
9. Interventional studies – ultrasound- and CT-guided
10. Excretory Urography
11. Radionuclide studies

Plain Films
Chest x-ray
Chest radiography will serve as the baseline for further assessment of the chest. It will also show other chest conditions that may appear-like intestinal obstruction like:

Cardiac failure: Cardiomegaly, pulmonary oedema, hilar fullness and pleural effusion.
Lower lobe pneumonia: Area of inhomogeneous opacity with air-bronchogram in the lower lobe.

Table 3.42: Other causes of intestinal obstruction

Neonate/children	Adynamic obstruction
Intestinal atresia	Postoperative
Meconium ileus	Visceral spasm
Midgut rotation	Electrolyte imbalance
Annular pancreas	Diabetes mellitus
Ladd's band	Neuromuscular disorders
Antral mucosal diaphragm	Shock – septic / hypovolaemic
Imperforate anus	Chronic hepatic/ renal diseases
Hirschsprung's diseases	Retroperitoneal abscess
Intussusception	Drugs – morphine, atropine etc.
Inguinal hernia	Bowel ischaemia
Appendicitis	Trauma – spine, ribs, hip, etc.
Midgut volvulus	Renal disorder – colic, failure
Hypertrophic pyloric disease	Chest conditions – CCF,
Large intra-abdominal mass	pneumonia.

Pulmonary infarction or pulmonary embolism: Wedge-shaped opacity with the pleural-based base and an apex located medially. Radionuclide ventilation / perfusion studies with perfusion defect will confirm the diagnosis.
Leaking dissecting aortic aneurysm: There is mediastinal widening and MRI will confirm the diagnosis.
Pneumothorax: Area of lucency devoid of lung markings is identified close to the lateral chest wall. The edge of the collapsed lung is observed as curvilinear line medially.
Pleurisy: Small pleural effusion with pleural thickening in one or both costophrenic angles may be identified.
Pericarditisis shown as irregularities of the heart margins.
Myocardial infarction may be signified by pleural effusion and cardiomegaly.

Abdominal Radiography – Erect and Supine
Dilated air-filled loops of bowels: The small bowel dilatation above 2.5 cm is abnormal and large bowel dilatation above 5.5 cm in diameter is abnormal.

Air-fluid level: Even though there are many normal causes of air fluid level, three or more air-fluid levels greater than 2.5 cm in diameter is abnormal and indicate small bowel dilatation.

Dilated sausage-shaped oval or round soft tissue densities: These opacities change position in different views may represent fluid-filled small bowel dilatation.

'String of beads' sign: Small gas bubbles trapped in rows between valvulae conniventes on horizontal ray film signifies almost completely fluid-filled dilated small bowels.

Completely fluid-filled small bowels: This will show ground-glass appearance of abdomen without any bowel gas. The bowel sounds are absent on clinical examination.

Increased bowel-diameter or bowel wall thickness: The bowel diameter or wall thickness may increase in patients suspected to have obstruction due to bands and adhesions signifying progressive bowel obstruction and the need to abandon conservative 'drip and suck' regimen for surgery.

No-gas obstruction: In certain high intestinal obstruction, affecting the first one-foot or so of the small intestine, gas-distended loops and fluid levels may be completely absent. This is because of regurgitation and vomiting of intestinal contents. This may occur after gastroenterostomy when small loops may invaginate into the lesser sac. Strangulation frequently results and failure to recognise it leads to grave prognosis.

'Stretch sign': Stretched-out and erectile valvulae conniventes completely encircle bowel lumen.

'Step-ladder appearance': Fluid levels, appearing in rows in step-ladder pattern are conclusive evidence of low small bowel obstruction. The more the number of dilated bowels the more distal the site of the obstruction.

Hyperactive peristaltic wave: This is seen as dilated air-filled bowels with curved serpiginous pattern and striking valvulae conniventes.

Paucity of gas in the rectum: In complete intestinal obstruction, no gas and no faecal matter is found in the rectum or colon after 12 – 24 hours.

Bowel lumen disparity: There exists a great disparity in size between obstructed dilated loop proximally and the contiguous distal unobstructed segment.

In large bowel obstruction, if the ileo-caecal valve is competent, the small bowel will not dilate but if the ileocaecal valve is incompetent, the small bowel will also be dilated.

Table 3.43: Small versus large intestinal obstruction		
Parameter	**Small bowel**	**Large bowel**
Valvulae conniventes	Present in jejunum	Absent
Number of loops	Many	Few
Haustral marking	Absent	Present
Distribution of bowels	Central	Peripheral
Radius of curvature	Small	Large
Diameter	3-5 cm	= + 5 cm
Solid faecal matter	Absent	Present

Pneumoperitoneum: Free air within the peritoneal cavity as a result of perforated hollow viscus. It can appear as air under the hemidiaphragm. They also can appear as triangular lucencies between three adjacent bowel loops.

Gastric outlet obstruction: Markedly dilated stomach occupying most of the abdomen with large diameter, air-fluid levels and with food debris.

Sigmoid volvulus: Large ahaustral dilated bowel with inverted U-shape, apex above D_{10}, overlying the left flank (left flank overlay sign) and inferior convergence of loops are noted in sigmoid volvulus.

Double-bubble sign: Double large air lucencies within dilated stomach and dilated proximal part of duodenum signify duodenal obstruction. This is common in neonate and children.

'Triple bubble sign': Three large air lucencies within the stomach, duodenum and proximal jejunum signify jejunal obstruction.

Gall stone ileus: Gas within the gall bladder and branching air lucencies in the biliary tree often centrally located over liver area are noted in gallstone ileus. Calculus may be found over the sacrum.

'Target sign' in intussusceptions: Two concentric circles of fat density lying to the right of the spine, which is often superimposed on the kidney. These are possible layers of peritoneal fat within the wall of intussusceptum alternating with layers of mucosa and muscle seen end-on (fig. 3.41 a and b).

Dilated gas-filled bowel with valvulse conniventes: This is observed in small bowel obstruction (fig. 3.41 c).

Dilated gas-filled bowel with haustral marking: This is observed in large bowel obstruction (table 3.43).

Appendicolith: Laminated calcific density in the right lower quadrant found in 6 – 15% of patients with appendicitis. This is calculus of the appendix.

Caecal volvulus: There will be a left hypochondrial mass due to twisted and inverted caecum and appendix. The mass may contain faecal material and may occasionally be centrally located if there is twist without inversion. Existing haustral marking excludes sigmoid volvulus.

Ileosigmoid knot: Dilated loop of pelvic colon usually located in the right side of abdomen. Signs of small bowel obstruction, retained faecal material in undistended proximal colon are found.

Anal atresia: Inability to pass meconium, proximal dilated bowel loops with anal dimple that does not allow passage of catheter for barium enema.

Ascariasis: Multiple linear air-lucencies central in the abdomen with whirlwind gas pattern.

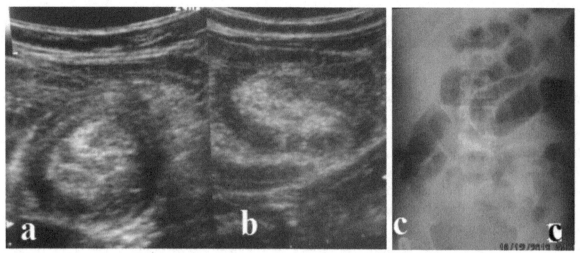

Figure 3.41: Imaging appearances in small intestinal obstruction. Sonogram of a patient showing target sign in intussception; transverse view (**a**) and longitudinal view (**b**). Plain abdominal radiograph showing centrally-placed dilated gas-filled small bowel loops with prominent valvulae conniventes and paucity of gas in the rectum (**b**).

Pneumatosis cystoides intestinalis: Linear gas streaks or cyst-like lucencies in bowel wall due to gangrene. They occur as a result of vascular compromise with bowel wall necrosis e.g. mesenteric thrombosis.
Gas in the portal vein: Branching lucencies due to gas in the portal vein overlying the hepatic area. The lucencies are peripherally located as against gas in the biliary tree which are medially located. They are also found in mesenteric thrombosis.

'Coffee bean' appearance: Large dilated bowel loop separated by thickened intestinal wall seen in strangulated hernia. Gas within the bowel wall signifies gangrene.
Pseudotumour: Soft tissue mass seen in strangulated hernia because the closed loop of bowel which maycontain fluid.

Gas below inguinal ligament: In strangulated inguinal hernia, gas may be found below the inguinal ligament within the hernia sac. Trichobezoars may also present this appearance.
Constipation: Thick faecal materials with mottled air lucencies are noted in the rectum and pelvic colon in faecal impaction and in patient with Hirschsprung's disease. The proximal bowels are dilated and filled with air/gas.

Ultrasound
Haemoperitoneum: Ultrasound can identify free intraperitoneal fluid appearing transonic within the abdomen outside bowels or vessels. This may signify blood in cases of trauma, or perforation or in patient leaking ectopic pregnancy.
Tumour mass: Antral carcinoma, carcinoma of head of pancreas, colonic tumours, lymphomas, etc causing obstruction can be identified as solid masses distal to the dilated bowel.
Abscess: Hypoechoic mass with multiple internal echoes. Internal septations may be present.

Hypertrophic pyloric stenosis: There is thickened muscle mass in the pylorus with hyperperistaltic wave of stomach wall seen on ultrasound. There is gross dilatation of the stomach filled with fluid, the gastric wall is thickened and there is elongated pyloric canal. Two parallel hypoechoic thickened pyloric muscles are seen on ultrasound of the pylorus, and the pyloric canal is marked by two echogenic line of the mucosa.

Acute pancreatitis: There is enlarged hypoechoic pancreas and fluid within the pancreas may signify necrotic area or abscess formation. Pancreatic pseudocyst is transonic and a complication of acute pancreatitis and is usually found under the stomach in the lesser sac.

Fluid-filled dilated bowel: These are seen with ultrasound as fluid within bowel which is transonic (figure 3.42 a). If the bowel contains food debris or if there is dehydration, the food debris may appear as semiliquid material within the bowel (figure 3.42 b). It is observed in fluid-filled intestinal obstruction when gas is almost completely absent. Plain film may show ground glass appearance and the intestinal obstruction may be missed.

Fibroid mass: Degenerative fibroid causing adhesion of bowel loops and intestinal obstruction are seen as hypoechoic masses with whorl-like echogenic concentric rings within it. Areas of degenerative changes may appear hypoechoic or cystic in cases of red degeneration or cystic degeneration respectively. Calcific degeneration will be echogenic with distal acoustic shadow. Matted adherent bowel loops are seen if the bowels contain fluid.

Barium studies

Failure of barium passage: Failure of barium to enter the stomach is seen in complete gastric volvulus. The left hemidiaphragm is elevated.

Failure of barium to pass the pyloric canal with dilated stomach is seen in gastric outlet obstruction and incomplete gastric volvulus.

Ulcer crater in duodenum: This is seen in peptic ulcer disease.

Thumb-printing: Sharply marginated finger-like indentations at colonic bowel wall or small bowel or nodular filling defects in bowel walls. These are due to haematoma or bowel wall oedema due to vascular insufficiency. They are seen in mesenteric artery thrombosis, volvulus, infections, ulcerative colitis, pseudomembranous enterocolitis, lymphoma and haematogenous metastasis.

Intestinal malrotation: Rotated bowel seen in complete or incomplete obstruction.

Intussusception: 'Coiled spring' appearance. The intussusceptum may produce concave defect in the head of barium column. There may also be abrupt cut-off of barium column.

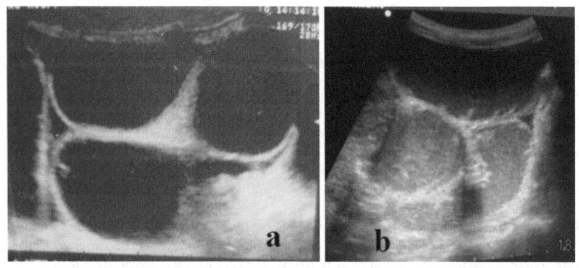

Figure 3.42: Sonograms of the abdomen showing in (**a**), multiple clear fluid-filled dilated bowel loops in small intestinal obstruction, and in (**b**), multiple dilated bowel loops filled with semiliquid material in small intestinal obstruction.

Hirschsprung's disease: Change in calibre between narrowed distal aganglionic segment and dilated proximal segment with a transition zone more commonly seen in the rectosigmoid region. An irregular serrated outline of aganglionic segment may be seen. Much of the contrast is retained in 24 hours delay film unlike in normal persons when nearly all would have been expelled.

Ascariasis: Linear filling-defects within the bowel-filled barium column due to the ascarids. Barium may outline the alimentary canal of the worm.

Small bowel enema: This distinguishes complete from incomplete obstruction. In complete obstruction, there is cut-off of barium column at the point of obstruction.

Signs of specific disease causing the obstruction: Bowel out-pouching in diverticular disease, granular bowel appearance in continuity in ulcerative colitis, aphthoid ulcer, cobblestone formation and skip lesions in Crohn's disease, filling-defect, shouldering and apple core deformity in carcinoma.

'Double barium sign': Barium in the stomach and proximal duodenum in duodenal obstruction.

Intraluminal - or intramural mass lesions. Intraluminal mass lesion appearing as filling-defects are identified. Such mass lesions include polyps, fibromas, leiomyomas, bezoars, haematoma, tuberculomas, helmenthomas, and malignant tumurs. Carcinomas may show narrowing, filling defects with apple-core deformity.

Computed tomography scan

Intra-abdominal abscess: Hypodense mass with attenuation value of 15 – 35 HU. Gas is present within the mass. There is ring enhancement following intravascular contrast administration. Percutaneous drainage under CT or ultrasound guidance is possible.

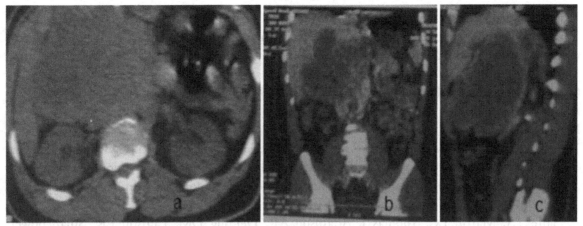

Figure 3.43: Cholangiocarcinoma. CT images of **a**, non-enhanced abdominal scan, **b**, Coronal reformatted contrast scan, **c**, Sagittal reformatted contrast scan images showing a large intrabdominal mass originating around the porta hepatis and causing small intestinal obstruction.

Trauma: Rupture of hollow and solid viscus, fractured vertebrae, intraperitoneal haemorrhage and pneumoperitoneum are visualised.

Bowel wall thickening: Can detect bowel wall thickening seen in bowel ischaema and obstruction more than plain films.

Gall stone ileus: CT can detect the gall stone as well as gas in the biliary tree.

Appendicolith: Calcified density within appendix can be detected by CT.

Bowel dilatation. CT studies will show dilated bowels and can identify the site and cause of the obstruction.

Large intrabdominal mass: An significantly large intrabdominal mass may by pressure effect on the bowel cause intestinal obstruction (figure 3.43).

Spiral CT and CT angiography
It can detect thrombosis of mesenteric artery/vein.

Angiography
Occlusion of mesenteric artery: Thrombus appearing as filling-defect lodged at the major branching point distal to 3 cm of superior mesenteric artery.

Bleeding peptic ulcer disease can be detected by identifying the point of bleed in real time by visual observation.

MR imaging
1. *Haematoma:* MRI can diagnose intraperitoneal blood collection.
2. *Dissecting aortic aneurysm:* MRI can diagnose aortic aneurysm. Blood within wall of vessel is hyperintense while flowing blood is hypointense.

Scintigraphy
Meckel's diverticulum: This is a diverticulum formed by persistence of a remnant of the embryonic omphalomesenteric into adult life of about 2% of the population. However, only a minority produce clinical symptoms seen commonly in adult life but could also be seen in any age. Most symptoms are due to peptic ulceration of retained gastric mucosa within the diverticulum. The symptoms include

abdominal pain, occult bleeding or signs of intestinal obstruction. Chronic ulceration produces scarring and is the major cause of small bowel obstruction in this disorder. The retained gastric mucosa within the diverticulum aid scintigraphic detection of the diverticulum.

(Adam & Dixon, 2008; Dahnert, 2011; Sutton, 2003; Swischuk, 2004; Palmer & Reeder, 2001).

Reference

1. Sala E, Watson CJ, Beadsmoore C, Groot-Wassink T, Fanshawe TR, Smith JC, Bradley A, Palmer CR, Shaw A, Dixon AK. A randomized, controlled trial of routine early abdominal computed tomography in patients presenting with non-specific acute abdominal pain. Clin Radiol 2007; 62: 961-9.

2. Jaffe TA, Martin LC, Thomas J, Adamson AR, DeLong DM, Paulson EK. Small bowel obstruction: Coronal reformation from isotropic voxel at 16-section multi-detector row CT. Radiology 2006; 238: 135-142.

3. Suri S, Gupta S, Sudhakar PJ, Venkataramu NK, Sood B, Wig JD. Comparative evaluation of plain films, ultrasound and CT in the diagnosis of intestinal obstruction, Acta Radiol 1999; 40: 422-428.

4. Yagan N, Auh YH, Fisher A. Extension of air into the right perirenal space after duodenal perforation: CT findings. Radiology 2009; 250: 740-748

5. Lagundoye SB, Itayemi SO. Tension pneumothorax. British Journal of Surgery 1970; 57: 576-580.

3.5 RADIOLOGICAL FEATURES OF CARCINOMA OF HEAD OF PANCREAS

Definition
This is defined as malignant transformation of some epithelial tissues in the pancreatic head.

Composition:
Pancreatic ductal adenocarcinoma, 80% – 99%
Pancreatic acinar cell carcinoma, 10%–20%
Tumour of unknown cell of origin within pancreas, 5% – 10%.

Pancreatic ductal cell adenocarcinoma arises from ductal cell epithelium (ductal cells make up only 4% of pancreatic tissue, but over 95% of the cancer arises from them). For practical purposes, discussion of radiological features of pancreatic carcinoma is mainly centred on ductal cell adenocarcinoma.

Sex Ratio: M: F = 2: 1
Age of affectation = 55 years and above, the peak is at 70 years

Areas of affectation
1. Head of pancreas = 60 – 70%, body = 20 – 30% and Tail < 10%
Size: 2 – 10 cm in diameter (But most are above 5 cm)

Clinical features
Jaundice, weight loss, upper abdominal pain, back pain (radiation from upper abdominal pain), anorexia, fatigue, malaise, steatorrhoea, thrombophlebitis, vomiting and late-onset diabetes mellitus.

Radiological investigative modalities
Plain film: The abdomen, chest, spine, skull, extremities
Ultrasonography – 3.5 MHz transabdominal ultrasonography.
Endoscopic ultrasonography/intra-operative
Barium meal, hypotonic duodenography and barium enema
Conventional tomography
Computed tomography: Non contrast, contrast and helical scan
Magnetic resonance imaging
Magnetic resonance angiography
Conventional angiography
Cholangiography (percutaneous and endoscopic retrograde cholangiography)
Endoscopic retrograde cholangio-pancreatography
Interventional studies (Ultrasound-guided biopsy/drainage of abscess, CT scan, ERPC and Cholangiography)
Percutaneous transhepatic venous sampling
Ultrasound guided percutaneous pancreatography
Fine needle biopsy

Radiological features
Plain film
Large cancer may show as soft tissue mass displacing the gas shadow of stomach and intestines inferiorly.
Gastric outlet obstruction: Dilated stomach filled with fluid or gas with air-fluid level due to extrinsic mass impression obstructing the 2nd part of duodenum.
Ascites: This may show as ground-glass appearance and is caused by peritoneal spread of the mass.
Osteolytic or osteoblastic changes in the spine due to metastatic spread may rarely be seen.
Pneumorrhachis: This means air within the spinal canal or spinal sub-arachnoid space. It is found in severe emphysematous pyelonephritis or severe bowel infarction with gangrene. Carcinoma of the prostate may occasionally induce diabetes mellitus, which could present with *emphysematous pyeleonephritis* and pneumorrhachis. It has poor prognosis.

Ultrasonography
There is a pancreatic mass which is hypoechoic in texture.
Target lesion: Mass is hypoechoic with high echo level at the centre resembling target lesion
Pancreatic mass disorganizing the gland: Mass is focal and often well defined, but over 10% may have diffuse enlargement of gland with disorganization of internal architecture.

Deformed pancreatic gland: The contour of the mass may be deformed and the uncinate process appear round.
Irregularity of pancreatic mass: The margins of focal benign tumours are well-defined and this is characteristic. Any associated irregularity strongly supports the diagnosis of malignancy.
Dilated common duct and main pancreatic duct: The common bile duct and main pancreatic duct are dilated in over 80% of cases causing jaundice.
Double duct sign: Visualisation of dilated common bile duct and main pancreatic duct
Enlargement of para-aortic glands: Para-aortic lymph node enlargement may be identified.
Ascites: Free anechoic intraperitoneal fluid due to peritoneal spread of the mass.

Metastases are hypoechoic and will be detected in the liver and lymph node (lymphadenopathy) in only one quarter (¼) of cases.
Calcification in the gland occurs only rarely.
Splenomegaly: Tumour invasion of spleen and portal veins produces splenomegaly.

Endoscopic Ultrasonography (7.5 – 10 MHz transducer)
Better demonstration of pancreatic body and tail: This is used in order to avoid bowel interference. This will show tumour of body and tail better than transabdominal ultrasound scan which demonstrates mainly tumour of the head.

Improved demonstration of retroperional and lymph node spread: This demonstrates tumour spread to the liver, lymph node and retroperitoneal tissues better.
Early portal invasion: It also demonstrates early portal vein invasion.

Colour Doppler ultrasonography
Tumour invasion of portal vein: This shows tumour invasion of portal vein with dilation of portal vein above 1.3 cm with flow disturbance including turbulent flow, sluggish flow and collateral circulation.

Portal vein occlusion with reversal of flow: Complete tumour occlusion of portal vein with reversal of flow may occur in 15% and identified by colour Doppler ultrasonography.

Portal vein thrombosis: Thrombosis within portal vein can be identified due to tumour cell infiltration.

Gastric varices: Gastric fundal varices may be identified sometimes with involvement of oesophagus due to complete occlusion of portal vein.

Barium swallow

Horizontal oesophagus: Elongation and straightening of the distal oesophagus (intra-abdominal oesophagus) to lie in horizontal position may occur due to pseudocyst or tumour mostly from tail of pancreas affecting distal oesophagus.

Distal oesophageal narrowing: Invasion or obstruction of distal oesophagus with rat-tail appearance

Lower oesophageal varices: There is splenic or portal vein invasion or occlusion and this may occur following gastric fundal varices.

Barium meal

Gastric fundal varices: Occlusion of splenic vein by malignant invasion and thrombosis of the vein by acute pancreatitis which occurs due to ductal occlusion may lead to gastric fundal varices. Nodular filling defects in gastric fundus are seen.

Widening of retrocardiac space (in shoot-through lateral view). The tumour displaces the stomach anteriorly and superiorly widening the retrocardiac space.

Antral pad sign: There is extrinsic mass impression on the posteroinferior margin of gastric antrum from the carcinoma of the body/tail of pancreas with widening of gastric mucosal fold.

Invasion of inferior stomach: Invasion of the inferior aspect of the stomach with mucosal fold irregularities, gastric ulceration.

Fixation of gastric wall. This is due to tumour invasion with abnormal peristalsis.

Thickened gastric mucosal fold due to spreading inflammation caused by the tumour resulting to oedema of mucosal fold and spasm.

Deformed duodenal C-loop: Irregular or smooth filling-defect on the C-loop of duodenum caused by ampullary carcinoma.

Hypotonic duodenography

Widened duodenal C-loop with mucosal irregularities.

Blunted, spiculated nodularity of mucosal fold or localised stricture may be observed resulting from direct malignant tumour invasion of the duodenum with infiltration, fixation and desmoplastic reaction.

Frostberg's "reversed-3 sign": Double contour on medial aspect of the c-loop of duodenum due to indentation by the mass.

Indented/deformed duodenal cap: An enlarged gall bladder due to common bile duct obstruction may indent and deform the duodenal cap.

Annular constriction of second part of duodenum with preserved mucosal pattern caused by carcinoma of the head of pancreas.

Barium enema
Mass-impression with padding of haustral marking, narrowing, or flattening with irregular zigzag contour at the posterior and inferior aspects of the transverse colon/splenic flexure.
Colonic fixation and tethering: Irregular diffuse fixation or tethering of the colon due to intraperitoneal seeding or metastasis.

Computed tomography (over 95% of tumour detected by CT)
There is a well-defined pancreatic mass but it may occasionally be diffuse causing diffuse enlargement of the gland.
Non-enhancing mass with isodensity and central area of reduced density giving the target lesion appearance

Double duct sign: Both the pancreatic and the common bile ducts are dilated. This is associated with visible mass within the pancreatic head but rarely the mass may not be visible.
Thickened coeliac axis: This is caused by tumour invasion of the peri-vascular lymphatics.
Thickened Gerota fascia

Obliteration of retropancreatic fat in up to half of the cases.
Pancreatic pseudocyst formation: Obstructed pancreatic duct may lead to enzymes digesting the pancreatic tissue to the exterior forming pseudocyst. This may also be seen in both acute and chronic pancreatitis.
Calcification is rare: Seen in only 2%. Extensive calcification strongly supports benign lesion.
Liver metastases: Metastatic nodular hypoechoic areas may be seen in the liver.

Lymph node enlargement: Lymphadenopathy is easily visualised and is due to metastatic spread to lymph nodes.
Pleural effusion is due to metastasis to the pleura.
Occlusion of bile duct: Bile duct occlusion with irregular stricture from malignancy is demonstrable. Multiple pulmonary nodules: multiple pulmonary nodular opacities due to metastasis can be shown by high resolution CT of the lung. Occasionally lymphangitis carcinomatosa in lung bases can be shown.
Cystic pancreatic head mass: Cystic mass in pancreatic head with dilated pancreatic duct, common bile duct and gall bladder can be caused by pancreatic cystadenocarcinoma.
Calcification in lymph node can occasionally be shown and is not necessarily caused by calcified pancreatic carcinoma.
Encasement of vessel: Encasement of superior mesenteric vein, portal or splenic vein may occasionally be demonstrated.
Atrophy of distal pancreatic tissue: Tumour mass with dilated distal pancreatic duct devoid of calculus and with atrophy of distal pancreatic tissue is characteristic.

Magnetic resonance imaging
Hyperintese mass on T1-weighted images: The mass is identified and on T_1-weighted imaging, the tumour is hypointense.
Avascular tumour: Since the tumour is avascular, on dynamic contrast imaging there is reduced enhancement.

In lymph node and liver metastasis due to pancreatic ductal cell adenocarcinoma, the signal is hyperintense on T_2-weighted imaging.

Invasion, occlusion and encasement of portal vein, superior mesenteric and splenic veins are often shown and indicate that tumour resection is unlikely.

Hypervascular islet cell tumour: Islet cell tumour and their liver metastases are hypervascular with low signal T_1WI and high signal on T_2WI.

Percutaneous transhepatic cholangiography

Gloved finger appearance: Dilated intrahepatic biliary radicles due to obstruction at distal common bile duct by pancreatic head.

Meniscus sign: Where an ampullary tumour obstructs the main pancreatic duct a meniscus sign is shown.

Long, irregular stricture of the distal common bile duct is shown in carcinoma of the head of the pancreas.

Magnetic resonance cholangio-pancreatography (MRCP)

Better demonstration of anatomy: It shows the pancreatic duct anatomy even in tight strictures or total obstruction of pancreatic duct where endoscopic retrograde cholangiography shows only the distal part.

Alternative to ERCP: It is useful also where previous gastric and pancreatic surgery or tumour invasion renders endoscopic pancreatography impracticable and in the same session as conventional MRI. However, stents, metallic clips from previous surgery, respiratory motion, poor resolution and inability to see terminal parts of ducts and side branches reduces or limits its use.

Endoscopic retrograde pancreatography

Pancreatic duct obstruction: Complete/eccentric obstruction of pancreatic duct is shown. Complete block is the commonest finding and if seen in the head often accompanied by complete block of the distal part of the common bile duct. The side branches are usually normal as opposed to chronic pancreatitis where they are abnormal.

Pancreatic duct stricture: there is rat-tail appearance of obstructed pancreatic duct. This is associated with displacement of main and side ducts around the tumour mass.

Cavities/scrambled egg appearance: In necrotic tumour, contrast enters necrotic defects within the tumour forming cavities; when this is multiple 'scrambled egg appearance' results.

Solitary main pancreatic duct devoid of side branches: there is destruction of normal pancreas by carcinoma with non-filling of side branches contained in the destroyed tissue.

Pre – stenotic dilatation: This is caused by localised encasement of pancreatic duct by tumour.

Duct tortousity and kinking: Tortuous elongated duct with kinking in some portions are identified in many cases and is highly suggestive.

Angiography

Hypervascular tumour: The tumour is hypervascular in most cases except islet cell tumours which are hypovascular.

Neovascularisation may be seen in up to half of the cases.

Tumour encasement of superior mesenteric, splenic, coeliac, hepatic and gastroduodenal arteries may be shown and all the arteries may not be involved simultaneously.

Obstruction of superior mesenteric and splenic veins and portal vein occur and may lead to splenomegaly.

Venous encasement: Encasement of superior mesenteric, splenic and portal veins may be identified.

Tumour blush: Dense tumour blush may be demonstrated with superselective catheterization and multiple view angiographies in islet-cell tumour.

Percutaneous transhepatic venous sampling

Multiple venous sites are used. Samples are taken from splenic vein, pancreaticoduodenal vein and the other pancreatic draining veins to check for several polypeptide hormones such as insulin, glucagon, gastrin, somatostatin, ACTH, vasoactive intestinal polypeptide and melanocyte stimulating hormones. Islet-cell adenocarcinoma metastasizes early and their metastases secret hormones. Insulinoma and gastrinomas are common with gastrinomas having high malignancy rate of 60%.

Interventional studies
Angiography

1. In angiography, tumour embolization of large inoperable tumours to cause relief (palliation) of symptoms is feasible.
2. Palliative embolization of hepatic artery in cases of hepatic metastasis helps reduce symptoms.
3. Intra-arterial cytotoxic drug injection is also done to shrink the tumour especially Islet-cell tumour.

Ultrasound

Ultrasound-guided biopsy of liver, lymph node and pancreas for histology is done with high success rate.

Ultrasound percutaneous drainage of pseudocyst is also done.

Endoscopic ultrasound-guided drainage of pseudocyst through the stomach is frequently done.

Ultrasound-guided percutaneous pancreatography to outline the pancreatic duct has high success rate especially when endoscopic retrograde pancreatography is not feasible due to presence of tumour of head of pancreas.

CT scan

CT scan-guided biopsy of liver, pancreas and lymph nodes for histology.

CT guided percutaneous drainage of pseudocyst.

ERCP

Drainage of pseudocyst: Endoscopic retrograde cholangiopancreatography guided drainage of pseudocyst. This can be done through the stomach.

Stent placement: Stent placement in both common bile duct and pancreatic duct can be done via endoscopic retrograde cholangiopancreatography.

Differential Diagnosis

1. Acute pancreatitis
2. Chronic pancreatitis
3. Metastases
4. Annular pancreas.

(Adam & Dixon, 2008; Dahnert, 2011; Sutton, 2003; Swischuk, 2004; Palmer & Reeder, 2001).

References

1. Müller MF, Meyenberger C, Bertschinger P, Schaer R, Marincek B. Pancreatic tumor: evaluation with endoscopic US, CT and MR imaging. Radiology 1994, 190: 745-751.

2. Catalano C, Laghi A, Fraioli F, Pediconi F, Napoli A, Danti M, Passariello R. High-resolution CT angiography of the abdomen. Abdom Imaging 2002;27:479-87.

3. Catalano C, Laghi A, Fraioli F, Pediconi F, Napoli A, Danti M, Reitano I, Passariello R. Pancreatic carcinoma: the role of high-resolution multislice spiral CT in the diagnosis and assessment of resectability. Eur Radiol 2003;13:149-56.

4. Megibow AJ. Pancreatic adenocarcinoma: designing the examination to evaluate the clinical question. Radiology 1992; 183; 297-303.

3.6 RADIOLOGICAL FINDINGS IN THE GASTROINTESTINAL TRACT OF PATIENTS WITH AIDS

Definition
AIDS means Acquired Immunodeficiency Syndrome and it is a disease caused by infection with human immuno-deficiency virus (HIV). Abnormalities in the gastrointestinal tract due to the pathological changes caused by this organism are found at multiple sites. Infection by several opportunistic organisms as a result of T-cell depletion leads to the most frequent changes. Multiple tumours are also found.

Investigative modalities
Plain x-ray of the chest (PA and lateral), extremities, abdomen, lateral neck, skull,
Ultrasound – conventional, Doppler, Echocardiography, Endoscopic ultrasound
Barium studies, (barium swallow, barium meal and follow-through and barium enema)
CT scan
MRI
Radionuclide studies
Interventional technique. Ultrasound-, CT-guided and endoscopic biopsy
Fibreoptic endoscopy

Lesions frequently identified are those from the following organisms:
Viral: Cytomegalovirus infection, Herpes simplex virus infection and HIV infection
Fungal: Candida infection, pneumocystis jiroveci (carinii), and histoplasmosis
Protozoan: Cryptosporidium and Gardia lamblia
Bacterial: Mycobacterium tuberculosis and Mycobacterium avium intracellulare
Other organisms: Isospora belli, Rickettsiales Bartonella henselae, strongyloides and Campylobacter

AIDS related neoplasia
1. Kaposi's sarcoma
2. Non-Hodgkin's lymphoma
3. Lymphadenopathy-associated Syndrome (LAS)

Areas of Affectation
Oesophagus: Oesophagitis, Kaposi's sarcoma, lymphoma.
Stomach: Gastritis, Kaposi's sarcoma, Lymphoma.
Small bowel: Duodenitis, malabsorption, Kaposi's sarcoma, lymphoma.
Large bowel: Colitis, procto-colitis, proctitis, ulceration, polypoid masses.

Candida Infection
Oesophagitis and the mouth
Candida infection is the most common opportunistic infection in patients with AIDS. It occurs in up to 20% in USA and over 80% in developing countries. It affects the mouth and oesophagus.
1. It leads to discrete linear/irregular or longitudinally oriented filling defects in the oesophagus on barium swallow.
1. Severe oesophagitis may lead to perforation
2. Severe oesophagitis may also lead to fistula formation

3. Stricture formation

    Note that absence of oral thrush does not exclude Candida oesophagitis.

Candida necrotising enterocolitis
1. High density intestinal contents are seen on plain film.
2. Ileal *pneumatosis cystoides intestinalis* are found
3. Air in the intrahepatic branches of portal vein is demonstrated.

Histoplasmosis
This is an opportunistic fungal infection with 10% involvement in the gastrointestinal tract. It forms disseminated disease in patients with AIDS.

Cytomegalovirus Infection
Oesophagitis
It is the most common cause of opportunistic life-threatening infection of viral origin in patients with AIDS.
It is demonstrated as a single or large discrete shallow ulcers in the background of normal mucosal pattern.
Giant or large superficial ulcers in the background of normal mucosal pattern may be seen.

Gastritis
It causes mucosal thickening with shallow ulcers.
The ulcers may be associated with malignancies (lymphoma) in patients with AIDS.
Non-specific changes due to gastritis are also noted.

Duodenitis
Causes duodenitis with thickening of mucosal fold, nodularity or effacement of mucosal pattern

Small intestines
Mucosal fold thickening and ulcerations are noted. It causes severe enteritis.
Ischaemic ulceration and perforation of the bowel due to invasion of endothelial cells of small vessels occur. There is narrowing of terminal ileum. There is submucosal nodule formation. Absence of lymph node involvement with uniform thickening of terminal ileum and caecum are seen in CT scan.

Colonic CMV infection
It causes local or diffuse colitis with involvement of pericolic fascia/fat. Colitis involves caecum and proximal colon. Sometimes extends to the terminal ileum. Discrete small ulceration in the background of normal mucosal pattern. Bowel wall thickening occurs and is often marked. It may manifest as diffuse lymphoid hyperplasia. Toxic megacolon may occur. Haemorrhage may occur causing haematochezia, crampy abdominal pain and fever.
Target sign or double ring appearance are seen on CT due to increased submucosal oedema. Perforation may be seen. Ascites may occasionally be seen.

Herpes Simplex Infection
Herpes simplex vesicles in the oesophagus produce filling defects on barium swallow.
When vesicles burst, they produce ulcers in a background of normal mucosa.

Similar changes are seen in the oral cavity, rectum and anus.

HIV Infection
HIV itself is capable of producing oesophageal ulcer which is often large and solitary. Multiple ulcers indistinguishable from those of CMV infection are also seen.

Actinomycosis
Oesophagitis with deep sinus tracts are found.

Cryptosporidium
This causes severe diarrhoea with fluid loss of over 10 litres per day.

Stomach
This causes antritis (inflammation of the gastric antrum). This appears as areas of thickening of gastric mucosa.
Ulcerations are occasionally seen.
Marked antral narrowing due to extensive inflammation is seen.

Duodenum
Duodenitis, mucosa fold thickening, nodularity, and effacement of mucosa occur.

Small intestines
There is dilated proximal small bowel especially the jejunum with intraluminal accumulation of fluid. The mucosa fold is thickened. There is also effacement, atrophy, blunting, fusion and loss of the villi. *"Toothpaste"* appearance of small bowels simulating tropical sprue.
Total mucosal atrophy may be found throughout the small bowel resembling acute graft versus host reaction.
There is dilution of barium due to extensive hypersecretion. Cryptosporidium is caused by a protozoön and small bowel biopsy from the brush borders may show the organism.
Oocyst of the organism may be found in the stool.

Colon
Rarely mucosal thickening may be seen in the colon
Focal or total atrophic changes may rarely be found.

Pneumocystosis (Pneumocystis jiroveci (carinii) infection)
This occurs in patients treated with aerosolized pentamidine.
Lesions are found in the liver, spleen and lymph nodes. Hepatic, splenic and lymph node calcifications are seen.
Foci of multiple tiny echogenic areas in spleen are shown. Varied sized multiple low attenuation areas in spleen which progress to calcification.

Isospora belli
A protozoan pathogen. The infection resembles cryptosporidium. Lesion occurs in the small intestine. Mucosal fold thickening or focal mucosal atrophy due to localised inflammation may occur.

Tuberculosis
Oesophagitis
1. Numerous discrete ulcers
2. Numerous extrinsic carinal filling defect due to carinal lymphadenopathy
3. Fistulations when caseous necrotic lymph nodes erode into the oesophageal lumen.
4. Scarring and stricture may occur

Stomach
Produces huge nodule/extrinsic mass/polypoid lesion in the antral region causing gastric outlet obstruction
Ulceration plus stricture formation
Peritoneum and lymph nodes also affected with polypoid lesions.

Small intestine
The features are more marked in the jejunum
Mucosal thickening with irregularity
Circumferential ulcers.
Varying lengths of segmental narrowing.
Polypoid lesions.

Colon
Ileocaecal valve area involved.
Circumferential ulcer
Mucosal thickening with irregularities
Segmental narrowing
Stricture formation
Polypoid lesions
Non-specific proctitis.

Mycobacterium avium intracellulare (MAI)
Oesophagitis
Lesions are similar to herpes simplex, cytomegalovirus infection and tuberculosis can be produced by MAI.
Gastritis
Mucosal thickening
Shallow ulcers
Changes may be associated with lymphoma.

Duodenitis
Duodenitis with thickening of the mucosa
Nodularity and effacement of mucosal pattern

Small intestine
The small intestine is the most common site of affectation, especially the jejunum.
It causes severe disease evidenced by:
Mucosal fold thickening which is diffuse

Nodular defects in bowel margins

Mild dilatation of the small bowel especially middle and distal parts.

Segmental separation of small bowel due to mesenteric and retroperitoneal lymphadenopathy; and hepatosplenomegaly

Multiple small echogenic foci but may occasionally be large, hypoechoic and seen in the liver and spleen.

1. MAI lesion resembles Whipple's disease
2. MAI is the most common bacterial opportunistic lesion.
3. Most common non-tuberculous mycobacterium lesion in AIDS patients.

Others

Gardia lamblia, campylobacter and strongyloides

These organisms produce diarrhoea, malabsorption and non-specific enteritis.

All these produce diarrhoea with malabsorption with lesion seen in the small intestines. There is mucosal thickening and irregularities with non specific changes.

Bacillary angiomatosis

This is caused by *Bartonella henselae* which is a bacterium in the order of *Rickettsiales*.

There is vascular proliferation within bacilli

It affects the liver, spleen and lymph nodes

Marked abdominal lymphadenopathies appearing as nodular filling defects in bowel walls are seen in barium studies and contrast enhanced CT scan

Peliosis is marked. These are blood filled cystic spaces in the liver/spleen.

AIDS-Related Neoplasia
Kaposi's sarcoma

This is tumour of blood vessels. It was a rare tumour before the advent of AIDS, found mostly in elderly men. Found in 50% homosexual men compared to 5% intravenous drug abusers with AIDS. Presently it is more frequently seen in AIDS patients who are homosexual men. GIT involved in 50% of cases. It is a polypoid mass often multifocal, producing submucosal tumour throughout the GIT. GIT is the third site of involvement after skin and lymph nodes. Areas involved in the GIT include the oesophagus, stomach, duodenum, small intestine and the colon. the oesophagus is the least frequently involved.

Oesophagus and stomach

Haemorrhagic patches seen in endoscopy at early stages in gastric mucosa

Barium studies show:

1. Large polypoid masses producing filling defects
2. Submucosal masses producing filling defects
3. 'Bull's-eye' lesions due to ulceration of large polypoid masses
4. *Linitis plastica* type of lesion in the stomach (Severe sclerosing-narrowing of the stomach with lack of gastric distensibility).
5. Submucosal infiltrative lesion thickens the mucosal fold.
6. Retroperitoneal lymphadenopathy as well as splenomegaly is seen on CT scan.

Small intestine

Large submucosal nodules with thickened mucosal fold

Plaques and central umbilication may be found in lymph nodes. This is more common in the stomach but may be seen in small bowel

CT shows lymph node enlargement and thickening of bowel wall.

Colon

Nodular tumours appear as filing defects on barium enema.

Found in submucosa and appear as extrinsic nodular tumours.

The tumour may progress and coalesce to form large bulky masses.

They are often multiple and found throughout the bowel.

Lymphoma

(Non-Hodgkin's lymphoma). It is the second most common AIDS-associated neoplasm. The stomach is most commonly involved. It occur in 4 – 10% of patients with AIDS. It is 60 times commoner in AIDS than the general population. The lesion is a b-cell lymphoma with high or intermediate grade of malignancy

It is also found in CNS, bone marrow and GIT. In the GIT the stomach and small bowel are most commonly affected.

Stomach

Mostly commonly affected. Accounts for 5% of all primary gastric malignancies

It occurs in younger age group and may involve the whole stomach more than cancer.

Barium studies

Lesions appear as well-defined spherical filling defects. They also appear as 'Bull's-eye' lesion due to central ulceration of polypoid lesion. Circumferential or focal thickening of gastric mucosa or wall or both may be seen.

CT scan

It appears as markedly lobulated gross wall-thickening (> 4 cm). There is severe lipoatrophy. Preservation of perigastric fat may rarely occur and is associated with better prognosis.

Small intestines

Hepatosplenomegaly causes bowel displacement. The distal ileum is involved in the small intestine. There is bowel wall thickening with polypoid masses. Ulceration with bowel perforation may occur.

Colon

The rectum is most frequently involved. There is bowel wall thickening, polypoid lesion, ulceration and perforation. Solitary or multiple liver lesions may be seen on ultrasound.

AIDS Cholangitis

Caused by CMV and cryptosporidium

1. Stenosis of common bile duct (CBD) papilla
2. Irregular dilatation of intra- and extra-hepatic bile ducts
3. Periductal fibrosis
4. Thickening of the wall of gall bladder and common bile ducts
5. Multiple intramural polypoid filling defects.

(Adam & Dixon, 2008; Dahnert, 2011; Sutton, 1998 and 2003, Palmer & Reeder 2001).

References

1. Pantongrag-Brown L, Nelson AM, Brown AE, Buetow PC, Buck JL. Gastrointestinal manifestations of Acquired Immunodeficiency Syndrome: radiologic-pathologic correlation. Radiographics 1995; 15: 1155-1178.

2. Rene E, Verdon R. Upper gastrointestinal tract infection in AIDS. Baillière's clinical gastroenterology 1990: 4: 339-359.

3. Haller JO. Imaging the gastrointestinal tract of children with AIDS. Paediatric radiology 1995; 25: 94-96.

4. Falcone S, Murphy BJ, Weinfeld A. Gastric manifestations of AIDS: Radiographic findings on upper gastrointestinal examination. Journal of Abdominal Imaging 1991; 6: 95-98.

5. Obajimi MO, Atalabi MO, Ogbole GI, Adeniji-Sofoluwe AT, Agunloye AM, Adekanmi AJ, Osuagwu YU, Olarinoye SA, Olusola-Bello MA, Ogunseyinde AO, Aken'Ova YA, Adewole IF. Abdominal ultrasonography in HIV/AIDS patients in southwestern Nigeria. BMC Med Imaging 2008;8:5.

6. Igbinedion BO, Marchie TT, Ogbeide E. Transabdominal ultrasonographic findings correlated with CD4+ count in adult HIV-infected patients in Benin, Nigeria. South African Journal of Radiology 2009; 13: 34-40.

3.7   RADIOLOGICAL MANIFESTATIONS OF ASCARIASIS

Definition
Ascariasis is the human infestation by the parasitic helminth, the round worm, known as Ascaris lumbricoides. This helminthic infection is the most common of all helminthic infections in humans. The worm measures about 15–50 cm in length, and 2-6 mm in thickness. The worm has a life span of about one year and produces about 200,000 eggs daily.

Age group affected: 1 – 10 years, most children.

Countries affected: About 25% of the world population (this is over one billion people) is affected. It is endemic (90% of children population affected) in the following regions Gulf coast, parts of Africa (especially Nigeria), South East Asia and South America.

Life cycle
1. Ingestion of contaminated vegetable/water/soil
   a. Eggs hatch in duodenum of the child.
1. Larvae migrate through the venules / lymphatic system of splanchnic organs and are carried to the lungs.
2. Larvae migrate to alveoli of pulmonary system and penetrate to the tracheobronchial system.
3. Larvae are coughed up and swallowed
4. They reach the upper gastrointestinal system and mature in the jejunum within 2 – 3 months.
5. The adult worms produce eggs which leave the body through the faecal route.

Symptoms in the intestinal phase
Asymptomatic, abdominal pain, vomiting, bowel obstruction, acute appendicitis and intestinal perforation

Symptoms due to the migration of a worm through the papilla of vater into the biliary tree include: Jaundice, biliary colic, recurrent pyogenic cholangitis, pancreatitis, hepatic abscesses and septicemia.

Symptoms and signs in the chest and other areas
1. Granulomatous peritonitis with significant malnutrition
2. Tuberculous pyopneumothorax with bronchopleural fistula
   (worm migrated from the intestines to lodge in the pleural cavity)
3. Acute respiratory distress syndrome with the worms obstructing the airways
4. Intrapleural ascariasis

Radiological manifestations
Plain abdominal x-ray
"Whirlpool effect": A whirlpool effect of mass of worms contrasted against the gas in the bowel usually in a distended segment resembling a tangled group of thick cords.
Partial or complete mechanical intestinal obstruction: This shows multiple dilated bowel loops with multiple air-fluid levels often in a typical stair – case or step-ladder configuration visible in erect plain abdominal radiograph

Bolus of sporge-like mass: The large bolus of coiled worms blocking the lumen of the gut may be visible at the most distal part of the dilated bowel.

Barium meal

Elongated radiolucent filling-defects within barium-filled lumen of bowels are shown especially in the small bowels. These are the outlines of the individual ascarids.

Long, cylindrical filling-defect: Characteristically long, smooth, cylindrical and often coiled filling-defects are seen due to the worms. Common sites in descending order where they are often visualised are jejunum, ileum, stomach (especially after vomiting) and the oesophagus.

White thread-like string: If the patient has fasted for at least 12 hours, the ascarid may ingest barium in which case its alimentary canals will be seen as white thread-like string within the length of its body which is seen in double contrast against the surrounding barium.

Barium enema

1. The worms may be found in the colon where they appear in barium enema as cylindrical or coiled radiolucent filling defects in the lumen of the colon especially in children.
2. Disordered bowel pattern with malabsortion.

Ultrasonography

Even though USS is cheap, rapid, accurate, readily available and does not use ionizing radiation, it has limitations, such as operator dependence of the accuracy and abdominal gas obscuring the biliary tree. However, the following findings have been demonstrated:

Echogenic tubular structure with 2–4 mm wide hypoechoic central line (digestive tract of worm). This is seen within the dilated common bile duct or common hepatic duct.

"Strip sign": One or more non-shadowing tube-like structures that may be straight or coiled.

"Spaghetti sign": This is shown when multiple, worms completely fill the bile duct.

Hyperechoic pseudotumour: When multiple worms are very densely packed in the bile ducts and appearing amorphous.

Intermittent biliary obstruction with features of thickened dilated gall bladder wall (cholecystitis) or echogenic common hepatic duct (cholangitis) seen together with worm in the common bile duct.

Enlarged hypoechoic pancreas suggestive of acute pancreatitis.

Hypoechoic area within the liver with multiple internal echoes within it suggestive of hepatic abscess/ emphysema.

Alternating areas of dilatation and stricture formation in the biliary tree.

Granulomatous peritonitis: Worms that have migrated within the peritoneal cavity may elicit granulomatous peritonitis when they die and this is associated with significant malnutrition, morbidity and mortality. The fluid is hypoechoic but with semi-liquid appearance.

Cholangiography (Intravenous, ERPC, Percutaneous)

Long filling-defect: Smooth cylindrical radiolucent filling defect in the gall bladder and biliary tree.

Better tomographic outline: Tomography with intravenous cholangiography will demonstrate the worms better with their outlines within contrast-filled biliary tree.

Reflux of barium through duodenum into the biliary tract when post-operative or otherwise incompetent sphincter of Oddi is present may demonstrate one or more ascarids in the common bile duct or biliary tree.

Mass with dilataion and stricture: Several worms tangled together within common duct and biliary radicules amid filling defects which are due to biliary sludge or stone or alternating dilation and stricture due to ascending cholangitis.

Duct necrosis, fibrosis and calculi formation: Worms that are in the sphincter of Oddi may become trapped, die, become macerated and fragmented and its components cause a severe inflammatory response leading to necrosis of the ducts, calculus formation, fibrotic stricture, and cholangitis

Chest radiography

Loffler's pneumonia (syndrome)
These are seen as scattered fleeting or transient, pin-point soft tissue opacities with patchy ill-defined asymmetrical infiltrates.
These are due to localised pulmonary inflammatory reaction or occasionally represent small areas of necrosis or pulmonary haemorrhages as the larvae migrate in the lungs.

Disseminated bronchopneumonia
In severe cases of larval infestation, there may be disseminated bronchopneumonia with diffuse small nodular infiltrates.

Lung collapse
Blockage of a bronchus by an adult worm may precipitate lung collapse, or segmental pneumonia distal to the point of obstruction. The pneumonia appears as area of consolidation with air-bronchogram.

Solitary pulmonary nodule
The death of a migrating larva within the lung may result in pulmonary granuloma. As fibrosis forms around it, the typical x-ray appearance of a solitary pulmonary nodule is seen.

Lung abscess
Migration of ascarids to the lung and blockage of a bronchus may lead to lung abscess if the distal blocked area is secondarily infected.

Pneumoperitoneum
Perforation of abdominal hollow viscus by adult worm penetrating the wall of the intestines may appear in chest x-ray as free gas under the hemidiaphragms.

Acute respiratory distress syndrome
This occurs when the worms obstruct the airway.

The worms can be seen with chest tube during thoracotomy
The worms can migrate through the chest drainage tube in a patient with pneumothorax or empyema that is being drained by thoracotomy.

MR imaging of abdomen

1. MR imaging using axial T2 weighted sequence shows hyperintense bile signals surrounding a dot or linear hypointense signal in the common bile duct.

Ascaris pancreatitis

Ascaris pancreatitis peripancreatic oedema.

Peripancreatic oedema alone without identification of the ascarid.

Diffusely dilated pancreatic duct containing a smooth linear filling -defect (ascaris worm).

Dilated and patent Ampulla of Vater (when the worm is just recently expelled).

MR cholangiography

The intraductal worms appear as linear hypointense filling defects.

Endoscopic interventional procedure

The worm can be extracted during ERCP without using forceps or baskets.

Endoscopic sphincterotomy and balloon extraction of the parasite and bile duct clearance has been done in some cases.

(Adam & Dixon, 2008; Dahnert, 2011; Sutton, 2003; Swischuk, 2004; Palmer & Reeder, 2001).

References

1. Lagundoye SB. Disordered small bowel pattern in ascariasis. Trop Geogr Med. 1972; 24:226-31.
2. Sanduok F, Haffar S, Zada MM, et al. Pancreatic- biliary ascariasis: experience of 300 cases. Am J Gastoenterol 1997;92:2264-2267.
3. Ferreya NP, Cerri GG. Ascariasis of the alimentary tract, liver, pancreas and the biliary system. Its diagnosis by ultraousound. Hepatogastroenterology 1998; 45: 932-937.
4. Kenamond CA, Warhauser DM, Grimm IS. Ascaris pancreatitis. Radiographics 2006; 26: 1567-1570.
5. Das CJ, Kumar J, Debnath J, Chaudhry A. Imaging of ascariasis. Australas Radiol 2007;51:500-6.
6. Khuroo MS, Zargar SA, Mahajan R. Hepatobiliary and pancreatic ascariasis in India. Lancet 1990;335:1503-6.
7. Rocha Mde S, Costa NS, Costa JC, Angelo MT, Lessa Angelo Júnior JR, Sonoda L,
8. de Andrade MR, Scatigno Neto A. CT identification of ascaris in the biliary tract. Abdom Imaging 1995; 20: 317-9.
9. Park MS, Kim KW, Ha HK, Lee DH. Intestinal parasitic infection. Abdom Imaging 2008; 33:166-71.

3.8 THE ROLES OF RADIOLOGY IN THE DIAGNOSIS AND MANAGEMENT OF PATIENTS WITH BLUNT ABDOMINAL TRAUMA

Definition
Blunt abdominal trauma is defined as any injury to the abdomen and its contents caused by an external force directed at it and without an associated open wound or disruption of the skin in either the anterior or posterior abdominal wall.

Causes
1. Motor vehicle injury/Road traffic injury
   - Motor vehicles
   - Motor Cycles
   - Bicycles
   - Pedestrians
2. Fall from height
3. Fall at home/work
4. Assault
5. Sports injury
6. Trauma at work
7. Other types of accidents

Role of Radiology/Radiology team
Assists the trauma team leader in:
1. Imaging for diagnosis, management and follow up of each individual patient.
2. Interpreting the imaging studies
3. Providing other specialist diagnostic and interventional skill.
4. Identification of complications and complications of treatment requiring further interventions

Priority in trauma is not imaging but rather to take care of:
1. Airway (A)
2. Breathing (B)
3. Circulation (C). These three form the (ABC) of first aid.
4. Resuscitation of patient

However, in patients from whom reliable history cannot be obtained and whose vital signs cannot be assessed for adequacy and stability, or patients who are unconscious, comatose (due to head injuries, alcohol or drugs), imaging becomes indispensable immediately.

The radiologist must make an attempt to obtain good quality images and provide quality interpretation in the knowledge of history, symptoms and signs.

Significant reliable indicators of intra-abdominal injury are:

1. Abnormal physical examination
   - Abdominal pain
   - Abdominal tenderness
   - Signs of peritonitis
2. Presence of frank haematuria
3. Chest injuries
   - Fracture of the 3rd - 6th ribs
   - Multiple rib fractures
   - Widened mediastinum
   - Haemoperitoneum
   - Pneumoperitoneum
   - Signs suggestive of aortic injury

SECTION A

Investigative Modalities

Plain Radiograph

Plain radiograph lacks specificity and sensitivity. It uses ionizing radiation which greatly limits its use in pregnant women and children. However, it may define the following:

1. Fracture of lumbar vertebrae and lower ribs often associated with intra-abdominal injuries.
2. Pneumoperitoneum which suggest ruptured hollow viscus.
3. Haemoperitoneum with fluid level outside the bowel wall.
4. Fracture of pelvic bones which may suggest severe injury to the bladder, blood vessels, or pelvic organs.
5. Cervical spine, thoracic spine and the skull can be radiographed if there are signs of associated injuries to these organs.
6. Fractures of the extremities can also be assessed.

Ultrasound

Ultrasound is cheap, fast, readily available, cost-effective, easily performed, portable, non-invasive, complication–free and does not use ionizing radiation.

Uses

1. It has excellent imaging of free intraperitoneal fluid.
2. Excellent in imaging of paediatric and unstable patients where other modalities may be impossible.
3. It can assess pregnant patients for foetal viability, uterine rupture and liquor volume or foetal distress.
4. It can assess bladder, kidneys, spleen and liver for laceration, rupture or batter; however, its accuracy in assessing solid organs is not as good as for cystic organs.
5. It can excellently image the brain in children 0 – 6 months without the use of ionizing radiation.
6. Echocardiographic assessment of the effect of trauma on the heart, pericardium and pleura can be done by showing pericardial fluid and pleural effusions as well as intracardiac blood clots or ruptured cardiac tissues and tendineae.

Pitfalls

1. It is useless in detecting free intraperitoneal air.
2. It cannot adequately assess patients with bandaged wounds, monitor or suction tubes, intravenous or monitoring lines and patients with conditions rendering them immobile.
3. It is highly operator-dependent.

Computed tomography (Conventional, contrast CT and Helical CT scan)

This is non-invasive and very specific for injury identification and an excellent diagnostic tool for general survey of the abdomen for injury.

Uses

1. Simultaneous imaging of pelvis (bladder, prostate, ureters, uterus, and ovaries) abdomen and retroperitoneum (kidney, pancreas and adrenals) can be done.
2. Head and thorax can be assessed in the same session in patients with multiple traumas to detect skull fractures, subdural, epidural or intracerebral haemorrhage.
3. The lumbar, thoracic and cervical spines can be evaluated for fractures.
4. Helical CT urography can carry out IVU to demonstrate ureters, kidneys and bladder in the same CT session.
5. Helical CT scan can assess the spinal cord without the use of contrast and without the long imaging time associated with MRI.
6. It allows for surgical planning and serial scans which can be done to monitor progress and response to therapy.
7. It has very high specificity at specific organ injury identification.
8. CT-guided percutaneous intervention and therapy like abscess drainage, drainage of urinoma, hydronephrosis, biloma and haematoma can be undertaken.
9. Contrast-enhanced CT/Helical CT angiography can quickly and accurately demonstrate active bleeding so that appropriate intervention can quickly be done.

Pitfalls

1. It is time-consuming, requires large number of labour and highly trained manpower with knowledge of anatomy and variants and artifacts for accurate studies and image interpretation.
2. It can only be performed in co-operative, sedated or anaesthetised patients.
3. It has poor sensitivity in bowel, mesenteric and pancreatic injuries.
4. In unstable patients, it adds to the delay in performing laparotomy.
5. CT interferes with patient's resuscitation, monitoring, and patients that are dependent on life support devices cannot be adequately evaluated by CT scan.

Diagnostic peritoneal lavage (DPL)

This is not a radiological procedure but when done under CT or ultrasound guidance is performed in conjunction with the radiologists.

Uses

1. It is very sensitive in detecting haemoperitoneum.
2. It does not interfere with patient's resuscitation so that it can be done simultaneously as the patient is being resuscitated.
3. It can be done on unconscious, uncooperative or sedated patients including children.

Pitfalls

1. It is highly invasive.
2. It is not sensitive at detecting specific organ injury or extent of the injury.
3. It does not detect retroperitoneal and bowel injuries.
4. It is insensitive at detecting pneumoperitoneum.
5. It is oversensitive as tap may be taken from vessels, bowel lumen, small haemoperitoneum and haematomas.
6. Up to 29% of non therapeutic laparotomies are performed due to its oversensitivity.

Magnetic resonance angiography

Magnetic resonance imaging has excellent soft tissue definition and does not use ionizing radiation.

Uses

1. It is non-invasive.
2. Does not use ionizing radiation and can be used in children and pregnant women.
3. It can detect injury to the spinal column and spinal cord without the use of contrast.
4. Simultaneous imaging of pelvis, abdomen, chest, skull (brain) as well as the spine in one session is possible.
5. Multiplanar capability without the need to move, especially immobile patients.
6. MRI angiography is possible in the same session to detect blood vessel injury, bleeding vessels, intravascular blood clots or thrombus as well as arteriovenous connections.
7. It can assess the extent of the bleeding or blood loss by measuring the cross-sectional area of vessels and determining the volume of blood remaining in them. This can be substracted from normal blood volume to determine the amount of blood that was lost.

Pitfalls

1. Long imaging time leading to delay where intervention is necessary.
2. Difficult to image patients on life support monitors.
3. Difficult to resuscitate patients in MRI environments
4. Has no clear-cut advantage over CT scan.
5. Claustrophobia limits certain patients from benefiting from its useful contributions although open MR scanners are being developed.
6. Expensive, not readily available; interpretation is difficult due to many protocols that are used. Thus the utility of MRI is limited in acute abdominal traumas.

Angiography

This is a highly invasive procedure but the only reliable demonstration of vascular anatomy when interventional study is necessary. Interventional studies can be done under conventional angiography. The aims of angiography are:

1. Demonstration of the anatomy of vessels.
2. Demonstration of on-going bleeding.
3. Embolization therapy to stop bleeding vessel.
4. Embolization therapy for post-operative bleeding.
5. Embolization therapy to stop bleeding in viscera as a form of non-operative management.
6. Demonstration of on-going bleeding even when arising from sources different from patients with onther known chronic conditions.

Pitfalls
1. It is highly invasive.
2. Contrast medium reaction and hypotension may limit its use is some patients that may require its utility.
3. Patients must be adequately resuscitated so that the procedure must be delayed and leads to delay in interventional therapy.
4. Unco-operative and restless patients must be sedated (which is not required in abdominal trauma) otherwise, the image may be blurred and limited for therapy planning.

Intravenous urography/excretory urography
Uses
1. This is minimally invasive and it is excellent at demonstrating renal function even in haemodynamically unstable patients.
2. It does not interfere with patient's resuscitation.
3. Normal IVU almost always excludes significant injury to the kidney, ureter and bladder.
4. It is superior to ultrasound in all types of renal injuries.
5. It is the investigation of choice in macroscopic or isolated renal injury.

Pitfalls
1. Does not detect other visceral injury.
2. Less sensitive than CT in detecting renal parenchymal injury.
3. Hypotensive patients cannot be imaged and those with indeterminate IVU still require CT scan.
4. CT is more accurate in staging of renal injury.
5. It does not demonstrate renal vascular injury and such patients still require CT scan.
6. Non-viable renal tissues cannot be detected.

Urethrocystography/cystography
This is used to show intra- or extra-peritoneal bladder rupture by instilling contrast into the bladder through it. It is highly sensitive but does not detect other injuries.

Endoscopic retrograde cholangiopancreatography
This can show the integrity of hepatobiliary ducts for rupture.

Barium studies
This shows extraluminal leaks from bowel due to perforation or rupture. Water soluble contrast is used if rupture or perforation is suspected.

Isotope scintigraphy
Cholecystoscintigraphy can show biliary duct injury and leaks using red blood cell-labelled agents.

Interventional studies
1. Ultrasound-guided drainage of haematoma, abscesses, biloma and urinoma can be done.
2. CT-guided drainge of haematoma is feasible
3. Embolization of bleeding vessel during conventional angiography. This has been discussed.

SECTION B

Highlight of findings in specific organ
Splenic Injury
This is the most commonly injured organ in acute abdominal trauma.
Plain film: Left lower rib fracture detected by plain film is an excellent indicator of splenic injury. It also shows gas-distended stomach.
Ultrasound can detect haemoperitoneum but cannot adequately characterise the severity of splenic injury. It may show gross rupture or blood around the spleen.

CT scan
Demonstrates splenic injury excellently.
It can demonstrate intra-splenic and extra-splenic haematomas;
It can also detect fragmented or shattered spleen.
It can also demonstrate associated haemoperitoneum.
It can show areas of devitalization of tissue in the spleen.
Other intra-abdominal injuries can be demonstrated.
However, splenic lobulation, clefts, non-homogenous contrast enhancement especially with helical CT and beam hardening artefacts from ribs can cause confusion and degrade the image quality for diagnosis. Repeat CT scan is excellent in showing delayed splenic rupture which occurs most at about 3 weeks after injury but by definition after 48 hours of injury.

Angiography
Differential splenic perfusion image may indicate line of cleavage in transected injuries. This can demonstrate active splenic bleeding since conservative management of splenic injury is the current standard management; non-operative embolisation of bleeding splenic vessel is the current practice in radiology to stop the bleeding vessel. Radiolabelled red blood cell studies together with serial CT scan, diagnostic peritoneal lavage and visceral angiography are used to predict patient's outcome. In elderly multi-injured patients with splenic rupture, conservative management is less fashionable. CT grading of splenic injury is non-prognostic and therefore unreliable.

Hepatobiliary Injury
The liver is the second most frequently injured solid intra-abdominal organ after the spleen. Right lower rib fracture seen in plain film is an excellent indicator of right lower lobe liver injury and for this reason; the right lower lobe is more often injured. Vetebral fractures seen on plain film are often associated with liver injuries.
Injuries to the pancreas and duodenum are also associated with hepatobiliary injury.

Ultrasound
It can show haemoperitoneum.
It shows distorted liver margin in the area of injury.
Ultrasound will detect subphrenic haematoma or abscess.
Disruption of the inferior or superior liver margin due to laceration is well shown.
Ultrasound can detect complication and it is useful in follow up of patients after trauma with or without operation.

Isotope scintigraphy

1. Biliary duct injury and leaks can be shown by cholecystoscintigraphy
2. Biliary leaks and minor bleeding and haemobilia can be assessed using red blood cell-labelled agents.

CT scan

This can detect, define and characterise liver injury. It can detect haemoperitoneum close to the area of the bleed.

Bleeding hepatic vessels can be identified.

Artifacts can degrade the quality of image and lower the accuracy of interpretation.

CT does not predict patients that will require surgery but those with CT grade 5 injury of hepatic trauma are not suitable for conservative management. CT scan can detect laceration, rupture, haematoma, fragmentation and intrahepatic perivascular injuries. Exsanguination can occur if shearing injury of junction of inferior vena cava and hepatic vein occurs, as manifested by presence of haematoma it is explored surgically. Haemobilia and biloma are seen as associated complications of laceration extending into the portal region.

Angiography

This is performed if there is any clinical evidence of on-going bleeding, haemobilia, acute portal hypertension or before surgery for liver trauma if time permits.

Interventional studies

This is done during conventional angiography or after it has been performed. It is used in:

1. Control of recurrent post-operative haemorrhage
2. Control of haemorrhage that causes haemobilia
3. Active arterial bleeding confirmed within the liver capsule or parenchyma using transcatheter hepatic artery embolization
4. Hepatic arterio-portal fistula and other injuries

Gallbladder Injury

This is a rare injury in acute abdominal trauma. CT is the main diagnostic modality. The CT findings are:

1. Pericholecystic fluid
2. Gall bladder collapse
3. Mass effect on duodenum
4. Poor definition of gall bladder walls
5. High density intraluminal haemorrhage

Duodenal perforation, haematoma and pericholecystic laceration are the most common associated injuries.

Renal and Urinary Bladder Injuries

Over 10% of renal injuries are caused by blunt abdominal trauma though over 85% of these are minor. Blunt abdominal trauma also causes about 80% of urinary tract injuries. All adults with gross haematuria following abdominal trauma require imaging studies. Adults with microscopic haematuria alone do not require imaging studies. Imaging is required for all children no matter the degree of haematuria.

Excretory/Intravenous urography (EU/IVU)

Investigation of choice as it can be done quickly without interfering with resuscitation.

It can also be used to assess haemodynamically unstable patients.

No significant injury is likely if the IVU is normal.

It assesses the function of the contralateral kidney in occasion of severe injury to one kidney and when nephrectomy is considered.

It can define the anatomy of the renal outline, pelvicalyceal system, ureters and bladder in one film.

IVU can detect:

1. Perirenal urinoma
2. Ruptured renal pelvis
3. Fracture of the pelvic, lumbar bones and lower ribs.
4. Extrarenal contrast extravasation.
5. Non-functioning kidney.
6. Renal position for ptosis, abnormal locations or migrations.
7. Other lesions like congenital anomalies, renal stones, renal polyps, polycystic kidneys, hydronephrosis and PUJ obstruction.
8. Extravasation of contrast following bladder rupture.

CT scan

Helical CT scan can perform IVU (CT urography) demonstrating the kidneys, ureters and bladder.

CT scan can delay patient's resuscitation and may to give adequate room for resuscitation in a severely injured patient and the risk must be weighted against stabilizing the patient before its performance.

CT scan clearly defines the following:

1. Parenchymal laceration
2. Haematoma close to the kidney
3. Urinary extravasation
4. Clearly demonstrates non-viable tissue after contrast injection
5. Renal vascular injury
6. Demonstrates associated organ injury like fractured vertebra, ribs, laceration of spleen, liver, haematoma, pneumoperitoneum.
7. CT with full length plain abdominal radiography may combine the values of both IVU and CT scan.

Arteriography and interventional studies

Renal arteriography with interventional embolisation is used to treat persistent haematoma from the bleeding vessel or origin of blood to a lacerated area.

CT scan of pelvis and urinary bladder

This can show pelvic fracture

Both IVU and CT scan can show contrast extravasation into the pelvis from ruptured or perforated ureter or bladder.

Intra-peritoneal and extra-peritoneal rupture can be demonstrated by CT.

Urethrography/Cystography
Using urinary catheter to instill contrast into the bladder to distend it, the classical appearance of intra-peritoneal and extraperitoneal bladder rupture can be shown.

Percutaneous drainage of abscess
Urinoma, hydronephrosis, and haematomas can be drained percutaneously under ultrasound or CT guidance.

Adrenal Injuries
This is mainly unilateral in 25% of major abdominal traumas.
Adrenal insufficiency does not often occur even in bilateral cases.

CT findings
1. High density round expansion of the adrenals
2. Stranding of periadrenal fat
3. Associated injuries to the adjacent organs like spleen, kidney, and vertebrae may indicate injury to the adrenals.

Pancreas
This is relatively uncommon.
Use of seat belt increases the likelihood of injury.
Occur in only 3 – 12% of severe abdominal injuries.

CT scan
CT scan is the mainstay of diagnosis
CT is poor at detecting injury but is the initial imaging modality of choice. The CT findings imclude:
1. Presence of fluid between splenic vein and pancreatic tail
2. Pancreatic laceration with post-traumatic pancreatitis
3. Pancreatic oedema.
4. Areas of reduced or increased attenuation
5. Pancreatic haematoma
6. Fluid in the lesser sac
7. Thickening of the anterior renal fascia
8. Retroperitoneal fluid collection
9. Fracture of the vertebral column

Endoscopic Retrograde Cholangiopancreatography
This detects ductal integrity.

Ultrasound
Insensitive, unreliable and it is better used in children with poor retroperitoneal fat.
Haemoperitoneum may be shown around the area of pancreas.
Pancreatic width/thickness greater than 3 cm may indicate oedema.

MRI
Better soft tissue definition
Bowel motion degrades the image.
Outline of pancreas is however visible for identification of laceration.

Injury to the bowels and mesentery
This is found in only 5%. Small bowel mesenteric injury is five times as common as colonic mesenteric injury. Safe seat belt and displaced lumbar spine injuries are associated with ruptured intra-abdominal hollow viscus.
Retroperitoneal duodenum is the site most commonly ruptured following blunt trauma.

Plain film
This will show pneumoperitoneum and fractured vertebrae or ribs. Gas-distended stomach may indicate splenic injury, or seat belt injury. Pneumoperitoneum may indicate rupture of gas containing hollow viscus such as stomach, colon, small intestines, caecum or rectum. Ground glass appearance is often due to haemoperitoneum.

Ultrasound
This will show haemoperitoneum.

CT scan
Imaging modality of choice
1. Free intraperitoneal fluid (blood)
2. Thick bowel wall
3. Mesenteric infiltration
4. Pneumoperitoneum
5. Presence of large free intraperitoneal fluid (blood) without sign of ruptured solid organ in CT scan suggests ruptured hollow viscus or mesentery.
6. Bowel wall enhancement
7. Bowel dilatation
8. Extraluminal oral contrast extravasation
9. Intraluminal haematoma
10. The main role of CT is to exclude solid organ damage and fractured bones and to raise the suspicion of mesenteric or bowel injury in the presence of haemoperitoneum.

Ultrasound guided intervention
This is used to follow up blood collection, haematomas, confirm haemoperitoneum and post-operative leaks. It is also used in ultrasound-guided drainage of abscess, haematomas and biopsy of mass lesions.

Contrast studies
This is mainly used in follow up of extralumnal lesions following surgery. Water-soluble contrast media like gastrografin must be used instead of barium to avoid barium peritonitis and granuloma formation.

Barium swallow

This is used to diagnose:

1. Gastric volvulus following trauma both organoaxial and mesentero-axial volvulus.
2. Rupture of diaphragm with intrathoracic herniation of abdominal contents and bowels.

Female Patients
Ultrasound

This is the best diagnostic modality for pregnant women and females of reproductive age in which their pregnancy status is not known.

It can show

1. Ovarian cyst
2. Solid debris in ovarian cyst suggestive of bleeding within it
3. Ruptured ectopic pregnancy with large haematoma in the pouch of Douglas.
4. Abruptio placentae of a pregnant uterus with solid mass behind the detached placenta compressing the foetus
5. Foetal viability
6. Foetal demise mostly due to foetal head injury or abruptio placentae
7. Incomplete abortion in case of early pregnancy, with bleeding and retained product of conception.
8. Inevitable/threatened abortion when internal cervical canal diameter is above 2 cm measured by ultrasound.
9. Marginal placental bleeding due to partial placental separation.
10. Ruptured uterus: The foetus may extrude into the pelvis, abdominal cavity or bladder.
11. Ruptured urinary bladder
12. Foetal intracerebral injury or bleeding

Conclusion

In conclusion, it is very important that the casualty officers and other doctors referring patients to radiology departments be very conversant and knows exactly the test that is required in each circumstance and what is the expected result in the light of the current state of the patient. Referral to wrong investigation may produce normal findings (false negative result) simply because the correct investigative modality was not employed leading to time wasting, added cost to the patient and poor patient care. Even with limited facilities in developing countries the information that can be obtained from accurate referral to radiological studies is still very high in the presence of the existing level of training of manpower.

(Adam & Dixon, 2008; Dahnert, 2011; Sutton, 1998 and 2003).

References

1. Boulanger BR, Brenneman FD, Kirkpatrick AW, McLellan BA, Nathens AB. The indeterminate abdominal sonogram in multisystem blunt trauma. J Trauma 1998;45:52-6.
2. Boulanger BR, Brenneman FD, McLellan BA, Rizoli SB, Culhane J, Hamilton P. Aprospective study of emergent abdominal sonography after blunt trauma. J Trauma 1995;39:325-30.
3. Cox EF. Blunt abdominal trauma. A 5 year analysis of 870 patients requiring colostomy. Ann Surg 1984; 199: 467-474.
4. Brofman N, Atri M, Hanson JM, Grinblat L, Chughtai T, Brenneman F. Evaluation of bowel and mesenteric blunt trauma with multidetector CT. Radiographics 2006;26:1119-31.

5.   McGahan JP, Wang L, Richards JR. Focused abdominal US for trauma. Radiographics 2001;21 Spec No:S191-9

6.   Brody JM, Leighton DB, Murphy BL, Abbott GF, Vaccaro JP, Jagminas L, Cioffi WG. CT of blunt trauma bowel and mesenteric injury: typical findings and pitfalls in diagnosis. Radiographics. 2000;20:1525-37.

7.   McKenney KL. Role of US in the diagnosis of intraabdominal catastrophes. Radiographics 1999;19:1332-9.

8.   Roberts JL, Dalen K, Bosanko CM, Jafir SZ. CT in abdominal and pelvic trauma. Radiographics 1993;13:735-52.

9.   Umerah BC. Radiology of trauma. In: Umerah BC (Ed). (1989). Medical practice and the law in Nigeria. Longman, Ikeja, Nigeria, pp 88-94.

10. Lagundoye SB, Itayemi SO. Tension pneumothorax. British Journal of Surgery 1970; 57: 576-580.

11. Eze KC. The role of radiology in the diagnosis and management of a patient with blunt abdominal trauma. Annals of Irrua Medicine 2007, 1: 29-36.

3.9   RADIOLOGICAL FEATURES OF ABDOMINAL TUBERCULOSIS

Definition
Tuberculosis is defined as a multisystemic caseating chronic granulomatous infectious disease caused by *mycobacterium tuberculosis*. It is common in developing countries. Abdominal involvement occurs by swallowing of expectorated sputum containing the mycobacterium, or from haematogenous spread from tuberculous focus in the lung or by drinking infected unpasteurized milk.

Symptoms
Weight loss, abdominal pain, nausea, vomiting, constipation, diarrhoea, palpable abdominal mass, pain, pyrexia and abdominal distension

Radiological investigative modalities
1.   Plain film, chest x-ray, abdominal x-ray
2.   Ultrasound scan, 3.5 MHz curvilinear probe
3.   Barium studies: Barium swallow, meal and follow-through, barium enema
4.   CT scan and Lymphography

Radiological Features

Tuberculous Peritonitis/Ascites
Plain film (plain abdominal radiograph)
The bowel gas pattern may be normal.
Plastic peritonitis: Areas of distension, interspersed with areas of narrowing may indicate stricture or plastic peritonitis.
Diffuse haziness with ground glass pattern: This is accompanied by displacement of bowel gas distribution from peripheral to central location.
Enterolith: Multiple small bowel calculi found in bowels proximal to areas of tuberculous stenosis of small bowel. They may be densely opaque or lamellated or appear as *'pop corn'*.
Pneumoperitoneum: Free intraperitoneal air may occur from perforation of bowel due to tuberculous ulcers.

Ultrasound
Echo-free space with multiple, small, diffuse internal echoes suggestive of high density ascites.
Omental cakes: Thick omentum appearing cake-like with some of it found in fixed immobile bowels, with wide separation of the bowel loops.
Echogenic collapsed floating bowels: The bowels are seen as echogenic masses, most of them are collapsed with few gas-containing bowels floating on top; otherwise, most are in dependent position.

CT scan
High density ascites with CT number of 20 – 45 HU
Thick omentum appearing like cake with irregular soft tissue masses on it due to lymphadenopathy.

The Liver
Plain abdominal radiograph
Calcification: Calcified old tuberculous granulomas appear as multiple round radiodensities in the liver area.

Ultrasound
Granulomas: Spherical area of parenchymal change appearing as 5- 10 mm diameter nodules of well defined hypoechoic areas. These are tuberculous granulomas in early stages. In later stages, they appear hyperechoic due to fibrosis and calcification.
Abscess: Spherical large hypoechoic area of liver destruction with multiple thick internal echoes. It is rare. *Comet tail* appearance due to gas in the abscess may be observed.
Shrunken liver: Marked destruction, distortion or contraction of a whole lobe or segment leads to shrunken liver.
Hepatitis: Generalised inflammatory changes in the liver with multiple pin-point nodular change due to miliary spread of tuberculosis to the liver may be observed.

CT scan
Tuberculous granulomas: Calcified or uncalcified granulomas are identified even when missed by plain film and ultrasound.
Abscess: CT scan will clearly demonstrate liver abscess with the abscess wall; gas may be clearly identified within it. CT number will confirm the abscess.
The size of the liver can be accurately measured in cases of shrunken liver.
Miliary spread to the liver: This is clearly identified and appear as multiple small hypodense spherical lesions in both the right and the left lobes.

Lymphadenopathy
Plain film
Mass lesion: A soft tissue mass lesion displacing the bowel gas pattern to another side is significant for mass lesion.
Duodenum, stomach and large bowels may be so displaced as to confuse the mass with lymphoma or Burkitt's lymphoma.
Bowel compression: Gastric outlet obstruction may be observed in plain film due to compression of gastric antrum. Localised duodenal ileus may be observed due to compression of the duodenum.
Enlargement of duodenal loops: Retroperitoneal lymph nodes close to the pancreas can enlarge or widen the duodenal loop with dilatation of duodenal calibre and gas shadow in dilated duodenal loop clearly identified.

Ultrasound
Multiple spherical hypoechoic solid masses of enlarged lymph nodes in their usual positions. Para-aortic nodes are more commonly enlarged.
Massively enlarged lymph nodes may be confused with lymphoma, Burkitt's lymphoma and gastric carcinoma.
Normal pancreas identified: Ultrasound will identify normal pancreas and show the widened duodenal loop due to lymphadenopathy.

CT scan

CT scan will accurately identify and measure the sizes of the enlarged lymph nodes. CT will show also mediastinal lymphadenopathy.

Lymphography

Enlarged lymph nodes are detected with para-aortic lymph nodes more commonly involved.
Filling defects or central lucencies in enlarged lymph nodes. These are due to caseous areas of necrosis in the centres of the enlarged lymph nodes.
Obstructive features and areas in the drainage lymphatic channels are seen.
Collateral formations are also observed.
Varicose drainage channels are seen emerging from lymph nodes.

Adrenal Glands
Plain films

Calcification: Punctate bilateral calcifications were observed commonly in the West when tuberculosis was common. However this is rare presently.

CT scan

Tumours / mass lesions: Tuberculous granulomas when bilateral may cause Addison's disease. There is deficiency of glucocorticoid and mineralocorticoid hormones. These deficiencies may present variable radiological features in different tissues or organs due to their action on these tissues or organs.

The Oesophagus

Barium swallow will show the following features:
Extrinsic mass effect or compression: This is due to tuberculous mediastinal lymphadenopathy.
Ulcers: Deep ulcers may occur due to tuberculous mediastinal lymphadenopathy eroding into the oesophagus.
Fistulae: Deep ulcers may progress to form fistulae by eroding through the wall of the oesophagus.
Sinus tracts: Intramural dissection of the ulcers may form sinus tracts.

Stricture and scarring: A chronic ulcer scarring the oesophagus and causing short- or long-segment narrowing and stricture.
Oesophagitis: Multiple discrete shallow ulcers are caused by *mycobacterium avium intracellulare* (MAI).
Mortility disorder: Abnormal oesophageal peristalsis from secondary motility disorders also occur and is seen in fluoroscopy or videofluoroscopy.
Tracheobroncho-oesophageal fistula may develop. This is rare.

The Stomach

Barium meal will demonstrate the following findings:
Antral narrowing: Extrinsic tuberculous adenopathy may cause extrinsic mass compression on gastric antrum. The image may mimic gastric cancer or linitis plastica.
Hyperplastic infiltration: This may appear as intramural mass lesion with shouldering and apple-core deformity, similar to what is seen in carcinoma.

Mucosal ulceration: Frank mucosal tuberculous ulcerations may be seen. They are often large and deep ulcers. This may be confused with peptic ulcer disease. Occasionally there is granulomatous mass lesion on which the ulcer develops and this may be misdiagnosed as carcinoma.

Gastric outlet obstruction: Dilated stomach with air-fluid and fluid-fluid levels due to barium and gastric content. Antral narrowing is the cause. Visible gastric peristalsis may be observed and if it occurs in a child may be misdiagnosed as hypertrophic pyloric stenosis especially if there is lymphadenopathy in the area of the gastric antrum. These changes may be of significance in distinguishing it from carcinoma of the stomach.

Thickened gastric mucosa
Linitis plastic: Caused by hyperplastic infiltration, ulceration and annular lesion. It is rare.
Widened retrogastric space: Caused by enlarged retroperitoneal tuberculous lymph nodes.
Fistulas: Antral fistulations are occasionally seen.

The Duodenum
Barium meal and hypotonic duodenography are used to demonstrate the following features:
Thickened duodenal mucosal folds: Distortion, nodularity, thickening and effacement of mucosal pattern are seen in infection by MAI in patients with AIDS.

Extrinsic compressive mass lesion: Due to retroperitoneal lymph node enlargement causing gastric outlet obstruction.
Widened duodenal loops: Carcinoma of the head of pancreas may be simulated.
Post-bulbar ulceration
Small Intestines
Findings in barium follow-through and small bowel enema are as follows:
Circumferential ulcers: Seen in lower ileum and caecum. Single or multiple small or large non-stenotic ulcers. They are transverse ulcers, associated with spasm of ileum and proximal ascending colon.
Aphthoid ulcers: This is not common. However, when seen in tropics where Crohn's disease and Yersinia colitis which are the commonest causes are uncommon should arouse the suspicion of tuberculosis.
Thickened bowel mucosal folds: Irregular, thickened fold with or without dilatation.
Tethered mucosal fold: This indicates desmoplastic reaction. There may also be angulation, kinking and separation of bowel loops.
Wide separation of bowel loops: Due to inflammatory infiltration of bowel wall and mesentery by tuberculous granulomas.
Multiple stenotic lesions: There may be normal intervening bowels between the stenoses.
Small bowel distension with stasis: This occurs proximal to narrow stenotic areas.

Enterolith: Radio-opaque, lamellated or radiolucent enteroliths may cause filling-defects in barium column. Enteroliths are formed in the areas of bowel stasis. Enteroliths are also observed in diverticula and Meckel's diverticulum and these differentials must be excluded as the cause.
Stricture: The fibrosis which follows the ulcers results in narrowing which may be diffuse. There is shortening of the caecum.

Fistulation: This may occur in matted adherent bowels.

Perforation: This may occur due to tuberculous erosion or ulcer perforation. There may be extravasation of barium and/or pneumoperitoneum. Water soluble contrast should be used if this is suspected.

Ileo-Caecal Region
Barium enema will demonstrate the following findings:
Commonest site of tuberculous lesion of gastrointestinal tract observed in over 80 – 90% of cases.
Rapid emptying of terminal ileum: Due to irritability of terminal ileum caused by tuberculous inflammation.
Thickened ileo-caecal valve with mass effect: This may be confused with carcinoma.
Rigid pipe-stem caecum: This is associated with cicatricial shortening.
Inverted-umbrella sign: Change in angle of ileocaecal valve with wide patulous and patent ileocaecal valve caused by narrowing of the immediate adjacent terminal ileum and associated rigidity of caecum.
Caecal filling-defects. This is due to Peyer's patches and granulomas.
Ulceration: Caecal ulceration is often multiple, transverse and circumferential. It is commonly diffuse.
Ileocaecal fistulas, sinus tracts and *ileocaecal perforation*
Enterocutaneous fistulas: Deep ulcers, fissures, and sinus tracts or perforation may lead to enterocutaneous fistulas.

The Colon
Barium enema: The disease involves right colon and is often segmental.
Coned Caecum: Spasm and transmural fibrosis lead to rigid contracted cone-shaped caecum.
Ulceration: Transverse or circumferential ulcerations which may be diffuse or annular are seen.
Thumb-printing: Mucosal irregularity with spiculation and thumb-printing may occur.

Thickening of colonic wall: It is caused by granulomatous infiltration and caseation.
Stricture: There is segmental narrowing involving variable length of the colon. Short-segment narrowing with apple-core deformity and shouldering simulating carcinoma may also be observed.
Pseudopolyps: Single or multiple inflammatory pseudopolyps are observed.
Shortening: Numerous areas of ulcers, fibrosis and stricture lead to shortening.
Hour-glass stricture: This may develop and grossly narrowing the lumen or calibre of the colon.

The Rectum
Fistula-in-ano: Both high and low types. May need fistulography for accurate differentiation and diagnosis.
Ischiorectal abscess: This is diagnosed with CT scan.

CT Scan of Colon and Small Intestine
1. This detects glandular enlargement with peripheral enhancement due to central necrosis. It also detects the presence of ascites it detects bowel wall thickenings and enteroliths.

Other Important Sites
Genitourinary System
Even though the organs are contained in the abdomen, their involvement by TB is more accurately discussed under genitourinary system TB. However a summary of features seen include:
Calcification: Calcification of urinary bladder wall, the ureters and kidneys may be seen.

Calculi: this develops in the bladder, ureters and kidneys.

Cavitation: In kidney resembling renal papillary necrosis.

Stenosis: Ureteric stenosis, renal pelvis or calyceal stenosis.

Filling-defects: In the ureter, kidney or bladders due to granulomas appearing like polyps.

Stricture: Ureteric stricture occurs and the ureter may have a beaded appearance.

Hydronephrosis: Hydronephrosis due to ureteric stricture narrowing the lumen and causing back pressure effect are seen in many patients.

Other findings: These include small size kidney, autonephrectomy and small contracted urinary bladder.

The Chest

The focus of infection is the chest and it spreads to the abdomen from swallowed sputum and haematogenous spread from the lung. Therefore, chest x-ray is mandatory to exclude the presence of active or healed tuberculous lesion. Features that may be seen include:

Lung fibrosis: This is thickened irregular strands of lung tissue.

Cavitation: This denotes active lesion

Reduction in lung volume due to lung fibrosis and fibrocystic changes.

Mediastinal shift often from lung fibrosis or obstruction of bronchi leading to atelectasis.

Other findings are *destroyed lung syndrome, fibrocystic changes, nodular changes* due to tuberculous infiltrates, *pleural effusion, bronchopneumonia* and *miliary tuberculosis.*

(Adam & Dixon, 2008; Dahnert, 2011; Sutton, 1998 and 2003, Palmer & Reeder 2001).

References

1. Pereira JM, Madureira AJ, Vieira A, Ramos I. Abdominal tuberculosis: imaging features. Eur J Radiol 2005; 55:173-80.
2. Levy AD, Shaw JC, Sobin LH. Secondary tumors and tumorlike lesions of the peritoneal cavity: imaging features with pathologic correlation. Radiographics 2009;29:347-73.
3. Burrill J, Williams CJ, Bain G, Conder G, Hine AL, Misra RR. Tuberculosis: a radiologic review. Radiographics 2007;27:1255-73.
4. Tan KK, Chen K, Sim R. The spectrum of abdominal tuberculosis in a developed country: a single institution's experience over 7 years. J Gastrointest Surg 2009;13:142-7.
5. Vanhoenacker FM, De Backer AI, Op de BB, Maes M, Van Altena R, Van Beckevoort D, Kersemans P, De Schepper AM. Imaging of gastrointestinal and abdominal tuberculosis. Eur Radiol 2004; 14 Suppl 3:E103-15.
6. Andronikou S, Wieselthaler N. Modern imaging of tuberculosis in children: thoracic, central nervous system and abdominal tuberculosis. Pediatr Radiol 2004; 34:861-75.
7. Ihekwaba FN. Abdominal tuberculosis: a study of 881 cases. J R Coll Surg Edinb 1993;38:293-5.
8. Akinkuolie AA, Adisa AO, Agbakwuru EA, Egharevba PA, Adesunkanmi AR. Abdominal tuberculosis in a Nigerian teaching hospital. Afr J Med Med Sc 2008;37:225-9.

3.10 RADIOLOGICAL DIFFERENTIAL DIAGNOSIS OF RECTAL BLEEDING

Definition
Rectal bleeding also known as haematochezia is the passage of blood through the rectum. It is also called bleeding per rectum. Usually, the blood is bright red and fresh signifying a bleeding source which origin must be made known to exclude malignancy or the risk of anaemia from repeated bleeding or shock from possible severe bleeding.

Other names
Blood in stool, haematochezia, blood in faeces, bloody stool or blood-mixed stool.

Site of bleeding:
The bleeding site for bright red rectal bleeding is usually located distal to the ligament of Treitz in the jejunum in the lower gastrointestinal tract and most frequently much lower down when the transit time of the blood is very short and in the order of a few minutes or a few hours. However, massive severe bleeding from the higher gastrointestinal tract can also appear as bright red rectal bleeding especially if there is associated diarrhoea or proximal intestinal obstruction that prevents vomiting of such bleeding.

Causes of the bleeding

Colorectal region
This constitutes over 70% of the source of the bleeding, which is usually massive bleeding
Diverticula (most common) (25%),
Colonic angiodysplasia (2nd most common cause), haemorrhoids, anal fissure.
Iatrogenic injuries, mostly biopsies (low rate of bleeding and small bleeding)
Crohn's disease, ulcerative colitis, infective colitis
Polyposis, benign and malignant tumour
Ischaemic colitis, vascular thrombosis/infarction and mesenteric varices

Small intestine
Polyposis, leiomyoma, hemangioma, metastases and other benign and malignant tumours
Ulcers, diverticula, Meckel diverticulum, Crohn's disease, ulcerative colitis,
Vascular malformation, visceral artery aneurysm, aortoenteric fistula

Appearances of different types of rectal bleeding
Rectal bleeding can take many varieties of appearances. It can be bright red, reddish purple, clotted blood, black and tarry, or occult (when the bleeding is not visible to the unaided eye).
The colour of the bleeding is determined by the location of origin in the gastrointestinal tract, the quantity or severity of the bleeding and the time the blood has stayed within the colon.
Location of origin in the colon: The closer the bleeding site is to the anal orifice, the more chances the blood will be a brighter red and vice versa. Therefore, bleeding from the anus, rectum, and the sigmoid colon tend to be bright red, whereas bleeding from the transverse colon and the right colon, which are several feet away from the anal orifice, tend to be dark red or reddish purple coloured.

Location of origin in the GI tract: Melaena stool is said to occur when the bleeding is seen as black, tarry and foul smelling materials or blood-mixed stool. Melaena usually signifies bleeding is from the upper gastrointestinal tract proximal to the ligament of Treitz in the jejunum, ileum or proximal colon. Bleeding from oesophageal varices, peptic ulcer, gastritis, Mallory Weiss syndrome and duodenitis may be seen as melaena.

Transit time within GI tract: Blood from the sigmoid colon and the rectum usually does not stay in the colon long enough for the bacteria to turn it black so it is bright red or frank blood. Melaena occurs when the blood has been in the colon for long time, long enough for the bacteria in the colon to break down haemoglobin in the blood into its chemicals components (haematin) that are black in colour. It is an oxidation process. Such time is in the order of about ten to fourteen hours.

Massive bleeding from peptic ulcer, duodenitis, gastritis, enteritis in the right colon, small intestine, or gastric ulcer, or duodenal / colonic lesion can cause rapid transit of the blood through the gastrointestinal tract by the mere strength of its volume and result in bright red rectal bleeding. In this case, the blood is moving through the colon so rapidly that there is not enough time for the bacteria to break down the blood to its components and alter it black.

Treatment

Endoscopic treatment

Intra-arterial vasopressin infusion therapy

Transcatheter embolization treatment using superselective catheterization

Laparoscopic surgeries for removal of lesions

Open surgeries for removal of the tumours and securing haemostasis.

Differential diagnosis of the causes
Diverticulitis

Diverticulitis is the most common complication of diverticula disease, seen in about 10 per cent of affected persons. Faecal retention within the diverticulum resulting to ischaemic necrosis with micro-perforation is responsible for the inflammation. Pericolic fat-walled abscess cavities may result. Eccentric rupture of area of wall weakness and intimal thickening of vasa recta over the dome of the diverticula is the cause of the bleeding. Rectal bleeding is however, more common on the right side even though diverticula are more common at the rectal region. On sonography, pericolic abscess is observed as a low reflective collection close to the bowel wall and surrounded by inflamed hyperechoic fat. On CT scan, there is the combination of diverticular changes with signs of inflammation with '*fat stranding*' and oedema producing a generalized increased attenuation. Abscess with gas is seen in over 30% with extravasations of intraluminal contrast due to perforation or fistula.

Colonic angiodysplasia

This is degenerative changes in normal vessels in the intestinal submucosa caused by normal daily colonic contractions, leading to its dilatation and formation of arteriovenous fistulae due to increasing age. It is the most common vascular lesion of the GI tract. The descending colon and rectosigmoid are involved in about 25% of cases while caecum and ascending colon is affected in about 75%, involving mainly the antimesenteric border. The lesion may be identified in colonoscopy but is not seen in barium enema examination as they become collapsed due to their soft nature. On radionuclide study, there is increased tracer accumulation of technetium 99 m-labelled red blood cells. On angiography, there is demonstration of arterial tufts, which are tangles, or network of vessels seen in arterial phase of the study and along the antimesenteric border. Contrast extravasation into the lumen of the bowel confirms and shows the site of the bleeding. There may also be observed early filling of draining ileocolic veins with densely dilated tortuous ileocolic veins seen in the late venous phase.

Colorectal carcinoma

Double contrast barium enema will show fungating polypoid mass appearing as filling-defect, annular ulcerating mass with apple core deformity, saddle lesion and signet ring appearance signifying scirrhous carcinoma. Curvilinear calcification within the mass on plain abdominal radiograph signifies mucinous adenocarcinoma and this may be better demonstrated on CT scan. On CT study, mucinous adenocarcinoma will appear as a hypo-attenuating mass with co-existing hypodense enlarged lymph nodes.

Haemorrhoids

Haemorrhoids, or piles, are distended, valveless veins at the lowest part of the portal system consisting of prolapsed varicose veins lining the anal submucosa through the anal canal. They are typically sited at the 3, 7 and 11 o'clock positions when the patient lies supine. Raising intra-abdominal pressure that tends to slow venous return rate and engorges the anal mucosa network of veins is believed to trigger piles. Straining while defecating due to fibre-free diet and pregnancy raise intra-abdominal pressure. Diseases that cause portal hypertension such as cirrhosis or hepatic congestion also cause haemorrhoid. The presenting symptoms are anal itching; aching, pain, tenesmus, rectal bleeding or permanent prolapsed of the piles. Males are more affected and present longer history of duration. Physical examination is adequate for diagnosis of haemorrhoids. However, abdominal sonography and CT may be required to diagnose the underlying cause.

Haemangioma

This is another rare colonic mesenchymal tumour. They are often multiple and located in the more distal part of the colon and are reported to be always multiple. On plain films, calcified phleboliths are seen in the rectal area. The lesion is asymptomatic but the commonest observed symptom is rectal bleeding. Endoscopy will diagnose the lesion and it is different from degenerative angiodysplasia.

Dieulafoy's lesion (*exulceratio simplex Dieulafoy*)

This is the occurrence of a large dilated and tortuous arteriole in the wall of the stomach but may also occur in other parts of gastrointestinal tracts such as duodenum, jejunum, colon and oesophagus and surgical anastomotic sites. The arteriole erodes and bleeds causing massive life-threatening haematemesis, recurrent haematemesis with melaena, or melaena without haematemesis. Massive haematemesis from this lesion or those in the colon may be seen as rectal bleeding. It is diagnosed using angiography, endoscopy or endoscopic ultrasound; and sclerotherapy, photocoagulation and embolisation can be performed to obliterate it.

Anal fissure

An anal fissure is defined as a tear in the anal lining. It usually extends into the internal anal sphincter for significant rectal bleeding to occur. As the fissure increases, the internal anal sphincter goes into spasm, causing widening of the tear, leading to impairment of healing process and pain after defecation. The fact that the tear is exposed to faecal matter also slows healing. Patients with an anal fissure may present with rectal bleeding, tearing sensation, burning pain, and dull prolonged pain after defecation or itching around the anus. Passage of hard or large stool or severe diarrhoea is usually the cause of the anal fissure. Anal fissures are diagnosed clinically based on the symptoms and physical examinations. A fissure most frequently appears in the 12 or 6 o'clock position when the patient lies supine and when located in other locations may mean associated underlying disorder is responsible.

Meckel's diverticulum

Meckel's diverticulum is a vestige of the embryonic omphalomesenteric duct. It is seen in about 2% of the population, is asymptomatic before 2 years of age, located within 2 feet of ileocaecal valve and measure about 2 feet in length. They are asymptomatic in up to 40%. The diverticulum is located within 6 feet of the terminal ileum and in the antimesenteric border containing all four layers of bowel. It contains ectopic gastric or pancreatic mucosa in up to 50%, which aids its visualization, and for those that bleed, 95% contain ectopic gastric mucosa. ^{99m}Tc-pertechnetate scintigraphy is diagnostic, has a low radiation dose and detection rate is improved with ranitidine premedication. On angiography, detection of vitelline artery which is an anomalous distal branch of superior mesenteric artery is characteristic.

Solitary rectal ulcer syndrome

This is a condition in which an area of ulceration is observed characteristically on the anterior wall of the rectum during recto-sigmoid endoscopy study. It is believed to be part of a spectrum of abnormalities seen in rectal prolapsed. The presentation includes difficulty in passing stool, prolonged straining, bleeding per rectum and the passage of excess mucus. On barium enema study, there is an ulcer crater, adjacent mucosal irregularity due to hyperaemia or nodularity due to formation of granulation tissue and deformity of the bowel wall at the site of the ulcer due to stricture. *Colitis cystica profunda*, which is a polypoid change at the margins of the ulcer due to retention cysts, is observed in both barium study and sigmoidoscopy. Rectal bleeding may be severe as to require blood transfusion in some cases. Defecography often demonstrate previously unrecognized intra-anal intussusception as the cause of the mucosa injury.

Juvenile polyposis

This is a rare autosomal dominant disease is characterized by growth of multiple juvenile polyps in the gastrointestinal tract. The polyps consist of both harmatomas with cystic epithelial tubules growing beyond the lamina propria giving the '*Swiss cheese effect*', and adenomas, and over 80% are found in the rectosigmoid area. Over 75% are seen in children and by 20 years, over 85% has manifested. The patients present with diarrhoea, rectal prolapsed, intussusception, anaemia, protein-losing enteropathy and rectal bleeding which could be intermittent and chronic. The condition is diagnose clinically when any number of polyp is seen in a patient with family history or there are multiple polyps throughout the GI tract of usually 50-200 in number or polyps of size above 5- 10 cm is observed in the colon. The polyps are diagnosed with double contrast barium GI studies where they appear as multiple oval filling-defects. On CT scan, the polyps are identified as oval densities with smooth round contour. On MRI, active growth is suggested by high signal intensity on T2-weighted images.

Amoebiasis

Infestation by cystic form *Entamoeba histolytica* which releases invasive cytolytic enzyme that invades the bowel wall and cause segmental or diffuse colitis with granular or ulcerating bowel mucosa appearing as aphthoid ulcerations. The ulcers have shaggy mucosal margins with granulation tissue, which may bleed resulting in rectal bleeding. It is common in the tropics and stool examination for the parasite is the definitive diagnosis. Barium enema will show shallow or deep ulcers with strictures. The granulomatous mass lesions may cause irregular strictures that resemble carcinoma. However, the mucosal outline is preserved in barium enema study unlike the appearance in carcinoma where it is destroyed. In about 15% of cases, colonic amoebiasis may embolise to the liver and cause amoebic liver abscess.

Kaposi's sarcoma

This is seen as diffuse or multifocal submucosal lumps that may combine into a single mass. GIT is the third most affected site after the skin and lymph nodes. The rectum is the most common affected area in the GI tract. There is high affectation of GI tract when the skin or lymph nodes are affected. The lesion may be asymptomatic but there may be rectal bleeding. On double contrast study, the lesion may appear as thickened nodular folds, or as multiple submucosal nodules, which may have umblicated centre. It may also appear as polypoid submucous mass which could reach 3 cm in diameter or as grossly narrowing the rectal lumen with linitis plastica appearance due to infiltrating nature of the lesion.

Tuberculosis

This could be from bovine origin through drinking unpasteurized milk and is endemic in tropical regions. The patient presents with ascites due to peritoneal involvement, lymphadenopathy favour TB and rectal bleeding. The bleeding is from the ulceration, which could erode into microvessels. On sonography, central caseous necrosis in lymph nodes gives it an appearance of a hypoechoic centre. Peripheral enhancement of such nodes of CT suggests tuberculosis. Tuberculous ulcers have a shaggy edge, hypertrophic or fibrotic forms have an inflammatory mass simulating lymphoma and stenosis of the bowel lumen demonstrable on barium studies. Barium enema signs of tuberculosis include a contracted conical-shaped caecum with a patulous ileocaecal valve, a dilated terminal ileum and transverse ulcers with hourglass stricture with well-defined transition from normal bowel.

Endometriosis

This is seeding of endometrial tissue of the uterus to distant organs and tissues. Gastrointestinal seeding occurs in about 10-37% of cases, involving mainly the sigmoid colon, small-bowel loops that extend to the pelvis, and rarely the caecum. Endometriosis is the third commonest cause of benign filling-defect within the colon after adenoma and lipoma. The patients present with cyclic rectal bleeding that is related to the menses. Serosal implants causing fibrosis, contraction of bowel wall, mass effect with preserved mucosal surface through which rectal bleeding occurs. High signal on T1-weighted fat-suppressed sequences, with 'shading' on T2-weighting due to residual blood products are seen if the mass contains a cystic component. Localized mass-effect with characteristic contracted mucosal folds is demonstrated by double-contrast barium enema study.

Villous Adenoma of Colon

This occurs with equal frequency in both males and females and is found in rectosigmoid colon in over 75% cases. It is associated with other GI tract tumour in 25%. The tumour is often broad–based measuring about 2 cm in diameter and has multiple frond-like mucosal projections. On barium meal, there is sponge-like appearance with barium entering many crevices due to villous nature of the tumour. The tumour may appear with brush border or change in size and may decrease in size in post evacuation films. On CT scan, the tumour shows heterogeneous hypodensity which is ascribed to copious mucin trapped within papillary projections. This tumour occurs in 7% of the population and 30% of it is associated with malignant transformation and invasion of surrounding tissues and organs.

Sacrococcygeal Chordoma

On plain abdominal films, there is a huge presacral mass, which does not extend posteriorly. There is lytic destruction of the sacrum and coccyx by a mass with peripheral calcifications and bone sclerosis in periphery of the tumour. On sonography, the tumour is solid with some cystic areas within it. CT scan shows a lobulated soft tissue mass with areas of hypodensity due to myxoid contents and areas of osteolysis. On MRI, the tumour is hypo- or isointense relative to the muscle on T1WI with hyperintense areas due to haemorrhage or mucinous content within it. The tumour is hyperintense on T2WI similar to nucleus pulposus. Contrast enhancement is heterogenous.

Colitis cystica profunda

Colitis cystica profunda is a disease characterized by multiple cysts that are filled with mucin and located within the mucosa and submucosa of the colon, mostly the rectum. The cause is unknown. The usual presentation is diarrhoea, abdominal pain, rectal bleeding, and prolapse of the rectum. Large cysts may occasionally cause rectal obstruction. Barium enema reveals, multiple polypoid filling defects within the colon with some elongated polyps. The mucosal pattern is remarkably normal.

Coloreactal lymphoma

Most primary colorectal lymphomas arise in the caecum and rectum and are usually of Burkitt or mucosa associated lymphoid tissue (MALT) subtypes. They are usually small, diffuse or segmental in distribution and tend to have intact mucosa. Solitary polypoid type may be seen usually in the caecum. There may be strictures, which are long-length, fissure and ulcerative changes within masses with fistulations. The patients presents with symptoms of bowel obstruction and rectal bleeding. Colonoscopy with biopsy for histology is diagnostic. Polypoid type appears as filling-defect on double barium enema studies histology is required to differentiate it from carcinoma.

Radiation colitis

Acute bowel injury due to radiation occurs where the total dose of radiation used exceeded 30 Gy (3000 rad). Radiation colitis is results from occlusive endarteritis in the company of thrombosis and fibrosis. The radiations that induces the colitis are to organs such as the prostate, the cervix, the uterus, urinary bladder or there gynaecological malignancies in which the rectum lies in the radiation field. On barium enema study, bowel wall deformity or fistulation are demonstrated. Radiation enteritis telangiectasia and ulceration, which are chronic changes of the radiation, are responsible for the rectal bleeding. On CT, there is diffuse rectal wall thickening, presacral space widening and thickening of the mesorectal fat and fascia.

Peutz-Jeghers syndrome

It is found mostly in the small bowel in 95%, colon (30%) and stomach (25%) in that order. In the rectum, it appears as multiple scattered small polyps of a maximum size of 3-4 cm in diameter, which are adenomatous premalignant polyps unlike the ones in the stomach, which are harmatomatous polyps. The respiratory tract and the urinary bladder may be involved by adenoma. Endoscopy is used for diagnosis of the polyps and removal of those measuring more than 5 mm in diameter. Barium studies will show the polyps as multiple scattered intra-luminal filling-defects. Both CT and MRI will also diagnose the polyps with its characteristic findings. It is associated with many types of cancer such as pancreas, breast, endometrial, ovarian, testicular and GI tract carcinomas.

Ulcerative colitis

Rectal involvement is the rule and the pattern of involvement is in continuity to the proximal spread without skip lesions. Rectal mucosal biopsy is essential for establishing the type of colitis while infective causes are excluded by laboratory tests. Endoscopy is highly sensitive as it shows vascular changes at the same time biopsy can be taken. CT scan is also a useful diagnostic modality. Wall thickening of about 4 mm or more is noted. Mucosal fat increase is characteristic of chronic ulcerative colitis. Erosions and submucosal haemorrhage are responsible for rectal bleeding. These give the mucosal a granular appearance on barium enema study.

Crohn's Disease

There is full thickness, asymmetrical involvement with skip-lesions unlike in ulcerative colitis that is continuous. Eventually a thickened, rigid segment of bowel, with creeping mesenteric fat results. Apthous ulcers, rose-thorn ulcers, fistulas and cobblestone pattern are observed in barium and CT studies. Adenocarcinoma and lymphoma may be seen representing a slightly increased risk of malignancy observed in this condition.

Ischemic colitis

In this condition, the normal blood flow decreases to about 20% of normal and is related to disease of small blood vessel leading to tissue hypoxia. This leads to mucosal congestion, tissue necrosis, mucosal ulcerations and oedema of submucosa and haemorrhage. There are many precipitating causes including thrombosis, intestinal obstruction, cardiovascular diseases, shock, bowel incarceration and vasculitis. On plain abdominal film, there will be segmental indentations of the colon. On barium studies film, there will be thumb-printing signifying mucosa haemorrhage. On colour Doppler sonography, the blood flow is absent or scarcely detectable with loss of arterial flow. CT may detect intra-arterial thrombus in superior or inferior mesenteric arteries. CT may also show shaggy mucosal appearance with obvious pericolic oedema and loss of haustral marking. On angiography, there will be mild quickening of arteriovenous transit time with or without small winding ectatic draining veins due to recanalisation of collaterals.

Prostate carcinoma

Carcinoma of the prostate is found in men aged 50 years and above and can present with rectal bleeding. Presenting symptoms of prostatic carcinomas frequently include signs of prostatism, hesitancy, haematuria, bone pain, pathological fractures from osseous metastases, uraemia, local haemorrhage and rectal bleeding from increased local fibrinolysin activity. Prostatic enlargement can be diagnosed by digital examination but sonography is accurate at measuring the size and volume. Both CT and MRI can conclusively diagnose prostatic enlargement. Histology is required to confirm that the prostatic mass is malignant.

Pneumatosis coli

Tear in the mucosa of bowels most likely allow gas or gas-forming microorganisms to enter the wall. Once started, a situation is reached when the lesion becomes self-maintaining. It may present with diarrhoea or constipation, and rectal bleeding from superficial bowel mucosal erosions. It can be asymptomatic. In plain radiography, there are multiple gas lucencies within the bowel. There are many causes including trauma, inflammatory diseases, recent surgery, radiation and ischaemic colitis.

Gardner syndrome

This has a variety of extraintestinal manifestations arising from mesenchymal cells. Such soft tissue tumours include sebaceous cysts, leiomyomas, fibromas, lipofibromas, lipomas, leiomyomas and neurofibromas. Other tumours include malignant fibrous tissue desmoid tumours and keloids. Gardner syndrome is a variant of familial polyposis syndrome. The presence of any one or more of these tumours associated with colonic polyposis is highly suggestive of Gardner syndrome.

Neurofibromatosis

Most of the reported colonic involvement by neurofibromatosis is in children. In this age group, the usual presentation is with intussusception or rectal bleeding. When the disease is disseminated, the gut is uncommonly involved. In some occasions, sole involvement of the gut can occur without any cutaneous manifestations and in such cases, biopsy of the lesion for histology is the arbiter. There is a slightly increased risk of malignant degeneration in colonic adenoma due to neurofibromatosis.

Typhlitis

This condition occurs in patients on treatment for malignancy, acute leukaemia on cytotoxic drug treatment, bone marrow transplantation in patients with aplastic anaemia, lymphoma, or AIDS. There are inflammatory changes leading to bowel necrosis and intestinal perforation. Multidetector CT (MDCT) reveals caecal distension and striking circumferential thickening of the caecal wall. This could be hypodense when oedema is present. Free fluid is noted when the terminal ileum is involved. Pneumatosis of the caecal wall is a very specific sign though rare sign, pneumoperitoneum, and pericolic collection can also occur.

Colonic lipomas

Colonic lipomas are slow-growing, benign and the most frequent submucosal tumours of the colon found most commonly in the right side of the colon. Majority of them are discovered as incidental finding or may be a cause of intestinal obstruction when they act as lead points for intussusceptions. In such conditions, the patient may present with abdominal pain, vomiting and rectal bleeding. The tumour is pliable and distensible and these are its distinguishing features. On barium enema, the mass is seen as a 3-5 cm smooth-surfaced filling-defect within the sigmoid colon. The mass is intraluminal and makes an obtuse angles with the normal colonic wall, without displacing the colonic lumen.

Stromal cell tumours (leiomyomas)

These are benign spindle or epitheloid tumours derived from mesenchyme. Colonic stromal cell tumours constitute less than 5% of these lesions seen in the gut and are rare in the anorectal region. Most patients are asymptomatic but rectal bleeding from mucosal ulceration, melaena, and intestinal obstruction may occur when they act as lead point for intussusception. On barium study, this tumour is seen as intraluminal filling-defect arising from the colonic submucosal. Biopsy for histology will differentiate it from numerous masses with such features. In adult, if seen with intestinal obstruction, malignant change should be suspected.

Viral haemorrhagic fever or viral pneumonia

Rectal bleeding initially is seen in this condition and may present with bleeding from other body orifices such as haemoptysis, haematemesis, vaginal bleeding or urethral bleeding. The implicated organisms are usually those that cause viral haemorrhagic fever and rectal bleeding may be an important diagnostic criteria. They include yellow fever, hansa fever, q-fever etc. Other viruses such as *cytomegalovirus, herpes simplex virus,* infectious mononucleosis and Rocky Mountain spotted fever, also cause bleeding from orifices such as rectal bleeding and haemoptysis.

Other infective colitis

There are many fungal, bacterial and viral organisms that can cause colitis with rectal bleeding. Infective colitis is defined as inflammatory bowel disease caused by infections. It is seen mostly in persons with poor hygiene or in immunocompromised patients. Clostridium difficiles causes pseudomembranous colitis, shigella dysentreiae causes shigellosis, which is a type of enterohaemorrhagic colitis, a group of Eschaericha coli O157:H7 also causes enterohaemorrhagic colitis. Actinomyces spp, Candida albicans, Aspergillus spp, Cryptococcus spp, Cocidioides spp, Pneumocystis jiroveci and atypical mycobacterium are also some of the implicated infective organisms. Some of these organisms secrete cytolethal distending toxins that cause cell apoptosis and mucosal ulcers. On colonoscopy, there could be redness of colonic mucosa, mucosal ulcer, and petechial bleeding or bleeding ulcers. Microbiological studies of rectal mucosal swab are required for accurate diagnosis.

(Adam & Dixon, 2008; Dahnert, 2011; Sutton, 1998 and 2003, Palmer & Reeder 2001).

References

1. Brandon JL, Schroeder S, Furuta GT, Capocelli K, Masterson JC, Fenton LZ. CT imaging features of eosinophilic colitis in children. Pediatr Radiol 2013;43(6):697-702.
2. Bento J, Magalhães A, Moura CS, Hespanhol V. Henoch-Schönlein purpura: a clinical case with dramatic presentation. BMJ Case Rep. 2010;2010.
3. White JS, Skelly RT, Gardiner KR, Laird J, Regan MC. Intravasation of barium sulphate at barium enema examination. Br J Radiol 2006;79(943):e32-5.
4. Chaptini L, Nammour F, Peikin S. Rectal bleeding and abdominal mass. Gut. 2006;55(1):15, 40.
5. Michalski JM, Gay H, Jackson A, Tucker SL, Deasy JO. Radiation dose-volume effects in radiation-induced rectal injury. Int J Radiat Oncol Biol Phys 2010;76(3 Suppl):S123-9.
6. Olde Bekkink M, McCowan C, Falk GA, Teljeur C, Van de Laar FA, Fahey T. Diagnostic accuracy systematic review of rectal bleeding in combination with other symptoms, signs and tests in relation to colorectal cancer. Br J Cancer 2010;102(1):48-58.

3.11 RADIOLOGICAL FINDINGS IN PNEUMOPERITONEUM

Definitions
Pneumoperitoneum is defined as free air or gas within the peritoneal cavity.

Importance
Over 90% of cases of pneumoperitoneum seen in acute abdominal cases will require emergency surgery.

Causes of Diagnostically Important Pneumoperitoneum
Disease of Gastrointestinal Tract
Perforated peptic ulcer, perforated gastric ulcer, perforated appendix, ingested foreign, body perforation, ruptured diverticulum, necrotising enterocolitis with perforation, toxic megacolon perforation, intestinal obstruction with perforation, meconium ileus, Hirschsprung's disease, imperforate anus, intestinal volvulus, neoplasm, bands and adhesions, strangulated hernia and necrotising enterocolitis

Trauma
Blunt trauma to bowels, compressed air towards anus, perforating foreign body e.g. thermometer and cardiopulmonary resuscitation with gastric perforation

Iatrogenic perforation
Laparoscopy, laparotomy/previous surgery, leaking surgical anastomosis / effect of diathermy, enema tube tip injury, endoscopic perforation, diagnostic pneumoperitoneum, vaginal cuff perforation and vaginal delivery with vaginal tear

(This must be remembered in postpartum period to avoid unnecessary laparotomy).

Others causes
Penetrating abdominal injury, ruptured urinary bladder, ruptured abscess, idiopathic gastric perforation Congenital gastric muscle defect), endoscopic biopsy, abdominal catheter perforation, perforated uterus /vagina, diaphragmatic eventration and emphysematous cholecystitis.

Causes of Pneumoperitoneum without Peritonitis
Air within post-operative abdomen, peritoneal dialysis, laparoscopy, emphysema, pneumonia, metastases, pneumomediastinum, entry through female genital tract/coitus/skying, pulmonary-peritoneal fistula, intermittent positive pressure ventilation, silent perforation which sealed off, perforated jejunal diverticulosis, intra-abdominal therapeutic embolization and gas from pneumatosis intestinalis.

Causes of False Pneumoperitoneum
Chilaiditi's syndrome (interposition of gas filled colon between the right hemidiaphragm and the right lobe of the liver), subdiaphragmatic fat, curvilinear pulmonary collapse, uneven diaphragm, distended viscus between liver and diaphragm, omental fat between liver and diaphragm, subpulmonary pneumothorax, intramural gas seen in pneumatosis cystoidis intestinalis and apposition of walls of two gas distended bowels resembling Rigler's sign.

Radiographic Sign of Pneumoperitoneum
Cupola sign
This is the collection of gas under the hemidiaphragm. This is most frequently seen in erect chest radiograph but may also be seen in erect abdomen if the gas is in large amount and patient sits or stands for at least 10 minutes before the radiographic exposure.

Rigler's sign
There is visualisation of the inner and outer walls of the intestine due to gas existing outside the intestinal wall. Caution is necessary in the interpretation of this sign as adherence of two bowel walls may make their inner walls visible and may be erroneously interpreted as inner and outer walls.

Football sign
Free gas, rounded or oval in shape may collect in the centre of abdomen usually over some fluid collection. The oval shaped gas appears as lucent football in the centre of the abdomen. However very large amount of gas may outline the whole of the abdominal cavity.

Triangle sign
Triangle-shaped pocket of gas collects outside the outer walls of three different bowel loops.

Urachal sign
Middle umbilical ligament (urachus) visualized as free gas outlines it. Lateral view is required for improved identification.

Doges cap sign
Triangle-shaped gas collection is seen in the Morrison's pouch in the posterior renal space.

Peritoneal reflection visualisation
Visualisation of the peritoneum in the inner surface of anterior abdominal wall. Reflection of peritoneum in the inner surface of anterior abdominal wall when large amount of gas lies on either wall of the peritoneum.
The medial umbilical ligament which is the obliterated umbilical arteries may be outlined by free gas when large amount of gas collects in the peritoneal cavity.

"Inverted V" sign
Both lateral umbilical ligaments can be outlined by large amount of gas. The lateral umbilical ligaments contain the inferior epigastric vessels.

Visualisation of inferior edge of the liver
Free gas in the subhepatic space may outline the inferior edge of the liver. It is seen in over 50% of large pneumoperitoneum.

Ligamentum teres sign
Visualisation of legamentum teres. Free air/gas appearing as linear area of hyperlucency or sharp vertical hyperlucent slit. This marks visualisation of posterior free edge of falciform ligament.

"Mustache" sign
Gas trapped below central tendon of the diaphragm appearing as mustache.

Parahepatic air collection
Free gas bubbles trapped lateral to the right edge of the liver. This is seen between the liver and the anterior abdominal wall.

Liver overlay sign
Large quantity of gas overlies the anterior surface of the liver.

Outline of diaphragmatic muscle slip
Two or three 6 – 14 cm and 6 – 10 mm-wide soft tissue, directed vertically, towards diaphragmatic dome, is outlined in the superior part of the abdomen.

Ligamentum teres notch
There is visualisation of inverted V-shaped area of hyperlucency located at the under surface of the liver.

Post-operative pneumoperitoneum
During laparotomy, air normally enters the peritoneal cavity but this is absorbed within 3 to 5 days. If identical radiographic technique is used any increase in volume of free gas identified within the abdomen after 72 hours postoperatively denotes another perforation or anastomotic leak. Another perforation may be due to umbilical vein catheterization, nasogastric tube, infection, ulcers, endoscopic procedures or other invasive procedures

Pneumoperitoneum in Ultrasound
Ultrasound appearance of pneumoperitoneum is as a result of scattering of the ultrasound waves at the soft tissue and air interface which is accompanied by reverberation of the waves between the air and the transducer. The end result of these is the usual increased echogenicity of the air or air-structure interface which is usually peritoneal stripe (high-amplitude linear echo). There is also accompanying posterior acoustic reverberation echoes with features of comet-tail appearance and the ensuing image changes with change in position of the patient. The collection of air itself is appearing echogenic and dirty.

Reverberation echoes
Free intraperitoneal air will appear as echogenic structure with reverberation. Reverberation is increased echogenicity of the peritoneal strip with posterior dirty moving echogenic artefacts

Comet tail appearance
Comet tail appearance of posterior artefactual echogenic echoes is seen appearing as dirty trailing comet tail sign of Harley's comet.

Murky appearance of underlying structures
Reverberation artefact will obscure the underlying organs and structures with dirty irregulars echoes. If seen surrounding a thin structure such as ligamentum teres, it may appear as thickening of the structure with increased echogenicity.

Changing position

The obtained hyperreflective images of comet tail and reverberation artefact change with change in the patient's position due to shift in the position or volume of air.

Patchy reflections within fluid

Free intraperitoneal air bubbles that are trapped within ascitic fluid or in a localized fluid collection will give rise to echogenic foci within the background of anaechoic fluid.

Why Pneumoperitoneum can be Missed in imaging Studies
Demonstrations

As little as 1 ml of free gas can be demonstrated on erect chest radiograph or lateral decubitus abdominal film using very patient and careful radiographic techniques. Patient must be in the radiographic position for at least 10 minutes before the radiograph is taken. Using ultrasound, the detection of pneumoperitoneum is operator dependent and practice in large number of patients is required for high proficiency in ultrasound detection of free intraperitoneal air.

Reasons for non-demonstration of pneumoperitoneum in radiography

Only about 75 – 80% of perforation of hollow viscus will have free gas demonstrated for the following reasons.

1. The perforation is promptly sealed off by oedema before significant free gas can escape.
2. Gas may not be present at the site of perforation.
3. There may be adhesions around the site of the perforation.
4. Patient's other serious medical or surgical conditions may over shadow pneumoperitoneum.
5. Radiographer may not have waited for 10 minutes with patient in erect position for air to rise under the hemidiaphragm.
6. Overpenetrated view or poor radiographic technique may obscure the pneumoperitoneum.

Accuracy of different radiographic methods

Plain film is very significant for demonstration of intestinal obstruction or pneumoperitoneum. However, CT scan can show pneumoperitoneum excellently.

For plain films

1. Combined erect and left lateral abdominal decubitus film show free gas due to perforation in about 90% of cases.
2. Erect chest radiograph is superior to erect plain abdominal radiograph and it demonstrates pneumoperitoneum in only 76%.
3. Supine abdominal radiograph which may be the only radiograph obtainable in very ill patients may demonstrate pneumoperitoneum in only 56% of cases.

Complication of penumoperitoneum

Pulmonary embolism
Cerebral infaction/embolism
Compartment syndrome

(Adam & Dixon, 2008; Dahnert, 2011; Sutton, 1998 and 2003, Palmer & Reeder 2001).

Reference

1. Roh JJ, Thompson JS, Harned RK, Hodgson PE. Value of pneumoperitoneum in the diagnosis of visceral perforation. Am J Surg 1983;146:830-3.
2. Chavez CM, Morgan BD. Acute appendicitis with pneumoperitoneum. Radiographic diagnosis and report of five cases. Am Surg 1966;32:604-8.
3. Lagundoye SB, Itayemi SO. Tension pneumothorax. British Journal of Surgery 1970; 57: 576-580.
4. Kasznia-Brown J, Cook C. Radiological signs of pneumoperitoneum: a pictorial review. Br J Hosp Med (Lond) 2006;67:634-9.
5. Baker SR. Diagnosis of minimal to moderate pneumoperitoneum. Abdom Imaging 1995;2:492-4.
6. Levine MS, Scheiner JD, Rubesin SE, Laufer I, Herlinger H. Diagnosis of pneumoperitoneum on supine abdominal radiographs. AJR Am J Roentgenol 1991;156:731-5.
7. Chiu YH, Chen JD, Tiu CM, Chou YH, Yen DH, Huang CI, Chang CY. Reappraisal of radiographic signs of pneumoperitoneum at emergency department. Am J Emerg Med 2009;27:320-7

Chapter 4

GENITO-URINARY SYSTEM

4.1 RADIOLOGY OF HAEMATURIA

Definition
Haematuria can be defined as passage of blood in the urine or bloody urine.

Classification
There are two major classifications.

Depending on the stage of urination when the blood is seen:
Early or initial haematuria: The blood appears at the onset or early, during the process of urination and is seen with the first few drops of urine. The causes are often in the urethra or bladder base.
Total or mixed haematuria: This occurs at the middle of urination and the blood may be mixed with the urine and the urine appears bloody or red. The causes are often in the bladder or due to blood dyscrasias.
Terminal haematuria: The blood is seen late or at the terminal aspect of urination. The causes are often in the ureter, kidney or bladder.

Depending on the quantity of blood seen:
Microscopic haematuria: Only a small amount of blood is seen or it may be red blood cells that are seen usually during urinalysis or urine microscopy. Microscopic haematuria is not seen with the naked eyes as it is unable to colour the urine. It is confirmed by examination of a fresh midstream urine using microscopy.
Macroscopic haematuria: This is haematuria seen with the naked eyes. It may originate anywhere along the kidney or urinary tract or be caused by blood dyscrasia.
Frank or total haematuria: The urine contains blood with appearance of watery blood and the patient is said to be urinating blood. This is caused by profuse active bleeding from the kidney or urinary tract.

Differentiation of causes by symptoms and signs
1. Passage of blood in the urine which is called haematuria results in a pink or bright red appearance of urine.
2. Blood coming from the kidney often caused by glomerulonephritis, or hypertension or blood coming from upper part of the ureter often caused by pyelitis or pyelonephritis is usually thoroughly mixed with urine, giving it a brownish or smoky appearance.
3. Passage of small amount of blood in the urine (often caused by cystitis) may lead to a smoky tint of urine.

4. Intake of rifampicin, a drug used in the treatment of tuberculosis may lead to watery red discolouration of urine, thus drug history is vital to exclude this. Phenazopyridine and to a lesser extent sulphonamides, quinine and phenytoin also cause red discolouration of urine.

5. Large consumption of beetroot or rhubarb can lead to an orange or red colour of urine by betanin pigment and is different from haematuria.

6. Patients with porphyria or myoglobinuria may have their urine discoloured red by porphyrin or myoglogin respectively.

7. Acute arsenic poisoning can lead to haematuria.

Causes of Haematuria
Urethral Lesions
Urethral erosions: Abrasions, erosion or rupture from any cause including sexual experimentation, urethral, catheters, instrumental dilatation and examination procedure.

Infections: Gonococcal and non-gonococcal uretheritis, Staphylococcus saprophyticus and E. Coli.
Urethral traumas: Straddle injury, pelvic fractures, torture instrumentation, urethra rupture.

Urethral stones: Rare and may appear where there is previous diverticulum.

Iatrogenic injury: Cystoscopy, catheter insertion, bougie, Transurethral resection of prostate (TURP).

Urethral stricture: Fibrosis from tuberculosis, schistosomiasis, gonococcal infections, non-gonococcal infections, instrumentation, trauma, surgery.

Urethral diaphragm: Posterior urethral valve, anterior urethral valve especially when infected by urinary tract infection.

Chemical instillation: Sodium permanganate, podophylin, 5 – fluorouracil, silver nitrate.

Bleeding tumours: Squamous cell carcinoma, transitional cell carcinoma, papilloma, fibrosarcoma.

Urethral polyp: Bleeding polyp of verumontanum, other polyps.

Bleeding urethral diverticulum: urethral diverticula, iatrogenic fistulas and diverticula.

Bleeding from prosthesis injury: Kaufman prosthesis, Brantley-Scot prosthesis.

Blood dyscrasias: Viral haemorrhagic fever, disseminated intravascular coagulation, excessive anticoagulant therapy.

Prostatic Lesion
Prostatitis: Infective, inflammatory and traumatic prostatis.

Prostatic enlargement: Benign prostatic hyperplasia (BPH), prostatic carcinoma, prostatic metastasis, metastasis from rectal carcinoma and others.

Prostatic abscess: Infective

Prostatic diverticulum: ureterocoele, abnormal opening of the duct of seminal vesicle or vas deferens.

Trauma to the prostate: road traffic injury, falling astride, transurethral resection of prostate, open prostatectomy.

Bladder Lesion
Cystitis or infection: This is caused by schistosomiasis, pyogenic cystitis, emphysematous cystitis (Diabetic or immunocompromised, gas forming organisms), tuberculosis via kidney or ureters, interstitial cystitis.

Infestation: Schistosomiasis, worms
Vesical trauma: Fracture of pelvic bones, abdomino-pelvic trauma, and intra-peritoneal rupture occurs in 20% while extraperitoneal rupture occurs in 80%.

Benign tumours: Vesical polyps, cysts, adenomas, fibromas

Vesical diverticulum: Congenital, acquired (60–70 years), infection, stone formation, carcinoma.

Iatrogenic injury: Catheter insertion, suprapubic catheterization, indwelling catheter, cystoscopy, bouginage, injury during surgery of pelvic organ e.g. uterus – Caesarean section, hysterectomy, myomectomy.

Ureterocoele: Ectopic, simple

Malignant tumours: Rhabdomyosarcoma, transitional cell carcinoma, adenocarcinoma, metastatsis from cervical, ovarian, colorectal, prostatic or endometrial carcinomas.

Vesical stone: Obstruction from posterior urethral valve, ureterocoele, bladder diverticulum from duplicate ureter; infection.

Vascular lesion: Haemangiomas, arteriovenous malformations, haemangiomas, venous thrombosis.

Vesical fistulas: Vesico-vaginal fistula, vesico-uterine, vesico-scrotal and vesico-perineal fistulas. *Blood dyscrasia* or bleeding disorders

Ureteral Lesion

Infections: Tuberculosis, schistosomiasis, leukoplakia, ureteric cystic, ureteric stone.

Trauma: Abdominal trauma, vertebral fracture.

Iatrogenic injury: Surgical injury during hysterectomy, retrograde pyelography, endoscopic instrumentation, other pelvic and obstetric surgeries.

Strictures: Tuberculosis, schistosomiasis, radiation injury, ureteric stones, granulomas.

Tumours: Ureteric sarcoma, lymphoma, spread from retroperitoneal tumours, transitional cell carcinoma, squamous cell carcinoma, metastasis, lymphangioleiomyomatosis.

Ureteric polyps: Fibroepithelial polyp.

Uretero-ileal conduits: Infections, stones, carcinoma

Congenital anomalies: ureteral reflux, ptosed kidney with redundant ureter, prune belly syndrome, ectopic vesicae.

Renal Lesion

Pyelonephritis: Infection from *E. coli*, renal stone, Emphysematous pyelonephritis due to diabetes, Fungal infection, xanthogranuloma elasticum, malakoplakia, leukoplakia, cholesteatoma.

Glomerulonephritis: Systemic lupus erythematosus, Goodpasture syndrome, Wegener's granulomatosis, polyarteritis nodosa, infection from group A b-haemolytic streptococcus, Nephrotic syndrome

Renal tuberculosis: Debris from renal papillary necrosis, renal scarring leading to ureteral scarring, ureteral calcification

Renal stones: Staghorn calculi, nephrocalcinosis, medullary stone

Trauma: Blunt abdominal trauma, penetrating trauma, trauma to pelvic kidney, renal transplant kidney, shattered kidney, PUJ junction avulsion (road traffic injury, assault, fall, and sports).

Tumours: Wilm's tumour, renal cell carcinoma, adenocarinoma (hypernephrosis), transitional cell carcinoma, lymphoma, leukaemia, sarcoma, metastasis.

Renal cysts: Simple renal cyst, multiple renal cysts, adult polycystic kidney, multilocular cyst, tuberous sclerosis, von-Hippel-Lindau syndrome, medullary sponge kidney.

Renal polyps: Leukoplakia, cholesteatoma, tuberous sclerosis, von Hippel-Lindau syndrome, oncocytoma, lipoma, myoma, fibroma, adenoma.

Iatrogenic injury: Interventional techniques, extra-corporeal shock wave lithotripsy, biopsy of tumours, renal vein sampling, radiation nephritis, percutaneous nephrolithotomy, stone manipulation into the kidney during extracorporeal shock wave lithotripsy.

Renovascular lesions: Renovascular hypertension (arteritis, neurofibromatosis, renal artery aneurysm, aortic aneurysm, renal vein thrombosis, acute cortical necrosis.

Angiomatous lesions: Arteriovenous malformation, haemangioma.

Renal papillary necrosis: Diabetes, analgesic abuse, pyelonephritis, infant in shock, sickle cell disease, obstruction, tuberculosis.

Metastasis: Lymphomas, leukaemias, pancreas, adrenals, breast, GIT, multiple myeloma.

Renal parenchymal disease: Acute pyelonephritis, renal abscess, acute tubular necrosis, acute cortical necrosis, focal reflux nephropathy, renal tuberculosis, acute glomerulonephritis, nephritic syndrome.

Congenital anomalies: Renal duplication, renal malrotation, renal ectopia, renal fusion, renal dysplasia, renal hypoplasia, renal agenesis, PUJ obstruction. They are more prone to trauma.

Systemic Causes

Haemoglobinopathies: Sickle cell anaemia, sickle cell trait, thalassaemia,

Blood dyscrasias: Haemophilia, disseminated intravascular coagulation, vasculitis, polyangitis, aneurysm, polyarteritis nodosa, Henoch-Schonlein purpura.

Systemic congenital anomalies: Tuberous sclerosis, neurofibromatosis, Haemorrhagic telangiectasia, Osler-Weber-Rendu syndrome, Sturge Weber syndrome, pelvic lipomatosis, renal artery aneurysm,.

Haemorrhagic fever: viral haemorhagic fever, Lassa fever, Hanta fever, dengue fever.

Others: Child abuse, factitious haematuria.

Clinical History and Physical Examination

These are extremely important as they can help to narrow the differentials and the range of investigation.

Simple laboratory tests

Urinalysis, midstream urine microscopy, culture and sensitivity, genotype, and blood film – may identify parasites, offending organisms or abnormal blood cells seen in tumours.

Table 4.11. Radiological investigative modalities	
Plain radiography	Abdomen, pelvis, lumbosacral spine, chest
Ultrasonography	7.5 MHz, 3.5 MHz, Endoscopic, urethral, vaginal, and abdominal surface transducers.
Excretory Urography (IVU)	Standard techniques, high dose urography, CT urography.
Computed Tomography:	Computed Tomography, Non- contrast, contrast, CT urography, CT angiography, CT-guided cyst puncture, CT colonoscopy, CT guided drainage
Urethrography	Micturating cystography urethrography, retrograde urethrocystography.
Excretory urography	Excretory pyelography: retrograde pyelography, loopography, antegrade pyelography.
Nephrostomy	Percutaneous nephrostomy, percutaneous nephrolithotomy, CT-guided, ultrasound guided percutaneous nephrostomy.
Angiography and interventional studies	Phlebography, renal venoplasty, phlebography, renal vein blood sampling.
Radionuclide studies	Renography, renal scanning, Cysto-urethrography.
Magnetic resonance imaging	Simple MRI, contrast MRI, MRA, MR urography.

Imaging overview of haematuria

Radiological evaluation of a patient presenting with haematuria may involve plain radiography, intravenous urography, ultrasound, CT and MRI with or without cystoscopy (table 4.11). Increasingly, multidetector CT (MDCT) is presently being used as the primary imaging investigation in some centres because of its high sensitivity for detecting malignant lesions, calculi and traumatic injuries. Infection, coagulopathy and instrumentation are diagnosable using clinical history and blood and urine testing. MDCT is also used for surgical planning due to its great anatomical details, particularly, urologists can definitely assess whether partial or complete nephrectomy of a malignant lesion is required while accurate renal vasculature image of potential organ donors are obtainable noninvasively. Due to the fact that CT urography (CTU) is now very refined and has very high sensitivity for recognition of small renal cell carcinoma, urinary tract stones and transitional cell carcinoma it has virtually replaced IVU in some centres. In patients with renal transplantation or pregnancy history is useful and allows tailoring the investigation to the particular case.

Differential diagnosis, radiological Assessment and Findings
Renal trauma

Plain film will demonstrate fracture of pelvic bones, ribs, lumbosacral vertebrae and other parts of the body (table 4.11). The trauma is usually as a result of road traffic accident, fall from height, sports injury, assault or home accidents. Ultrasound will show gross rupture or tear of the kidney appearing as lack of cortical continuity of the kidney with free fluid around the kidney in the retroperitoneal space but it may miss mild or moderate laceration or contusion. IVU will stage the renal trauma. On CT, there will be demonstrated, parenchymal contusion with disruption of renal capsule, peri- and intra-renal hematomas, injury to pelvic pedicle and urinomas depending on the type and extent of the injury. CT will also assess injuries to adjacent organs such as the liver, spleen, bowel and pancreas.

Renal vein thrombosis

In the acute stage, using ultrasound, the kidney is hypoechoic and becomes hyperechoic after about 10 days. There is also loss of cortico-medulary differentiation, poor visualization of renal pyramid and disorganisation of intrarenal parenchymal architecture. An echogenic mass within the lumen of dilated and expanded renal vein and absence of normal venous signal is shown in Doppler ultrasound in renal vein thrombosis. Following excretory urography, there is poor nephrogram and as the severity increases there may be complete absence of nephrogram or a striated nephrogram. There is also stretching-out of the calyces due to parenchymal odema in the 5 to 10 minutes or delay films. The kidney may shrink and atrophy as time progresses. Venous collaterals from renal capsular or accessory renal veins may produce ureteric notching which could aid the diagnosis. On phlebography, there may be tubular filling defect (which is actually the thrombus) extending into the inferior vena cava. Selective renal vein phlebography is done if the inferior vena cavogram is normal. On CT, it is seen as enlarged hypodense kidney with dilated renal vein that contains a filling defect that is better demonstrated at contrast enhancement.

Renal artery thrombosis

There is associated abnormal coagulopathy, particularly disseminated intravascular coagulation (DIC), trauma, sepsis, haemoglobinopathies, and abnormal pressure on the vessel by lymphnodes, nephritic syndrome and glomerulonephritis. There is an echogenic mass within the renal vein lumen, swollen hypoechoic kidneys with loss of normal Doppler venous signal and non functional kidneys on IVU in acute stage. Due to some degrees of thrombolysis in subacute stage, the kidneys will be enlarged and IVU will show dense persistent nephrogram with some degree of calyceal compression due to swelling. Also seen are wedge-shaped hypoechoic areas within the renal parenchyma due to infarction in most cases. Dilated venous collateral may cause ureteric notching. Loss of corticomedullary pattern with marked generalised reduction in renal echogenicity is shown by ultrasound. On CT the renal attenuation is reduced and both CT and MRI will demonstrate the thrombus within the lumen of the renal artery. In chronic stages, severe cases will show small atrophic kidney.

Renal arterial infarct
Renal artery occlusion with infarction of the area of renal parenchyma supplied by the occluded artery results from thrombosis (atheroma), atrial fibrillation, trauma, renal artery dissection, embolus and arteritis.

The occlusion occurs because the renal artery and its major branches are end arteries. Ultrasound will show hypoechoic and swollen kidneys. There is lack of Doppler tracing arising from any of the major branches of the renal artery on Doppler studies. On IVU, at early minor infarct, there is a defect in renal parenchyma without any calyceal deformity and unenhanced CT will be normal while contrast CT will show a wedge-shaped perfusion defect. In severe cases, IVU will not show any nephrogram and the kidney will be non-functioning even in delayed films and CT and MRI will show enlarged oedematous kidneys in acute phase without any sign of contrast enhancement. However, marginal rim enhancement (cortical rim sign) may occasionally be seen from the preserved capsular arteries supplying the capsule and immediate adjacent cortex. Chronic stages will show small, fibrosed kidney which may be difficult to identify in severe cases due to its small size.

Renal artery stenosis
Stenotic narrowed area in the artery can be identified directly and post-stenotic turbulent flow with colour change or increased bruit area are shown. The dilated post-stenotic area can also be visualised. A velocity of over 180 cms^{-1} in the renal artery is diagnostic of renal artery stenosis. A ratio of over 3.5 between the velocities of blood in the renal artery and aorta is also diagnostic of significant renal artery stenosis. Acceleration time above 0.1 second means significant stenosis. Loss of early systolic complex as a change in the waveform signifies a proximal stenosis.

Arteriovenous malformation or fistula
They are usually acquired from renal trauma usually renal biopsy. Sonographically, they may be echo poor or echogenic depending on the size of vascular spaces. Doppler studies, CT, MRI or angiography can demonstrated the vascularity including the feeding arteries and draining vessels. CT study is best at demonstrating marginal calcifications. The definitive diagnosis is by angiography and the feeding vessels can also be embolized through the procedure. Angiography is also best for demonstrating arteriovenous fistulas when it shows large early venous filling of arteriolar vesels with large venules. Pulsatile venous flow and increased flow in the supplying artery to such fistula may produce audible bruit.

Angiomyolipoma
This consists of benign hamartomas made of changeable proportions of blood vessel, muscle and fat tissues. They are often large at presentation but small angiomyolipomas are also diagnosed incidentally with CT or sonography. They are more common in females and over 80% are seen in adults often appearing solitary, small and asymptomatic. About 80% of patients with tuberous sclerosis has angiomyolipoma and 20% of those with angiomyolipoma has tuberous sclerosis and are often multiple and bilateral. The lesions are shown in ultrasound as a well-defined mostly echogenic mass. When

small they are homogenous, becoming heterogeneous as they increase in size. Fat content within the tumour are better demonstrated by CT or MRI. The tumour is very vascular and there is characteristic aneurysmal dilatation of abnormal vessels and early venous filling on angiography. Bleeding into the tumour mass is common and may be life- threatening in some cases for which embolization of the renal artery could be life-saving.

Renal cell adenocarcinoma

The tumour is hypervascular with venous lakes, early venous filling and neovascularization. Only 10% are hypovascular. They make up over 85% of adult renal malignancies and there is increased incidence in von Hippel Lindau syndrome and patients of long term dialysis. In ultrasound they appear as small solitary soft tissue mass bulging the renal outline. They may be hypo- or hyperechoic but large tumours are heterogenous while small ones tend to be homogenous. Microcalcifications show as areas of hyperechogenicity with distal acoustic shadowing. On CT and MRI a soft-tissue mass that is partly solid, often lobulated and associated with loss of the normal renal architecture is shown. On CT scan, they are generally isodense or hypo- dense compared to normal renal tissue, but only rarely hyperdense. They enhance variably with intravenous contrast but this is almost always less than normal renal tissue enhancement. Renal arterial embolization may be done as a palliative treatment for severe haematuria.

Transitional cell carcinoma

The tumour is hypovascular or avascular. There is early venous encasement and enlargement of the pyeloureteric artery. It arises from transitional epithelium of the renal pelvis, ureter or bladder with a ratio of 25:2.5:1. It is associated with hydronephrosis or hydrocalyx and presents with haematuria. It is an adult disease and rare in childhood. It constitutes approximately 5-10% of renal malignancies. Extensive parenchymal involvement may lead to non-functioning kidney. Renal calcification on plain film is a rare exception. In the kidney, the tumour is usually confined to the collecting system and only on about 25% or less are the renal parenchyma invaded. On ultrasound it appears as hypoechoic mass within the central hyperechoic area. Ill-defined hypoechoic area expanding the renal cortical tissue indicates parenchymal invasion. Inflammatory debris, calculi and keratin presence may give it a complex appearance. On CT, the tumour is small, ill-defined, hyperdense to the urine and hypodense/isodense to the renal parenchyma. CT is used for differentiating the tumour from poorly echogenic calculi and for staging.

Glomerulonephritis

There is reduction in renal cortical thickness of the kidney due to cortical scarring. Focal area of reduction in the thickness is due to focal area of scarring. In IVU, it is seen as enlarged kidney in early stages, but later bilateral symmetrical renal cortical atrophy results.

Polycystic kidney

The major congenital types are seen as autosomal dominant condition (adult polycystic kidney disease), porter type III or autosomal recessive polycystic kidney disease of the childhood Porter type I. They show as multiple bilateral, asymmetrical, non-communicating cysts of various sizes within an enlarged kidney. Initially, the cysts are simple surrounded by normal parenchyma, but as the disease progresses they increase in number and size producing increase in renal size, and the cortical mantle may be critically reduced in thickness or disappears. The cysts may become thick-walled, septated and with echogenic debris or marginal calcifications due to the effects of secondary infection and bleeding (figure 4.11 a). There is a link of this disease with tuberous sclerosis. On IVU, there may be widespread displacement of the renal calyceal pattern with spider web appearance. They appear as multiple round hypodense areas that do not enhance following contrast administration on CT scan. Cyst haemorrhage is responsible for the haematuria.

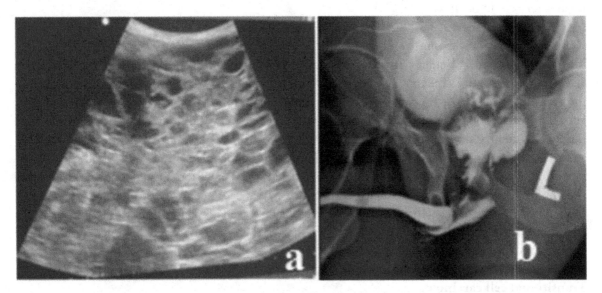

Figure 4.11: Sonogram of polycystic kidney (**a**) showing varied size multiple well-defined non-communicating cysts occupying almost the whole kidney. Retrograde urethrocystogram (**b**) showing irregularities of the area of membranous urethra with contrast outlining the prostate gland, the urinary bladder and entering into a pelvic vein due to injury to the urethra and prostate gland as a result of road traffic injury.

Renal lymphoma

Enlarged kidney with single or multiple mass lesions appearing as radiolucent areas disrupting the renal outline. Ureteric compression by retroperitoneal lymphadenopathy may lead to hydronephrosis. On CT scan, the tumour is shown with diffuse infiltration and loss of normal renal architectural outline resulting in bilateral renal enlargement. It is isodense and poorly enhancing mass on CT. Areas of haemorrhage may appear hypoechoic. *Chloroma* may be demonstrated which is a focal soft tissue mass in which histology proves to be composed of leukaemic cells. Retroperitoneal and mesenteric lymphadenopathy as well as metastasis to the liver and spleen are also shown by CT scan.

Urolithiasis

Plain abdominal radiograph or KUB will show radiopaque calculi in the renal, ureteral or bladder area. Renal stone is seen on ultrasound as echogenic spherical mass within the kidney or renal pelvis with distal acoustic shadow. In the ureter, it is seen as a spherical echogenic structure with distal acoustic shadowing. Small stones less than 5 mm in diameter may not be visualised. The stone is found in the dependent part of the bladder unless it is adherent to the wall by fibrosis and inflammation. Inflammation induced by the stone causes the haematuria. Urethral calculus is seen as spherical echogenic mass within the urethra with distal acoustic shadows. Urethral calculus is rare. CT will also demonstrate renal or vesical calculi as hyperdense structure in non-contrast film.

Renal/urinary tract tuberculosis

Chest x-ray may show fibrocystic changes or fibrotic scars with or without cavitary changes due to tuberculosis caused by Mycobacterium tuberculoisis. There may be calcified tuberculous nodules in the kidneys. Renal urogram or nephrogram may be normal in early stages. However, in advanced cases there will be deformity of renal outline by abscess, fibrosis or atrophy. Cavitation with irregular walls and stricturing of the calyces and renal pelvis are also shown. Calcifications, often punctate are seen and in extreme cases, autonephrectomy may occur with or without calcification *en block*. Ureteric tuberculosis is often as a result of renal tuberculosis. Ulceration and healing by fibrosis cause 'corkscrew' ureter due to multiple ureteric strictures and is demonstrable on IVU together with changes in the kidneys. Renal papillary necrosis and focal cortical loss may be demonstrated. Among diabetic patients an acute form is seen. Chronic form is more common in those with analgesic abuse. Up to three quarter of the affected patients develops macroscopic haematuria.

Renal papillary necrosis

The causes of this are analgesic abuse, obstruction with infection, sickle cell disease, diabetes mellitus, pyelonephritis and in infancy any severe illness. On IVU, normal or slightly reduced renal size with cortical thinning over affected papillae is seen. Papillary swelling followed by shrinkage, partial and then total sloughing are noted. Egg-in-cup appearance is an abnormal radiodensity seen between papilla and the pyramid due to partial detachment and is characteristic. Loss of the normal cupping of the calyx with the formation of abnormal ring shadow seen in complete detachment is another characteristic feature. Clubbed, blunted or trauncated calyces are seen but are non-specific features. If the papillae remain in the upper collecting system, the necrosed papilla may calcify. It may cause obstruction to urine flow with resulting hydronephrosis.

Wilms' tumour

Wilms' tumour is seen in children aged 3 months to 11 years with a peak age of 3-4 years. A great majority of cases are observed before ten years of age but it can also be diagnosed in the adolescent and adult. It occurs equally in both sexes and is rare in the neonate. It is usually large at presentation with expansile growth with sharp margins due to pseudo-capsule demonstrated on plain abdominal radiographs. On sonography it is seen predominantly as a solid spherical mass with heterogeneous echogenicity but occasionally irregular anechoic areas due to central necrosis, or cyst formation or haemorhage are seen. On IVU, there is poor *or lack of excretion* of intravenous contrast medium resulting from invasion or compression of hilar vessels, distorted collecting system *or* widespread tumor infiltration of renal parenchyma (figure 4.12). On nonenhanced CT, it appears as a well-circumscribed heterogeneous mass with hypodense areas due to necrosis, cyst formation or haemorrhage. Invasion with obstruction of the renal vein or inferior vena cava, renal pelvis and ureter or nodal or hepatic metastasis is demonstrated on contrast enhanced CT scan. On MR imaging, the tumour is hypointense on T1WI and shows high *or* variable intensity on T2-wheadacheeighted images. Haematuria is due to haemorrhage from the tumour.

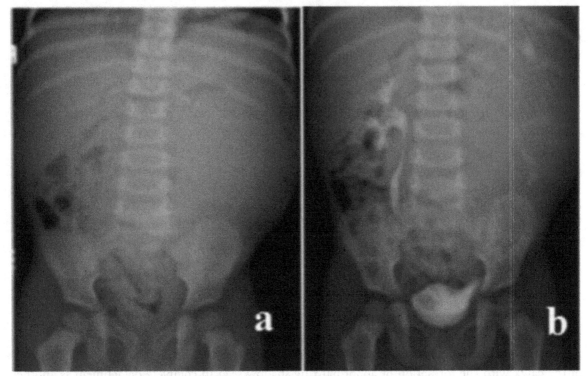

Figure 4.12: Plain film (**a**) and excretory urography (**b**) of a patient with Wilms tumour. In (**a**), note soft tissue opacity in the left flank due to a mass that pushed the bowels to the right. In (**b**), note the distorted and amputated calices on the left. Filling defect in the urinary bladder denotes ureterocoele.

Sickle cell disease

Sickle cell disease may show sclerosis of pelvic bones with radio-opaque density in the renal area due to calculi or calculi in the gall bladder may be shown. Typical femoral head destruction, infarction of the vertebrae and sclerosis of ribs and skull bones may be seen. Splenic calcification may suggest infarcted spleen. Autosplenectomy, hepatosplenomegaly, gall stone, splenic infarction, echogenic kidney due to renal failure, may be shown. Gross recurrent haematuria is observed and this is from multiple infarction of renal or genitoury tract organs.

Renal congenital anomalies or rotation and fusion

In *renal fusion*, which has an increased incidence of Wilm's tumour, the lower poles of the kidneys may be fused when the functioning renal tissues cross anteriorly over the midline giving the horseshoe kidney. The renal axis and orientation of pelvicalyceal system are abnormally altered. There is high incidence of obstructive hydronephrosis, infection, stone formation and trauma. In *crossed-fused ectopia,* one kidney crosses to the other side and fuses with the inferior pole of the kidney in normal position. The ureters are normal. Infection, trauma and obstruction are common because the kidneys are in a rather exposed positions. In *vesical ureterocoele*, there is dilated calyceal system with contrast columnization of the ureters. The distal aspect of the ureter is dilated with 'cobra-head' appearance. Simple ureterocoele is asymptomatic, seen in adults while ectopic ureterocoele is seen in children and is symptomatic and of congenital origin.

Metastasis

Solitary or multiple destruction due to metastasis, lymphoma, multiple myeloma, sickle cell disease or trauma (history is diagnostic) will be shown with disruption of normal bone shape. Metastasis to the pelvic or lumbosacral bone appearing as radiolucent (lytic), osteoblastic or mixed lesion will be shown. Prostatic metastasis shows as osteoblastic lesion with chalky-appearing sclerosis in pelvic bone and lumbosacral vertebrae. Lymphoma may show as solitary dense vertebra. Metastasis to the kidney, bladder and prostate can be shown by CT as multiple nodular masses. Metastasis to the lungs, liver, kidney, spleen and peritoneum is well shown by MRI because direct sagittal and coronal sections can be taken.

Hydronephrosis

Enlarged kidney with multiple dilated calyces which are shown as communicating cystic spaces within the kidneys. This may be as a result of distal obstruction from benign prostatic hyperplasia, bladder tumours, ureteric stone, or posterior urethral valve, etc. Calyceal dilatation, with dilated calyces filled with contrast may be seen in such lesions as PUJ obstruction, posterior urethral valve, prostatic enlargement. Renal mass causing obstruction, ureterocoele, etc.

Urinary tract infections

This includes pyelonephritis, glomerulonephritis, cystitis and urethritis. The kidneys are scarred and small with asymmetrical changes when there is bilateral affectation.

Wilm's tumour: It is seen commonly in the young. Solid irregular mass lesion of soft tissue density which will enlarge the affected kidney. Cystic degenerative changes will be seen within it if the tumour is large due to tumour cell necrosis. Metastatic changes into the liver, spleen, and enlargement of the lymph nodes may be demonstrated.

Pelvi-ureteric junction obstruction

Unilateral hydronephrosis, often on the right. Bilateral PUJ obstruction is extremely rare. The pelvis of the affected kidney is grossly dilated.

Haemangiomas

Echogenic mass with multiple cystic areas within it is seen on ultrasound. A few echogenic foci with distal acoustic shadows are caused by phleboliths. *von Hippel-Lindau syndrome:* Multicentric unilateral or bilateral renal cysts, renal cell adenomas or lesions suggestive of carcinoma are seen in this syndrome. In *tuberous sclerosis,* angiomyolipomas which are identified as tumours with solid areas, areas with features of haemangiomas, and echogenic fat-containing tumours are seen, co-existing renal cysts are also shown.

Other tumours

The malignant ones includes renal ureteral, bladder or urethral tumours. The commonly encountered tumours include transitional cell carcinoma, squamous cell carcinoma, lymphoma, leukaemia, sarcoma and metastasis. The benign tumours include adenoma, will show soft tissue mass in the renal area, displacing bowel gas to the contralateral side. Calcification may rarely be seen in some tumours. Curvilinear calcification in the wall of polycystic or multicystic kidneys may be seen or complete ring calcification in the wall of simple renal cyst may be visible. Up to 20% of them are avascular and little or no flow in the Doppler signal may be identified. *Transitional cell carcinoma of kidney:* This appears as echogenic mass and necrosis within it are shown and differentiated from calculi or blood clots. CT scan can stage the tumour. These are well shown by MRI and can be differentiated from tumours of adrenal and adjacent organs.

Mass lesion with mass-effect: Neuroblastoma which has infiltrated the kidney will show as soft tissue mass in the flank, with amorphous or punctate calcification within it and displacing bowel loops.

Tumour of bladder

Bladder tumours like polyps, fibromas, papilloma, and lymphomas can be seen as well defined spherical masses with regular capsule within the bladder. Transitional cell carcinoma, rhabdomyosarcoma and other carcinoma of the bladder will appear as an intravesical mass with lobulated and irregular margin. There may be cystic areas within the tumour due to tumour cell necrosis. The urinary bladder wall will be thickened above 3 mm due to tumour cell infiltration and inflammatory changes. Polyps will appear as spherical filling defects with regular margin in contrast- filled urethra.

Ureteral injury

Ureteral injury occurs at the pelviureteric junction when associated with trauma. On CT findings obtained in excretory phase, contrast material is seen accumulating in the inferior medial perinephric space. About 70% of the ureter is involved by penetrating injuries. Iatrogenic ureteral injuries due to gynaecological surgery for malignancies occur in 0.4–2.5%. Haemorrhage, uterine enlargement, endometriosis, cancer and adhesions increase the likelihood of ureteric injuries. Retrograde pyelography is used for confirmation and to establish the location and extent of the injury.

Foreign bodies

Radio-opaque foreign bodies in the ureter, bladder, kidneys or urethra can be seen with plain film. These may have been left in place as a result of torture or from treatment such as surgical blades, pins, catheters, gauze and may form gossypiboma particularly within the urinary bladder. Overzealous sexual practices may leave bizarre foreign bodies within the urethra or urinary bladder. They are usually identified by ultrasound scan as echogenic or mixed echo structures with distal acoustic shadowing. Plain films is useful in cases of metallic foreign bodies.

Iatrogenic injuries

Percutaneous nephrostomy, haematuria occurs in 5%, with about 2.4% needing transfusion. Retrograde pyelography, urethroscopy, extracorporeal shock wave lithotripsy, cystoscopy, boogie dilatation, urethral catheterization may all present with haematuria after the procedure. Prostate biopsy and biopsy of any genitourinary tract tumour may present with haematuria. History is vital for accurate diagnosis of the cause. Abrasion, laceration, pucture or injury to vascular tissue is responsible for the haematuria.

Cystitis or Emphysematous cystitis

On plain films, emphysematous cystitis due to diabetes mellitus or other immunocompromised lesions will show as curvilinear lucency within the urinary bladder, ureter or kidneys. The lucency is gas produced by gas-forming organisms such as *E. coli*, *Klebsiella*, *Aerobacter*, *Pseudomonas*, etc. Gas within the perinephric tissue, renal parenchyma, and air-pyelogram may also be seen. Ultrasound will show bladder wall thickening >3 mm in cystitis due to infection. In prostatitis, bladder wall may also thickened due to upward spread of infection to the bladder base. There may also be loin pain, fever, lower abdominal pain and pain during voiding.

Schistosomiasis

This is caused by *Schistosoma haematobium*. Curvilinear thin lines of calcification in the wall of urinary bladder from schistosomiasis will be well shown in plain film. Calcification of distal ureters with cow-horn configuration will also be shown as a result of schistosomiasis on plain films. Vesical, ureteric and renal granulomatous debris may calcify and appear as calculi and if sufficiently radio-opaque will be shown as dense shadows on plain x-ray but better shown by CT. Calcification with cow-horn configuration involving the distal ureters is seen. An entire ureter may calcify in continuity. Changes within the bladder are often shown. There may be hydronephrosis with vesicoureteric reflux on IVU, multiple filling-defects in the ureter and bladder due to ureteritis, cystis or granuloma. Squamous cell carcinoma is a complication that may develop and should be excluded in the work up of chronic cases.

Vesical diverticulitis

Bladder diverticula can be a focus of infection, calculus and neoplasm causing haematuria. They are out-pouchings of bladder mucosa. They are seen on bladder view of excretory urography but best in micturating cystourethrography when their narrow isthmus or neck is opened by pressure. They are spherical area of outpouching or contrast collection outside the urinary bladder profile.

Diverticulum will show as area of outpouching with contrast collection, a narrow neck and with regular margin on IVU.

Enlarged prostate

Prostatic enlargement due to benign prostatic hyperplasia and carcinoma of the prostate could present with prostatism and haematuria. On Ultrasound, the prostate may be inhomogeneous, nodular with lobulated margin and capsular destruction but prostatic carcinoma is hypoechoic on ultrasound. On excretory urography, there will be filling-defect within the bladder base with or without bilateral hydronephrosis. Smoothly marginated filling-defect in the bladder base is seen in cystography. CT can diagnose extraprostatic spread of tumour tissue into peri-prostatic fat, seminal vesicles and bladder base. CT can diagnose lymph node enlargement. MRI can resolve intraglandular prostatic tumour mass and can show focal thickening or bulging of capsule due to tumour infiltration. MRI can differentiate between ectatic pelvic vessels and enlarged lymph node without the need for intravascular contrast injection.

Posterior urethral valve

Grossly dilated bladder, dilated prostatic urethra and various degrees of bilateral hydronephrosis are shown on sonography. Abrupt narrowing of the urethra immediately distal to the area of posterior urethral valve is noted. On urography, there is dilated posterior urethra with *spinning top* appearance and abrupt sharp distal narrowing due to urethral valve or diaphragm. Hydronephrosis of the kidney and multiple bladder diverticula are seen in long-standing cases.

Bladder rupture and injury to Urnary tract

In intraperitoneal rupture there is contrast extravasation into the peritoneum outlining the bowels and often extending to the diaphragm. In extraperitoneal rupture there is extravasation of contrast medium into the perivesical space with the contrast filled bladder having a rain-drop appearance. Over 80% of bladder rupture are missed by IVU if cystography as an independent procedure is not done. About 75% of the bladder rupture is associated with pelvic trauma among which over 80% are occurring extraperitoneally. Ureteral injuries result from hysterectomy, endoscopic instrumentation for ureteric stone. Excretory urography confirms the function of the kidneys and shows any urine leak or fistula.

Urethral trauma

The membranous urethra are most commonly involved and at the urogenital diaphragm where it is relatively fixed. It occurs in 10% of patients with pelvic fractures. Contrast studies demonstrates contrast extravasation due to urethral tear which could be partial or complete.

In partial tear contrast medium is seen filling the urinary bladder which is absent in complete tears. Complete tears occur twice as often as partial tears and are more likely to develop a short stricture (< 2 cm). Complete tears require surgical repair, whereas partial tears are usually treated conservatively with catheterization. Urethral rupture will be diagnosed by extravasation of contrast outside the urethra canal. On urethrography urethral strictures, urethral diverticula and urethral polyps can be well shown in late stages. Strictures are seen as areas of narrowing, usually short-segment. In ruptures, there is breach in continuity of the urethra (figure 4.11 b).

Child abuse

Injury to the urethra at the vagina during sexual abuse may present with haematuria. If the patient intends to conceal the history, it may be very difficult to diagnose. However, extensive laboratory test and sometimes involving DNA may be required to conclusively diagnose sexual abuse. If in normal sexual relationship there is injury, the partner may present false history of trauma or injury from common objects in use. Imaging is usually unhelpful except to confirm that the genitourinary organs are of normal functions.

Anticoagulants

The use of anticoagulant drugs to prevent the formation of blood clots in patients at risk of deep vein thrombosis and pulmonary embolism has been associated with haematuria.

Catamenial haematuria

This results from endometrosis of the genitourinary tract and account for about 20% of atypical sites of endometriosis implantation. It is seen as cyclical, monthly haematuria in a woman of child bearing age when all other causes of recurrent haematuria has been excluded. The urinary bladder is more frequently involved and the focus is at the dome and projecting into the lumen. On MRI, there is high T1 and T2 signal seen due to the haemorrhagic nature of the lesion which helps in its diagnsosis.

Factitious haematuria

This is a genitourinary manifestation of Munchausen's syndrome. These patients intentionally formulates symptoms and signs. Children and medical staff are frequent involved. The patient may secure the blood that he uses to colour the urine red through a self-inflicted external skin wound. The patient may undergo extensive invasive investigations including renal biopsies or multiple surgeries before it is discovered that he has factitious haematuria produced by contaminating urine with blood. The importance of inclusion of factitious haematuria in the differential diagnosis is because its early detection is vital in order to avoid unnecessary, invasive and expensive investigations.

(Adam & Dixon, 2008; Dahnert, 2011; Sutton, 1998 and 2003, Palmer & Reeder 2001).

References

1. Joffe SA, Servaes S, Okon S, Horowitz M. Multidetector row CT urography in the evaluation of haematuria. Radiographic 2003; 23: 1441 – 1455.

2. Leyendecker JR, Barnes CB, Zagoric RJ. MR Urography: techniques and clinical applications. Radiographics 2008; 28: 23 – 48.

3. Muraoka N, Sakai T, Kimura H, et al. Rare causes of haematuria associated with various vascular diseases involving the upper urinary tract. Radiographics 2008; 28: 855-867.

4. Lowe LH, Isuni BH, Heller RM, et al. Paediatric renal masses: Wilm's tumour and beyond. Radiographics 2000; 20:1585-1603.

5. Adeyinka AO, Ibinaiye PO. Expression of adult polycystic renal disease in a 17-year-old male. West Afr J Med 2006;25:164-5.

6. Olapade-Olaopa EO, Agunloye A, Ogunlana DI, Owoaje ET, Marinho T. Chronic dehydration and symptomatic upper urinary tract stones in young adults in Ibadan, Nigeria. West Afr J Med 2004 ;23:146-50

7. Okafor PI, Orakwe JC, Mbonu OO. Cyclical haematuria sequel to uterine myomectomy: a case report. West Afr J Med 2002;21:341-2.

8. Anyanwu SN. Is routine urography necessary in all patients undergoing suprapubic transvesical prostatectomy? East Afr Med J 1995;72:78-80.

9. Osegbe DN. Haematuria and sickle cell disease. A report of 12 cases and review of the literature. Trop Geogr Med 1990;42:22-7.

10. Chugh KS, Harries AD, Dahniya MH, Nwosu AC, Gashau A, Thomas J, Thaliza TD, Hogger S, Ajewski Z, Onwuchekwa AC. Urinary schistosomiasis in Maiduguri, north east Nigeria. Ann Trop Med Parasitol 1986;80:593-9.

11. Adetiloye VA, Dare FO. Obstetric fistula: evaluation with ultrasonography. J Ultrasound Med 2000;19:243-9.

4.2 RADIOLOGICAL FEATURES OF TUBERCULOSIS OF THE URINARY TRACT (GENITOURINARY TUBERCULOSIS)

Definition
Tuberculosis is an infection caused by mycobacterium tuberculosis. Genitourinary tuberculosis is the involvement of the infection in the genitourinary tract.

Tuberculosis of the Urinary Tract
Urinary tract infections are often from haematogenous spread from foci in the lung, bone and gastrointestinal tract. The site or focus of infection is the renal cortex from where it spreads to the collecting ductal system through the renal tubules and papillae, causing caseating granulomatous lesions. The pattern of spread in the genitourinary tract is from the kidney to ureter to bladder to urethra, cervix, uterus, prostate and seminal vesicles (descending infection). This is unlike schistosomiasis which spreads from the bladder to ureter and kidney (ascending infection). There may be a history of previous clinical chest infection of tuberculosis. Even though the infection is often bilateral, unilateral lesions are more common radiologically because one side may have healed completely. If it is seen bilaterally, there is asymmetrical appearance. Most infections are subclinical, only few progress far enough to have radiological features.

Clinical features
1. Microscopic haematuria
2. Macroscopic haematuria
3. Pyuria (usually sterile when cultured)
4. Dysuria
5. Frequency
6. Urgency
7. Symptoms of chest, gastrointestinal or bone infections

Radiological Appearance

Plain Films
The Chest
Evidence of pulmonary tuberculosis (in less than 50%). There may be fibrocystic changes, or fibrotic strands in the lung. There may be features of destroyed lung syndrome suggestive of chronic active tuberculosis.
Cavity: Lung cavity suggestive of active tuberculosis is found in less than 10%.
Paraspinal mass/abscess: This is abscess on one or both sides of the spine due to tuberculous spondylitis of the dorsal spine.
Pleural effusion: This could be due to pulmonary tuberculosis, involvement of the pleura or renal lesion.

Abdomen
Calcification: Calcifications are noticed in the liver, spleen, lymph nodes and adrenal glands. These are calcified caseous granulomatous necrotic tissues.
Paraspinal abscess or mass: Abscess due to tuberculous spondylitis of the dorso-lumbar vertebrae will appear as paraspinal mass which can be unilateral or bilateral. It may calcify in late stages.

Wedge-shaped vertebral collapse: Collapse/fracture of vertebrae due to Pott's disease may be seen, showing site or focus of the primary disease.

Kyphosis / Kyphoscoliosis

Discitis: Disc destruction with narrowing and destruction of adjacent end-plates.

Renal calculi in 10%

Calcified autonephrectomy: Small, shrunken, calcified, non-functioning kidney.

Calcified beaded ureter: Solid calcification often in distal ureter. Less common than in schistosomiasis.

Calcification of the entire ureter

Calcified seminal vesicles inferior to the pubic bones. This may appear as honey-comb pattern.

Calcified vas deferens: Solid calcification. Uncommon.

Prostatic calcification

Calcified bladder or calcification of parts of bladder

Vesical calculus: Calcified necrotic granulomatous lesion.

Urethral calcification: Calcification in the posterior urethra.

Fallopian tubes: Amorphous calcification in tuberculous pyosalpinx; the pyosalpinx is confirmed by hysterosalpingography.

Excretory Urography

Kidney

Enlarged kidney shown as enlarged nephrogram: This is seen in early stages.

Normal or small sized kidney in late stages.

Tuberculoma: This causes local displacement of collecting ducts by spherical mass lesion.

Irregularity of the surface of the papillae

Moth-eaten appearance of the calyx: Erosion of calyx or papillae with moth-eaten appearance.

Cavitation: Large irregular cavities with parenchymal destruction.

Hydrocalycosis Dilated calyces with stricture/ narrowing of the infundibulum.

Putty kidney: Pyonephrosis from ureteral stricture

Abscess. Tuberculous renal/peri-renal abscess.

Hydronephrosis: Due to stricturing of renal pelvis or ureter in healed renal disease.

Renal papillary necrosis

Ureters

There is always evidence of renal involvement. Distal third of the ureter is commonly involved and it can be unilateral or bilateral involvement. When bilateral, it is most frequently asymmetrical. The pattern of involvement includes:

Filling defect: Filling defect in the ureter due to mucosal granulomas.

Saw-toothed ureters: Irregular contoured ureters due to multiple dilatation with mucosal ulceration and ureteric wall oedema.

Ureteral stricture: Single or multiple, often a late change.

Beaded ureter: Alternating areas of dilatation and narrowing or stricture.

Cork-screw ureter: Marked tortuosity of ureter with stricture and dilatation.

Pipe-stem ureter: Straight, aperistaltic, short, thick and rigid ureter.

Vesico-ureteric reflux: Distal ureteric orifice is fixed, patent and patulous allowing reflux.

Bladder
Thickened bladder wall: Inflammatory changes due to cystitis and bladder muscle hypertrophy.
Bladder ulceration: Bladder wall ulceration seen in double-contrast cystography or cystoscopy.
Shrunken bladder: Reduced bladder capacity due to scarring
Fistula formation: Vesico-perineal fistula, vesico-vaginal fistula, recto-vesical fistula, shown by cystography.

Prostate, testes and scrotum
Testicular mass
Hydrocoele
Scrotal abscess
Prostatic abscess

Ultrasonography
Calcification: Calcification noticed in the kidney and bladder as hyperechoic nodules with distal acoustic shadows.
Abscess: Renal abscess and perirenal abscess. Hypoechoic cystic mass with internal echoes.
Paraspinal abscess: Paraspinal hypoechoic mass lesion with multiple internal echoes.

Hydronephrosis: Calyceal dilatation filled with hypoechoic fluid
Autonephrectomy: Non-functioning shrunken kidney may be seen outside the renal area. It may be calcified or show calcification.
Pelvic abscess: This could be from pelvic inflammatory disease (PID). Small fluid with irregular margin of thickened uterus and adnexa (PID) or a frank pelvic abscess appearing as a hypoechoic cystic area with multiple internal echoes.

CT Scan
CT scan will identify Pott's disease or tuberculous cavity even when plain film is normal.
Paraspinal abscess: Better shown on CT scan.
Calcification: Calcifications in the kidney, ureter, bladder, vas deferens and epididymis are better shown on CT scan.
Calcification: Renal or vesical calculus are better shown on CT scan
Autonephrectomy: Small shrunken non-functioning kidney.
Pulmonary tuberculosis: CT scan will show the hidden areas of the chest and any lesion of tuberculosis like fibrosis, cavity, infiltrates or collapse.
Renal cavity: Renal cavitary lesion or tuberculoma may better be shown by CT scan.

Helical or Virtual CT Urography
Stricture: The stricture is better shown by spiral CT scan.
Shrunken kidney: Size of kidney is well shown with areas of scarring and the size can be accurately measured.

MR Imaging
It has multiplanar capability and it can be used in children and women of reproductive age without the risk of ionizing radiation.
It will show renal lesions better as it has better soft tissue resolution.

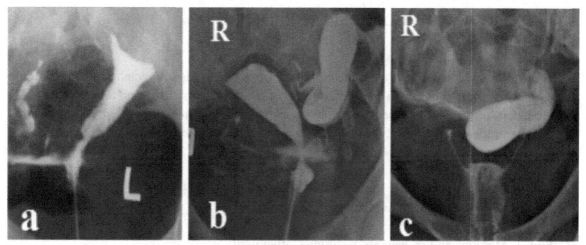

Figure 4.21: Hysterosapingographs showing multiple small filling defects within the uterus, beaded right fallopian tube and blocked left tube (**a**) caused by chronic tuberculous endometritis and salpingitis. Right tubal blockage with grossly dilated left fallopian tube (**b**) that is persistent in delay film (**c**), due to chronic tuberculous salpingitis.

Interventional studies
Ultrasound-guided drainage of renal, perirenal or paraspinal abscess can be done.
Ultrasound-guided renal biopsy
CT-guided drainage of abscess
CT-guided renal or pulmonary biopsy

Hysterosalpingography
Tubal blockage: Bilateral or unilateral tubal blockage in tuberculous salpingitis (figure 4.21 a and b).
Beaded tubes: Beaded, irregular-calibre tubes with filling defects and occasional dilatation of their distal parts (figure 4.21 a and b).
Hydrosalpinx: Contrast retained in the dilated distal parts of the fallopian tubes (figure 4.21 a, b and c).
Tuberculous endometritis: Tuberculous involvement of the uterine endometrium results in small irregular contracted uterus with multiple filling defects which may progress to marked reduction in the uterine cavity (figure 4.21 a).

(Adam & Dixon, 2008; Dahnert, 2011; Sutton, 1998 and 2003, Palmer & Reeder 2001).

References
1. Premkumar A, Lattimer J, Newhouse JH. CT and sonography of advanced urinary tract tuberculosis. AJR Am J Roentgenol 1987; 148:65-9.
2. Wang LJ, Wu CF, Wong YC, Chuang CK, Chu SH, Chen CJ. Imaging findings of urinary tuberculosis on excretory urography and computerized tomography. J Urol 2003; 169:524-8.
3. Gibson MS, Puckett ML, Shelly ME. Renal tuberculosis. Radiographics 2004;24:251-6.
4. Orakwe JC, Okafor PI. Genitourinary tuberculosis in Nigeria; a review of thirty-one cases. Niger J Clin Pract 2005; 8:69-73.
5. Matos MJ, Bacelar MT, Pinto P, Ramos I. Genitourinary tuberculosis. Eur J Radiol 2005;55:181-7.

4.3   OVERVIEW OF BIOPHYSICAL PROFILE

Definition
This is the objective and dynamic assessment of foetal well-being using sonography and an electronic foetal heart monitoring device to perform a group of measurements. It is a non-invasive APGAR score to assess for presence or absence of asphyxia in the intra-uterine period in order to determine whether continuing the pregnancy is likely to lead to the survival of the baby or whether delivery would be most prudent.

Aim of biophysical profile
The aim is to decrease perinatal morbidity and mortality.

Method: 1. Manning and co-workers' technique (often used).
1. Vintzileos and co-workers' method.

Gestational age at entry: 25 weeks, but it is more often done from 32 weeks.

Time of monitor: This is 30 minutes. However if the foetus is well, 5 – 10 minutes is adequate. Very sick babies may require up to 1 hour or more for accurate assessment. Full bladder is not required.

Variation: There is rhythmic variation in foetal activities depending on whether the foetus is awake or asleep but within an acceptable limit of normal.

Parameters assessed: 5 (table 4.31).

Scoring scale: A score of 2 is given for normal and 0 for abnormal observation (for Manning method, table 4.31).

Total maximum score: There is a total score of 10, expressed as 10/10. Minimum score is 0 or 0/10. If only the ultrasound parameters are used, total maximum score is 8, expressed as 8/8 as non stress test is omitted.

Interval between testing
Once the test has been initiated, it is continued, repeated bi-weekly or weekly until delivery. However, in very critical condition, it can be done twice weekly or daily till delivery or normalization of condition.

Time to obtain accurate score according to the state of the fetus
1. Awake and well foetus: 3 to 5 minutes.
2. Foetus in rapid eye movement (REM) sleep: 3 to 5 minutes.
3. Foetus in quiet non-REM sleep: 26.3 minutes
4. Sick foetus or those with IUGR or associated with high risk pregnancies: 30 to 60 minutes or more.

Table 4.31: Assessment of Biophysical Profile and score (Manning and co-workers' method)[1,2,4]

Parameter	Normal (Score = 2)	Abnormal (Score = 0)
Foetal breathing movement	One or more episodes of breathing lasting >= 30 seconds	Absent or no episode of breathing lasting >= 30 seconds
Gross body movement	3 or more separate episodes of discrete body/limb movements	Less than 3 separate episodes of body/limb movements
Foetal tone	One or more episodes of active extension with return to flexion of foetal limbs or trunk	Slow extension with return to only partial flexion, movement of limb in full extension, absent foetal movement
Amniotic fluid volume	One or more pockets of fluid measuring >= 2 cm in *both* vertical and longitudinal axes	Largest pocket < 2 cm in *any* of both axes
Non stress test (Reactive foetal heart rate)	(*Reactive*). 2 or more episodes of acceleration of >= 15 beat per minute and of > 15 second associated with foetal movement within 20 minutes	(*Non-reactive*). One or more episodes of acceleration of foetal heart rate of < 15 beat per minute within 20 minutes
Total score	**10**	**0-9**

There is an aternate method by Vintzileos and co-workers' which uses a score of 0, 1 and 2 (table 4.32).

Table 4.32: Asseement of biophysical profile Score (Vintzileos and co-workers' method)[1,3,4]

Parameter	Normal (2)	Abnormal (1)	Absent (0)
Foetal movement	Three or more episodes of simultaneous trunk and limb movement	One or two movements	No fetal movement
Foetal breathing movement	One or more episodes of breathing lasting for at least 60 seconds	One or more episodes of breathing lasting 30-60 seconds	< 30-60 seconds breathing or none.
Foetal tone	One or more episodes of extremity extension with return to flexion or spine extension and flexion.	One episode of extremity or spine extension and flexion	Extremity extended or movement without flexion; open hand; or no movement
Amniotic fluid volume	> 2 cm vertical pocket, fluid throughout the uterine cavity.	1-2 cm vertical pocket.	< 2 cm vertical pocket, fluid absent in most areas of uterus; extremity crowding.
Non-stress test	*(Reactive).* Two or more episodes of acceleration of >= 15 beats per minutes and of > 15 second associated with foetal movement within 20 minutes	*(Reactive).* One or more episodes of acceleration of foetal heart rate of < 15 beats per minute within 20 minutes	*(Non-Rective).* No episode of acceleration of foetal heart rate of < 15 beats per minute within 20 minutes
Total	**10**	**Variable**	**Variable**

Non-Stress Test

A non-acidotic foetus has normal functioning and intact autonomic nervous system. Such a foetus will have periodic acceleration of foetal heart rate. Normal acceleration of foetal heart rate is a rise that peaks at least 15 beats per minute above the baseline and lasts for at least 15 seconds from the beginning of the rise until the return to the baseline. Acceleration is associated with foetal movement. The foetal activity, like sleep, affects non-stress test. If all the ultrasound variable findings are normal, then non-stress test (NST) is excluded.

However, if one or more ultrasound variables are abnormal, it is a good practice to perform the non-stress test. Other people view non-stress test as the main independent parameter that determines normal foetal outcome and that the other parameters of biophysical profile are used to reduce the high false positive score rate of non-stress test. It is most useful between 32 weeks and term.

Table 4.33: Average perinatal mortality of various scores[1,2,4]

Score	Description	%	Mortality/1000
8 - 10	Normal	97.52	1.86
6	Equivocal	1.72	9.76
4	Abnormal	0.52	26.3
2	Abnormal	0.18	94.0
0	Abnormal	0.06	285.7

Interpretations of Biophysical profile

Breathing movement: Foetal breathing movements, when present, has the highest specificity in predicting an absence of foetal infection.

Foetal tone: Foetal tone is the most consistent variable for time interval at delivery.

Early effect of foetal acidaemia: In foetal acidaemia, foetal heart rate reactivity and foetal breathing movements are the first parameters to be compromised. Absent foetal tone and foetal gross body movement are late occurrences in foetal acidaemia.

Abnormal breathing movement: If there is normal breathing movement, the patient is managed according to the measurable volume of amniotic fluid.

Absent foetal activities: If all the foetal activity variables of biophysical profile (non-stress test, foetal breathing movement, foetal tone, gross body movement) are absent, the foetus is delivered as quickly as possible.

Absent non-stress test and foetal breathing movement: If there is only absent non-stress test and foetal breathing movement, then other extended testing is necessary to exclude foetal sleep.

Oligohydramnios at near term: In structurally normal foetuses, the presence of oligohydramnios at term or near term is an indication for immediate delivery, even if other variables are adequate.

Oligohydramnios at preterm: In structurally normal preterm foetuses, the presence of oligohydramnious is an indication for daily biophysical profile and if non-stress test becomes abnormal, delivery should be undertaken.

Progressive foetal hypoxia and hypercapnia: In progressive foetal hypoxia and hypercapnia, heart rate reactivity and foetal breathing movements are first compromised, followed by foetal tone and gross body movement.

All the variables do not have equal significance (table 4.33).

Most important parameters: The amniotic fluid volume, foetal breathing movement and non-stress test are the most important parameters.

Acute and chronic markers of foetal well-being: There are acute and chronic markers of foetal well-being. Acute markers are non-stress test, foetal tone, gross body movement and fetal breathing movement while liquor volume is a chronic marker.

Ante-partum foetal surveillance: It is used in ante-partum foetal surveillance including premature rupture of membrane, chorioamnionitis, post-date, oligohydramnios, prolonged labour, infection, etc. Identification of abnormalities should be followed by measures to prevent progressive metabolic acidosis which is what leads to foetal death.

Reliance on individual components: The management decision should not be based on the total score alone but also on the scores of the individual components.

Modified Biophysical Profile

Only amniotic fluid index and non-stress test are measured (however, the false negative score rate is increased). Modified biophysical profile was developed to reduce the time for performing the assessment in busy units.

Conditions requiring biophysical profile

1. Premature rupture of membrane
2. Premature or preterm labour
3. Placental abnormalities such as insufficiency, praevia, marginal bleed, etc.
4. Pregnancy-induced hypertension
5. Pre-eclampsia or history of previous pre-eclampsia
6. Small-for-gestational age or IUGR
7. History of Rh-incompatibility or non-immune foetal hydrops
8. Maternal renal, hepatic, hormonal or autoimmune diseases
9. Maternal diabetes mellitus, alcohol or drug intake.
10. Post-date, prolonged labour
11. Oligohydramnios or polyhydramnios
12. History of injury to the mother from trauma
13. Infection, SCD, high-risk pregnancies.

Advantages of biophysical profile

Inexpensive and non-inasive: It is non-invasive, simple and inexpensive.

High acceptability: It is the most acceptable non-continuous method of assessment of foetal well-being.

Does not require additional training: Each parameter measures an aspect of foetal well-being and can be performed without extensive further training.

It measures renal function: Amniotic fluid volume estimation indirectly measures foetal urine production and by implication renal perfusion and function.

Omission of non-stress test: Non-stress test may be omitted if other parameters are normal.

Reduction of cerebral palsy: The use of biophysical profile score in antepartum foetal monitoring has been associated with a major reduction in the prevalence of cerebral palsy when compared to an untested population.

Disadvantages of biophysical profile

High false positive rate: High false positive rate of 75% for score of six. (Foetal activities decrease in stress states because of the need to conserve energy and oxygen consumption and also due to slow CNS development in foetuses with IUGR).

False positive rate: False positive rate of 20% for a score of zero. This is because foetal activities decrease in stress states to conserve energy and reduce oxygen consumption (table 4.33).

Long performance time: Long performance time of at least 30 minutes for sick babies (slow development of the CNS with markedly decreased foetal activities).

Subjective interpretation: Interpretation of non-stress test is visual and subjective leading to high false positive interpretations.

Indirect information: The information on foetal cardiovascular health and renal perfusion are indirect.

Sleeping state: Sleeping foetus has a high false positive rate (in all except amniotic fluid assessment).

Reasons for high false positive scores

Endorphins: Maternal and foetal endorphins produced in stress states in pregnancy are potent depressants of foetal central nervous systems and foetal activities.

Sleeping state: A sleeping foetus has depressed activities and high false positive rate (in all except amniotic fluid assessment).

Subjective interpretation: Interpretation of non-stress test is visual and subjective leading to high false positive interpretations.

Congenital muscle dystrophy: It is of little significance in foetuses with congenital muscular diseases or central nervous system conditions that affect muscular function since movement or activities are affected by other conditions than what is tested by biophysical profile.

It is altered in congenital anomaly: Negative predictive value of a normal biophysical profile score in structurally normal foetus is not applicable to foetus with congenital anomalies, since other conditions can lead to unexpected death of these anomalous foetuses. If the congenital anomaly is not obvious it may lead to a situation where the biophysical profile score is wrongly adjudged to be erroneous (table 4.33).

Brain depressant drugs: Central nervous system depressant drugs taken by the mother may affect biophysical profile score and it may not be taken into consideration when interpreting the score because of failure to take the mother's drug history and the mother may not know that a CNS depressant is among her drugs.

Methods of reducing false positive scores
1. Use of all the five parameters at any given time.
2. The repeated testing at intervals to overcome the effect of sleep periods.
3. Use of vibroacoustic stimulators to wake the foetus or stimulate foetal activity.

(Dahnert, 2011; Sutton, 2003; Swischuk, 2004; Sanders & Winter, 2006).

References

1. Guimarães Filho HA, Araujo Júnior E, Nardozza LM, Dias da Costa LL, Moron AF, Mattar R. Ultrasound assessment of the foetal biophysical profile: what does an radiologist need to know? Eur J Radiol 2008;66:122-6.
2. Manning FA. Foetal biophysical profile: a critical appraisal. Clin Obstet Gynecol. 2002;45:975-85.
3. Oyelese Y, Vintzileos AM. The uses and limitations of the foetal biophysical profile. Clin Perinatol 2011 Mar;38(1):47-64, v-vi.
4. Lalor JG, Fawole B, Alfirevic Z, Devane D. Biophysical profile for foetal assessment in high risk pregnancies. Cochrane Database Syst Rev 2008;(1):CD000038.

4.4   RADIOLOGY OF INTRAUTERINE GROWTH RESTRICTION (IUGR)

Definition
Intra-uterine growth restriction (retardation) (IUGR) is defined as a condition in which the foetal or neonatal (perinatal) weight measures below the 10th percentile (5th percentile in the UK) for gestational age *occurring as a pathological process* that prevents the expression of normal (genetic) growth potential. The major causes are poor maternal nutrent reaching the baby and inadequate oxygen delivery to the foetus.

What does below 10th percentile for gestational age mean?
This means that the foetus / neonate weighs less than 90 percent (95 percent, UK for 5th percentile) of the average weight of all other normal (morphologically or in physical appearance) foetuses / neonates of the same gestational age.

What precaution must be taken before definitive diagnosis of IUGR after birth?
About 70% of foetuses with weight below the 10th percentile are *small for gestational age* (constitutionally or legitimately small and therefore physiological normal and not pathologic). Constitutionally small babies are well proportioned and developmentally normal. Foetus / babies with IUGR, however, are often malnourished or dysmorphic (asymmetry or abnormal physical appearance) and occupy the remaining 30%. IUGR is the pathological equivalent of small-for-gestational age. A foetus is diagnosed as small for gestational age only after a pathological process has been excluded, which requires examination of the newborn after birth therefore the diagnosis is made in retrospect to distinguish it from IUGR.

Prevalence of IUGR
1.   10% of all pregnancies are complicated by IUGR in the USA.
2.   3-5% of pregnancies in healthy mothers are complicated by IUGR.
3.   25%-30% of all pregnancies in mothers in high-risk groups (hypertensive, chronic kidney disease, advanced diabetes, heart or respiratory disease, malnutrition, anaemia, infection) present with IUGR.

What are the problems of IUGR
1.   Perinatal mortality for foetus/infants with IUGR is 6-10 times higher than those of a normal growth population.
2.   Severe perinatal infections leading to long-term residual complications.

The foetus may suffer from:
1.   Low umbilical cord pH.
2.   Intrapartum foetal distress (IUGR is a major cause).
3.   Intrapartum asphyxia (Low biophysical profile score).
4.   Intrauterine foetal demise (From hypoglycaemia, cerebral hypoxia, intraventicular haemorrhage, etc).

The new born may suffer from:
1.   Low Apgar scores, intraventricular haemorrhage, necrotizing enterocolitis, hypoglycaemia, hypocalcaemia, polycythaemia and meconium aspiration syndrome

What are the long term effects of IUGR?
1. Inability to achieve normal height.
2. Performance and attention deficit in the children.
3. Negative effect on brain growth and overall mental development.

Types of IUGR
There are 3 types (USA). (UK recognises only the first two types).

Type 1. Symmetrical IUGR
Severe form of IUGR where there is a proportionate decrease in all the foetal growth parameters (HC, BPD, AC, FL) maintaining normal HC/AC ratio. Detectable from 24 weeks of gestation.

Pathology
Early severe injury which occurred during the period of cell hyperplasia (cell division, organogenesis, embryogenesis) resulting in *decrease in cell number across all cell lines in the foetal tissues and organs.* Injury overwhelms the normal brain protective mechanism in which blood and nutrients are preferentially shunted to the brain and the heart at the expense of all other tissues and organs like the liver, muscles and fat.

Type 2. Asymmetrical IUGR
Asymmetric or disproportionate reduction of foetal growth parameters with relative normal or near normal BPD and HC compared to AC, and FL which are more markedly reduced. Detectable from 32 – 34 weeks of gestation

Pathology
The IUGR is caused by late onset injury occurring (uteroplacental insufficiency) during the period of cell hypertrophy (increase in size) resulting in *decrease in cell size (but not number) only and with normal number.* There are features of foetal starvation due to uteroplacental insufficiency but with preferential shunting of blood to the foetal brain and heart at the expense of muscles, fat and liver due to preservation of brain protective mechanism (brain sparing or vital organs sparing mechanism) from the cardiac output. It often occurs after 26 weeks of gestation and is detected frequently at 32 – 34 weeks. Sustained, long period of injury or the occurrence of early severe insult may lead to the development of symmetrical IUGR.

Type 3. Mixed type (USA alone, controversial)
Intermediate or near- normal IUGR with impaired foetal growth and asymmetry.

Pathology
IUGR occurs at a period of mixed hyperplasia and hypertrophy resulting in overlap of symptoms, signs, diagnostic features and outcome. When the insult causing asymmetric growth restriction occurs early in the pregnancy, is very severe, or sustained long enough, the foetus may be identified when in the process of losing the ability to compensate and will show features of both symmetrical and asymmetrical types

Causes of Asymmetrical IUGR

Asymmetrical IUGR is caused mainly by lesions that cause uteroplacental insufficiency

1. **Maternal physiological causes**

   Maternal demographic criteria *(which could be physiological) include* racial influence (Asians) and small stature women (maternal genes mainly influence birth weight).

   Other physiological causes are high altitude, nulliparous women, adolescent mothers, advanced maternal age, decreased supply of nutrients and multiple gestations

2. **Maternal illnesses / health conditions.**

   Severe anaemia, maternal starvation, drugs, illicit drugs, uterine abnormalities, maternal vascular conditions, pre-conceptual diabetes mellitus, pre-eclampsia, chronic heart or renal diseases and collagen vascular diseases (SLE)

3. **Placental causes**

   Placental infarction, placental separation (chronic partial), placenta praevia, placental infection (malaria), chorioangioma and placental metastasis

Causes of Symmetrical IUGR

This is caused mostly by serious foetal conditions that restrict the expression of full growth potentials and include:

a. Chromosomal abnormalities: aneuploidy, trisomy 13, trisomy 18, triploidy.

b. Congenital heart disease

c. Intrauterine viral infections. TORCH complex

d. Any of the causes of asymmetrical IUGR if it is severe and occurs early in the pregnancy.

Clinical features

Features of IUGR in the foetus / baby

Absence of foetal body fat

Decreased liver glycogen

Decreased muscle glycogen

Decreased fat in the buttocks/thigh with wrinkled skin.

Wizened baby / Baby with stary eyes.

Reduction/absence of foetal heel fat pad

Decreased paraspinal fat pad

Wrinkled skin especially over abdomen (due to decreased omental fat, decreased liver and skin fat).

Reduced abdominal size / flat abdomen due to reduced omental fat.

Features in the pregnancy

1. Small or reduced size of the pregnant abdomen relative to gestational age / date.
2. Reduced symphysiofundal height for date.
   a. Decrease by 3 cm from the expected measurement is highly suggestive of IUGR.
   b. Decrease by 4 cm or more from expected measurement is diagnostic of IUGR.
3. Polyhydramnios (mixed type, or symmetrical type)
4. Oligohydramnios (Asymmetrical type).
5. Decreasing or inadequate maternal weight than the expected for date.
6. 3-4-fold increase in risk in a mother with previous history of IUGR.

7. High maternal blood pressure (Due to pre-eclampsia).
8. Oedematous mother with puffy face (may show proteinuria).
9. Caesarean section scar due to operative delivery of previous IUGR.

Criteria for Accurate Diagnosis:
1. **Gestational age / Foetal date must be known for sure by:**
    a. Accurate date of last menstrual period (LMP) from mother in a woman with regular menstrual cycle.
    b. Early pregnancy test
    c. Early physical examination to assess the fundal height
    d. Early ultrasound examination. Ideally before 13th week and not beyond 20th week. The error margin before 13th week is below 10 days. Error margin in third trimester ultrasound dating is about 3 weeks).
2. **Determine (if possible) the underlying cause by:**
    a. Accurate history and physical examination
    b. Basic laboratory tests
    c. Continuous questioning on family and social history
    d. Foetal blood analysis
3. **Exclude hypertension:**
    Try to measure accurate maternal blood pressure at all times and on different occasions and mood and try to obtain a record of the patients previous blood pressure measurement.

Radiological Findings
The radiological investigative modalities are:
1. Ultrasonography using 3.5 MHz transducer (mainstay diagnostic modality).
2. Doppler ultrasound scanner.

Findings In Symmetrical IUGR
1. Decreased FL, HC, AC
2. Markedly decreased BPD
3. AC > 2 SD (SD = Standard deviation)
4. Normal HC/AC or near normal (Proportionately affected)
5. Normal FL/AC or near-normal (Proportionately affected)
6. Elevated umbilical artery systolic/diastolic ratio
7. Low total intrauterine volume
8. Low estimated gestational age
9. Normal liquor or polyhydramnnios (polyhydramnios is due to foetal hydrops).
10. Amniotic fluid index may also be reduced (if less than 5, delivery should be considered to avoid intrauterine demise).
11. Abnormal uterine artery wave form (in Doppler studies).
12. Slow BPD growth rate (In serial ultrasound scan at 2 weeks intervals).
13. Increased placental calcium deposits (may occur)
14. Biophysical profile – variable (depends on the stage of foetal well being).
15. Foetal blood analysis may detect cause (Foetal blood obtained by ultrasound guided amniocentesis and may detect hypoglycaemia, hypercapnia, hypercalcemia, elevated alpha feto-protein, etc)
16. Karyotyping to detect chromosomal abnormalities.

17. There will be wrong delivery date if the ultrasound date in third trimester is used for delivery. (This will lead to failure to recognise IUGR).

18. Foetal monster. (This is recognised by noting that there are difficulties in clearly identifying individual foetal parts or structures using ultrasound scan performed in late pregnancy).

Findings in Asymmetrical IUGR

1. Decreased FL, HC, AC
2. Decreased but near normal BPD
3. AC > 2 SD (SD= standard deviation)
4. High or elevated HC/AC (Most distinguishing sign from symmetrical IUGR)
5. High or elevated FL/AC
6. Elevated umbilical artery systolic/diastolic ratio
7. Low total intrauterine volume
8. Low estimated gestational age
9. Oligohydramnios
10. Abnormal uterine artery waveform
11. Slow BPD growth rate
12. Increased placental calcium deposit
13. Biophysical profile - variable
14. Foetal blood analysis (may detect hypoglycaemia, hypercapnia, hypercalcaemia, elevated alpha feto-protein, etc).
15. Wrong delivery date if the ultrasound date in third trimester is used for delivery (This will lead to failure to recognise IUGR).
16. Reduced amniotic fluid index (normal is 8 or more. If AFI is less than 5 or exists with oligohydramnios, delivery should be considered to avoid intrauterine demise).

(Adam & Dixon, 2008; Dahnert, 2011; Sutton, 2003; Swischuk, 2004; Sanders & Winter, 2006).

References

1. Ott WJ. Diagnosis of intrauterine growth restriction: comparison of ultrasound parameters. Am J Perinatol 2002;19:133-7.
2. Ott WJ. Sonographic diagnosis of foetal growth restriction. Clin Obstet Gynecol 2006; 49:295-307.
3. Divon MY, Guidetti DA, Braverman JJ, Oberlander E, Langer O, Merkatz IR. Intrauterine growth retardation--a prospective study of the diagnostic value of real-time sonography combined with umbilical artery flow velocimetry. Obstet Gynecol 1988;72:611-4.
4. Falo AP. Intrauterine growth retardation (IUGR): prenatal diagnosis by imaging. Pediatr Endocrinol Rev 2009;6 Suppl 3:326-31.
5. Brodsky D, Christou H. Current concepts in intrauterine growth restriction. J Intensive Care Med 2004;19:307-19.
6. Rizzo G, Arduini D. Intrauterine growth restriction: diagnosis and management. A review. Minerva Ginecol 2009;61:411-20.
7. Pardi G, Marconi AM, Cetin I. Placental-foetal interrelationship in IUGR foetuses--a review. Placenta 2002;23 Suppl A:S136-41.
8. Gardosi J. Intrauterine growth restriction: new standards for assessing adverse outcome. Best Pract Res Clin Obstet Gynaecol 2009;23:741-9.

4.5   RADIOLOGY OF EX UTERO INTRAPARTUM TREATMENT (EXIT) PROCEDURE

Definition
Ex utero intrapartum therapy (treatment) (EXIT) procedure is defined as a transient procedure during Caesarean Section, involving the delivery of the foetal head and neck only, so that the mother-placenta that is still attached, provides an *in situ* natural extracorporeal membrane oxygenation (ECMO) support for the foetus while foetal lesions are treated to the extent necessary to tolerate independence from maternal circulation.

EXIT procedure is also defined as a transient technique to secure the foetal airway during Caesarean section, while foetal oxygenation is maintained through preserved utero-placental circulation enabled by non-delivery of the placenta during the procedure. The procedure is performed simultaneously on both the mother and the foetus and both of them are at high risk of complications.

Other names by which it is known
Operation on a placenta support (OOPS), *Ex utero intrapartum* tracheostomy, *Ex utero intrapartum* therapy (EXIT), *Ex utero intrapartum* treatment (EXIT) and *Ex utero intrapartum* technique (EXIT) procedure.

Historical points
It was originally performed as a perinatal operation on a placenta support (OOPS) making it possible to create a surgical airway in a foetus with severe airway obstruction in which absence of such intervention will invariably result in early neonatal death. However, more extensive use is now done much more than what OOPS promised, applying uterine hypotonia and preservation of uterine volume so that more time is gained for the treatment of foetal condition while maintaining maternal utero-placental-foetal circulation.
Once the airway is secured, the umbilical cord is clamped and cut.

Aims and objectives of EXIT procedure[1-5]
Prevention of loss of uterine volume: To prevent uterine contraction, control uterine hypotonia and loss of uterine volume while foetal condition is being treated.
Preservation of uteroplacental circulation: To preserve uteroplacental circulation (by preventing placental detachment) with neonatal anaesthesia in order to gain time to reverse tracheal occlusion or establish a patent airway.
Increased Apgar score: To increase the Apgar score in a foetus with severe airway obstructing lesion and thus increase his survival.
Prevention of neonatal respiration: To prevent neonatal respiration and defer the transition from maternal-foetal circulation to neonatal circulation while foetal lesion is treated.
Reduction of foetal hypoxia: To slowly wean off a foetus with severe congenital heart abnormalities from the maternal circulation, and thereby reduce hypoxia to the fetus from the sudden discontinuation of placental circulation by changing to the extracorporeal bypass route.
Rapid control of airway: To allow for rapid control of the airway in cases in which surgery is indicated for survival, e.g. conjoined twins

Indications of EXIT procedure[1-3]
1. *EXIT-to-airway procedure*
   Neck masses (massive goitre, cystic hygroma, neuroblastoma, cervical teratoma, haemangioma, lymphangioma and other vascular or lymphatic conditions).
2. *Congenital high airway obstruction syndrome* (CHAOS).
   Trachea atresia, laryngeal atresia, micrognathia and other causes of upper airway obstruction.

1. *EXIT-to-resection procedure*
   Bronchopulmonary sequestration, congenital pulmonary airway obstruction, chest masses with intra-thoracic airway obstruction, mediastinal teratomas, pericardial teratomas, congenital hydrothorax, congenital cystic adenomathoid malformation of the lung (CCAM) and congenital pulmonary agenesis.

2. *EXIT-to-ECMO procedure*
   Severe congenital heart disease, severe congenital diaphragmatic hernia

3. *EXIT-to-separation procedure*
   Separation of conjoined twins

4. *EXIT-to-intervention procedures*
   Tracheoplasty, tracheostomy, ablation surgery for tumour and intrathoracic intubation.

Roles of radiology

Radiology and the radiologist are at the centre of EXIT procedure. The radiologist makes the prenatal diagnosis of the condition, is involved in the planning of the procedure, performs intrapartum imaging during the procedure, intra-procedure interventional procedure and post-procedure imaging and intervention for diagnosis, treatment, prevention and dealing with the complications. He also performs follow up assessment as the patient comes for post-operative clinic. The radiologist and radiology are the focal point of diagnosis, treatment and imaging information as outlined below:

Prenatal or antenatal diagnosis/imaging of the condition[1-7]

The radiologist uses two basic imaging modalities namely ultrasound and magnetic resonance imaging to make diagnoses and image the patients in EXIT procedure including interventional procedure.

Quick general survey: Sonography is used for quick survey of the foetus and since routine sonography is performed for most pregnancies it is the first imaging modality to draw attention to any unusual appearance and its real time imaging adds to its versatility.

State of respiration and swallowing: Sonography provides information of the respiratory function of the foetus and on foetal swallowing due to its real time capability.

Distinguish cystic from solid lesions: Sonography demonstrates cystic lesions and distinguishes it from solid lesions so that pre-EXIT procedure fluid aspiration could be done to reduce the size of the mass for easy and fast delivery of the head and neck before EXIT procedure.

Polyhydramnios: Sonography will also demonstrate polyhydramnios which could also be aspirated before Caesarean section (CS) to reduce the size of the incision for CS.

Vascularity of neck masses: Doppler sonography provides information on the vascularity of neck masses or the lesions.

Intracardiac abnormalities: Cardiac sonography (Echocardiography) can provide information on the functional state of the heart and haemodynamic cardiovascular abnormalities.

Calcification: Sonography is used to show calcifications for calcifying lesions better than MR imaging.

Conjoined twins: Both sonography and MR imaging are used to show conjoined twins, but MR has wider field of view and allows for better assessment of anatomical structures and is thus better than sonography in overall foetal assessment.

Foetal anomalies: Sonography is used to reveal the foetal anomaly but MR imaging is added to reveal complex anomalies due to its multiplanar capability.

Upper airway obstruction: MR imaging is used to show the severity, distortion, compression and structural displacement of upper airway obstruction by the mass or congenital lesion.

Cartilaginous structures: Prenatal MR imaging is used to show cartilaginous structures which are very difficult to identify with sonography.

Liver herniation and lung-to-heart ratio: On the whole, in prenatal diagnosis and imaging both sonography and MR imaging are complementary and both can show liver herniations to the thorax and lung-to-heart ratio, vital for assessment of foetal complications and survival.

Planning for EXIT procedure[1,2,3,6]

Diagnosis of an anomaly does not immediately translate to EXIT procedure. However, once the decision to perform EXIT procedure is taken, there is the need for multidisciplinary participation by various specialties for a hitch-free procedure. The radiologist should determine:

Foetal presentation: The foetal position, presentation and placental location. These determine the size and position of the incision.

Foetal altitude: The flexion or extension of the foetal head which will determine how the head and neck is delivered.

Cystic or solid lesion: Whether neck mass is solid or cystic. Cystic masses can be drained percutaneously under ultrasound or MR guidance before or during exit procedure for easy delivery of the head and neck.

Lesion characterization: Further prenatal MR of foetus just before EXIT procedure provides detailed views and current lesion characterization.

Blood supply: Current blood supply that must be preserved using Doppler sonography.

Placental edges: Ultrasound and MR imaging are used to show placental edges and polyhydramnios since polyhydramnios displaces placental edges from it true position.

Lung-to-heart ratio: The lung-to-heart ratio and any liver herniation to the chest.

Bowel herniation: Herniation of bowels to the chest especially in Bochdalek hernia, to differentiate the true pulmonary tissues in the left hemithorax and determine the extent of pulmonary hypoplasia.

Foetal hydrops: Hydrops fetalis which is necessary for assessment of prognosis.

Imaging during the procedure[1-7]

During the EXIT procedure the radiologist is also intimately involved in aseptic intraprocedural sonography to determine doing the following:

Position of hysterostomy incision: Placental edges to identify where hysterostomy incision should be. Position of head and neck: Position of the head and neck to discern the best position to deliver the head/neck that is best suitable for intubation.

Intraoperative amniotic fluid drainage: Intraoperative amniotic fluid drainage or cystic mass aspiration under ultrasound guidance to decrease the size of the mass for delivery and decrease incision size.

State of placenta: Placental position, location, state, attachment, abruption or retroplacental bleed during the intraoperative period.

Intracardiac abnormalities: Transoesophageal sonography/echocardiography of the foetus is done during the intraoperative period to determine intracardiac abnormalities.

Interventional radiology before or during the EXIT procedure[1-5]

Interventional procedure: Ultrasound-guided percutaneous tracheostomy can be bone in the second trimester for a foetus with CHAOS, for amelioration of the condition before EXIT procedure close to term.

Percutaneous angioplasty: Atretic and stenosed trachea and larynx could be dilated percutaneously *in utero* using angioplasty balloon catheter and placement of coronary stent all under ultrasound guidance at second trimester.

Sclerosant obliteration of feeding abnormal vessels: Ultrasound-guided percutaneous laser coagulation of feeding artery to sequestrated lung segment or injection of coagulative sclerosant to obliterate the feeding artery and atrophy the sequestrated segment performed in the second trimester and or at EXIT procedure.

Fluid aspiration from huge cystic mass: Aspiration of the fluid from huge cystic mass in the neck under ultrasound guidance to decrease the size of the mass for delivery and decrease incision size.

Intraoperative amniotic fluid drainage: Intraoperative amniotic fluid drainage of polyhydramnois under ultrasound guidance to decrease the size of the uterus in order to decrease incision size.

Insertion of inferior vena cava filter: Pre-procedure maternal insertion of inferior vena cava filter.

Post-EXIT procedure imaging[1,2,7]

Chest radiography: Maternal chest radiography to exclude aspiration pneumonia, pulmonary embolism and lung collapse.

Retained product exclusion: Maternal abdominal sonography to exclude intra-abdominal collection and intrauterine retained products or any forgotten foreign body.

Assessment of baby lung expansion: Baby's chest radiography to assess the state of the lung and lung expansion and ventilation.

Assessment of neonatal brain: MR imaging and ultrasound of the newborn's brain to assess for any brain abnormalities.

Assessment of chest complications: Repeated imaging of the newborn's pharynx and chest is necessary to assess for chylothorax, pneumothorax, emphysema, haematoma, laryngomalacia, trachea re-stenosis, etc.

Deep vein thrombolectomy: Post-procedure interventional maternal deep vein thrombolectomy.

Inferior vena cava filter insertion: Post-procedure maternal insertion of inferior vena cava filters to prevent subsequent embolic materials reaching the lungs.

Problems of EXIT procedure[1,2,3,7]

Multi-disciplinary participation and action: It requires multi-disciplinary participation of personnel and the decision, judgment and action (function) of each of them is critical to the survival of both the mother and the foetus.

Intrapartum haemorrhage: There is extended uterine hyoptonia leading to intrapartum haemorrhage.

Small space for manipulation: The space available for the whole treatment is very small as only the head and neck are delivered while the rest of the foetal body is within the uterus.

Foetal hypothermia: The foetal head and neck are exposed for long time and hypothermia often develops.

Anaesthesia for mother and perinate: Both the mother and foetus require anaesthesia with the associated risks.

Long term residual sequelae: Most of the conditions requiring EXIT procedure are in the head, neck or thorax with resultant long term residual sequelae for the foetus.

Future chronic conditions: It is a high-risk procedure on a high-risk pregnancy meaning that more babies with chronic conditions will emerge in future due to the procedure.

Complications
1. Malposition of endotracheal tube.
2. Failure to secure airway resulting in foetal death.
3. Foetal hypothermia
4. Intra-procedure abruptio placenta.
5. Intrapartum haemorrhage
6. Post-partum haemorrhage from uterine hypotonia.
7. Hysterectomy.
8. Impaired speech problem later in life
9. Prolonged respiratory problems.
10. Pulmonary embolism of the mother

References
1. Dighe MK, Peterson SE, Dubinsky TJ, Perkins J, Cheng E. EXIT procedure: technique and indications with prenatal imaging parameters for assessment of airway patency. Radiographics 2011;31(2):511-26.
2. Chu GM, Yue V, Abdullah V, Chan HB, To WK, Chan MY, Kwan A. Ex-utero intrapartum treatment: a controlled approach to the management of anticipated airway problems in the newborn. Hong Kong Med J 2006; 12(5):381-4.
3. Shih JC, Hsu WC, Chou HC, Peng SS, Chen LK, Chang YL, Hsieh FJ. Prenatal three-dimensional ultrasound and magnetic resonance imaging evaluation of a fetal oral tumor in preparation for the ex-utero intrapartum treatment (EXIT) procedure. Ultrasound Obstet Gynecol 2005;25(1):76-9.
4. Filipchuck D, Avdimiretz L. The ex utero intrapartum treatment (EXIT) procedure for fetal head and neck masses. AORN J 2009;90(5):661-72.
5. Shih JC, Hsu WC, Chou HC, Peng SS, Chen LK, Chang YL, Hsieh FJ. Prenatal three-dimensional ultrasound and magnetic resonance imaging evaluation of a fetal oral tumor in preparation for the ex-utero intrapartum treatment (EXIT) procedure. Ultrasound Obstet Gynecol 2005; 25(1):76-9.
6. Myers LB, Bulich LA, Mizrahi A, Barnewolt C, Estroff J, Benson C, Kim HB, Jennings R. Ultrasonographic guidance for location of the trachea during the EXIT procedure for cervical teratoma. J Pediatr Surg 2003;38(4):E12.
7. Abraham RJ, Sau A, Maxwell D. A review of the EXIT (Ex utero Intrapartum Treatment) procedure. J Obstet Gynaecol 2010 Jan;30(1):1-5.

4.6 RADIOLOGICAL FINDINGS IN A PATIENT WITH CARCINOMA OF THE PROSTATE

Definition
This is defined as malignant transformation of some epithelial cells within the prostate. The involvement of the epithelia tissues leads to:
1. Prostatic adenocarcinoma = 99%
2. Transitional cell carcinoma = 1%

Sites of origin of adenocarcinoma within the prostate
Peripheral zone (posterior, lateral and apical) 80%
Transitional zone (within the centre) 10 – 15%
Central zone (between peripheral and transitional zone) 5 – 10%

Site of origin of transitional cell carcinoma
It arises from the prostatic ducts.

Demographic factors
1. Affects only males (only males have prostate)
2. More common in blacks than whites, least in Asians
3. One out of every 11 Americans develops the disease.

Normal prostate gland dimensions
Size = (4 x 3 x 3.8) cm
Volume = 20 cm^3
Weight = 20 g
Prostatic carcinoma may co-exist with benign prostatic hyperplasia (figure 4.61 A and B).

Diagnostic methods
1. Rectal Examination for size, consistency, nodularity
2. Serum prostate specific antigen (PSA) estimation
3. Radiological examination.

All the three methods are complementary to each other as none is 100% accurate or sensitive. Screening examination employing these tools must commence in any black male aged 40 years and above.

Definitive diagnosis
Biopsy of the lesion for histological examination. Histology proves diagnosis.

Role of Radiology
1. Diagnosis and staging of tumour
2. Evaluation of bladder outlet obstruction
3. Evaluation of effect of bladder outlet obstruction on the kidneys
4. Diagnosis of metastasis to organs and surrounding structures.
5. Diagnosis of tumour recurrence by examination of prostatic bed

6. Monitoring of therapy for determination of remission including complications and complications of therapy.

7.

Radiological Features
Plain films (

Osteoblastic metastasis: Plain film of pelvis may show osteoblastic (osteosclerotic) areas (figures 4.61 A and B). Prostatic carcinoma is the commonest metastatic bone tumour in males and almost all are osteoblastic.

Metastasis: Round or oval areas of increased density especially in the pelvis and spine may be shown. These grow slowly and merge, producing wide-spread, diffuse increase in density or chalky opacity.

Periosteal reaction: Periosteal reaction or periosteal new bone formation may be seen in pelvic bones.

Table 4.61: Radiological investigative modalities	
Plain films, various sites	Cystography
Excretory urography	Urethrography
CT and CT urography	Lymphangiography
MRI, MR urography, MR Angiography	Bone radionuclide imaging (scintingraphy)
Ultrasound scan -transrectal 7.5 MHz linear or phased array probe, transabdominal 3.5 MHz probe, transurethral 7.5 – 10 MHz probe, endoscopic scan using7.5 – 10 MHz probe.	Interventional studies -Ultrasound-guided biopsy for histology, CT-guided biopsy, Fluoroscopy-guided biopsy of lymph nodes, Endoscopic ultrasound-guided placement of stent

Bone expansion: Expansion of the bone may follow periosteal reaction.

Expansile osteolytic lesion: Expansile osteolytic metastatic lesion may be seen in some patients.

Solitary osteolytic lesion: Solitary osteolytic or sclerotic lesion in the bone due to metastasis.

Soft tissue mass at the bladder base: Soft tissue mass with new bone formation at bladder base simulating osteosarcoma may be seen.

Chalky sclerosis: Generalised dense sclerosis of pelvis, spine, ribs and skull may occur.

Osteolytic lesion in the trochanter: Osteolytic lesion in the greater or lesser trochanter may occur in isolation.

Miliary seeding: Multiple nodular pin-point hyperdense opacities in the lung can be seen. These are miliary seedings of the metastasis and may give rise to respiratory symptoms.

Lymphangitis carcinomatosa: This is due to metastatic spread to pulmonary perivascular, interlobular and perilymphatic channels in the lung bases appearing as linear opacities.

Pathological fracture: Pathological fracture of pelvis, femur or other bones weakened by metastatic lesion.

Ultrasound Scan

Prostatic enlargement: Asymmetrical enlargement of the prostate gland far above 20 cm^3, 20 g and (4 x 3 x 3.8) cm.

Most of the tumour is hypoechoic (> 60% of cases). However, isoechoic tumours are seen in 10% and hyperechoic tumour in 10%. In up to 20% and above tumour is not identified as they are imperceptibly isoechoic.

Irregular bulge sign: Multiple nodular changes with lobulated margins and deformed contour but intact prostatic capsule.

Heterogeneously nodular mass: Heterogeneously nodular and irregular mass with breached capsule. This suggests advanced tumour.

Hydronephrosis and hydroureters: This is calyceal dilatation due to the effect of bladder outlet obstruction and the ureters may also be dilated.

Metastasis: Metastatic hypoechoic nodules in the liver, spleen and kidneys.

Pleural effusion: Pleural effusion appearing as echo free space within the pleural cavity may be due to metastasis to the pleura.

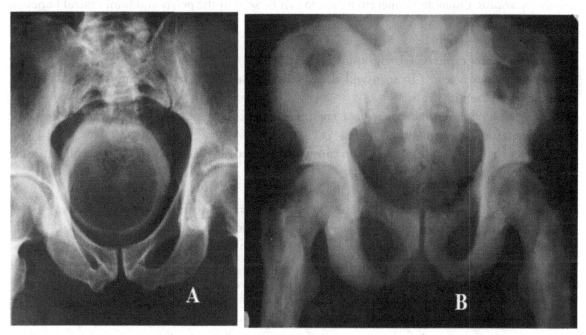

Figure 4.61. Imaging findings in carcinoma of the prostate. Bladder view of an excretory urography showing a large spherical filling defect within the bladder due to carcinoma of the prostate and also sclerotic metastasis in the pelvic bone (**A**). Plain radiograph of the pelvis in another patient showing chalky sclerotic metastasis due to prostatic carcinoma (**B**).

Ultrasound-guided Biopsy

This is done to biopsy the suspicious zone for histology as an adjunct to clinical examination and PSA chemistry assessment. It is not used as screening purposes.

Excretory Urography (EU) / Intravenous Urography (IVU)

Bladder filling-defect: Filling defect at the base of the bladder seen on bladder view. This is usually due to the enlarged prostate gland but could be due to prostatic carcinoma and both may co-exist together (figure 4.61 A).

Urinary bladder diverticulum: Bladder diverticulum, trabeculation, and wall thickening as a result of chronic urinary retention from bladder outlet obstruction.

Stone formation: This is seen in the urinary bladder, ureters or kidneys. It is due to urinary stasis from enlarged prostate encouraging stagnation of residue within the bladder and formation of stone.

Bilateral hydronephrosis: Enlarged kidney with bilateral hydronephrosis and hydroureter is demonstrated. There may be delayed nephrogram due to hydronephrosis. This hydronephrosis is later demonstrated with hydroureters bilaterally. This is caused by the prostate mass causing bladder outflow obstruction.

Elevation of vesico-ureteric junction by enlarged prostate: This also causes hydronephrosis and hydroureters bilaterally.

Distal ureteral invasion: Invasion of distal ureter with filling defect or lack of opacification of one or both distal ureter. Proximal hydronephrosis and hydroureter is also shown. The tumour stage at this time is stage 4.

Osseous metastasis: Osteoblastic metastatic lesion can be seen in the pelvis and lumbosacral bones on preliminary film.

Computed Tomography/CT Urography/Helical CT

Bladder base involvement: CT scan will detect extra-prostatic spread involving the bladder base, prostatic fat and seminal vesicles.

Lack of detection of lesion in normal-sized nodes: CT scan cannot detect intra-glandular tumour or tumour metastasis in normal sized nodes.

Measurement of lymph node size: CT scan can show enlarged external iliac lymph nodes and measure their size for tumour staging (table 4.61).

Improved anatomical details: CT urography/helical contrast CT scan will show the kidney, ureter, bladder and changes within them together with their relationship to surrounding organs.

Osseous metastasis: CT scan can detect osseous metastasis to spine and pelvis earlier than plain films.

Pulmonary metastasis: High resolution chest CT scan will show metastasis to the lung as multiple small dense opacities or linear opacities. These will be seen earlier than in plain films.

Magnetic resonance imaging

Perneural penetration: Focal thickening or bulging of posterior capsule of the prostate denotes tumour penetration to the perineural and adjacent tissues.

Vascular invasion: Tumour invasion of the perineural tissues and vascular structures at the angles of the prostate is better demonstrated by MR imaging than sonography or CT and could lend a clue to the possible extent of surgery.

Lymphadenopathy: T_1-weighted images will demonstrate lymphadenopathy.

Improved tumour staging: MRI can correctly stage the tumour in up to 70% of cases and is superior to ultrasound.

Non-specific heterogenous intensity: Heterogenous intensity which is non-specific is seen within the tumour; therefore, biopsy is used to confirm malignancy.

Measurement of tumour volume: Tumour volume can be measured by MRI which gives a guide to therapy, success of therapy and tumour recurrence.

Tumour recurrence: MRI can demonstrate tumour recurrence in prostatic bed by checking for presence of tumour and its volume after previous measurement. It is also used to check for emergence of new or larger enlarged lymph node.

Rectal infiltration: Obliteration of rectoprostatic angle is demonstrated by MRI and this shows tumour infiltration to the rectum.

Detection of distant metastasis: Distant metastasis to any organ can be found since MRI does sagittal and coronal sections of the whole body.

Cystography

Bladder filling-defect: This is used in the absence of ultrasound scan and MRI. It can show filling defect at the bladder base due to enlarged prostate gland.

Bladder wall thickening: Thickened bladder wall, diverticula and trabeculation formation.

Bladder stone: Vesical stone due to urinary stasis

Vesicorectal fistula: Fistulation between bladder and rectum shown on lateral view.

Osseous metastasis: Osseous (osteoblastic) metastatic lesion may be seen in pelvic bone and lumbosacral bone.

Urethrography

Both retrograde and micturating cystourethrography are performed.

Elevation of bladder base: Bladder base elevation is shown

Voiding hesitance: Hesitancy in micturition (voiding the contrast) is observed in micturating view due to urethral obstruction.

Bladder base filling-defect: Filling-defect at the bladder base.

Lymphangiography

External iliac lymphnode enlargement: External iliac chains of lymph nodes are enlarged and if they measure greater than 1 cm in diameter, it is a sure indicator of metastasis to lymph node.

Filling-defect within opacified lymphnodes: Opacification of irregular nodes with smaller filling-defects within them will enable their biopsy under fluoroscopy to be performed.

Bone scintigraphy

This detects metastasis with great accuracy and is the most sensitive method of its detection. Metastatic areas appear as hot areas on bone scan.

Interventional study

1. CT-guided biopsy
2. Ultrasound-guided biopsy
3. Fluoroscopy-guided biopsy after lymphangiography.
4. Ultrasound-guided endoscopic placement of expansible stainless steel stents for patients unfit for radical prostatectomy.

(Adam & Dixon, 2008; Dahnert, 2011; Sutton, 2003; Sanders & Winter, 2006).

References

1. Yablon CM, Banner MP, Ramchandani P, Rovner ES. Complications of prostate cancer treatment: spectrum of imaging findings. Radiographics 2004; 24 Suppl 1:S181-94.

2. Akbar SA, Sayyed TA, Jafri SZ, Hasteh F, Neill J. Multimodality imaging of paratesticular neoplasms and their rare mimics. Radiographics 2003; 23:1461-76.

3. Claus FG, Hricak H, Hattery RR. Pretreatment evaluation of prostate cancer: role of MR imaging and 1H MR spectroscopy. Radiographics 2004; 24 Suppl 1:S167-80.

4. Choi YJ, Kim JK, Kim N, Kim KW, Choi EK, Cho KS. Functional MR imaging of prostate cancer. Radiographics 2007 ; 27:63-75.

5. Anyanwu E, Anibeze CIP, Akpuaka FC, Mgbor S. Establishmentnent of normal prostate sizes within age groups in south eastern Nigeria. Journal of Experimental and clinical anatomy 2004;3: 42-44.

6. Marchie TT, Onuora VC. Determination of normal range of ultrasonic sizes of prostate in our local environment. West African Journal of Radiology 2001; 18: 54-64.

CHAPTER 5

HAEMOPOIETIC SYSTEM

5.1   RADIOLOGY OF SICKLE CELL ANAEMIA

Definition
Sickle cell disease is a congenital and hereditary disorder characterised by the presence of abnormal haemoglobin with reduced oxygen carrying capacity due to mutation of deoxyribonucleic acid (DNA).

Phenotypes
Heterozygous HbAS: Sickle cell trait without anaemia.
Homozygous HbSS: Sickle cell anaemia with symptomatic anaemia. It is rarely seen above 40 years as sufferers rarely live above this age.
Compound heterozygous variant: HbSC, HbSb-thalassaemia. These have normal life span and are less severe than HbSS. However, certain complications such as retinitis proliferans, osteonecrosis, and pulmonary embolism or acute chest syndrome appear to have a higher incidence in HbSC disease compared to HbSS

Prevalence: Black Africans particularly Central Africans (commonest) and West Africans, American Blacks 8 – 13%, Black Africans in Diaspora, Arabs, Italians, and Greeks.

Pathologic basis
The basic defects are as follows:
HbS: Mutation of DNA is due to substitution of glutamic acid with valine in position 6 of the b – chain.
HbC: In the DNA, there is substitution of glutamic acid with lysine in position 6 of the b – chain. In the presence of relative blood stasis in the capillaries due to sluggish flow, lowered oxygen tension leads to altering in the shape of the red blood cells to assume a sickle and unchanging or rigid shape. This increases the viscosity of blood leading to further stasis and vessel occlusion. Infarction of tissue may then develop.

Areas frequently affected by sickling include
1. Areas of slow blood flow in sinusoids, liver, spleen and medulla of bone and kidneys.
2. Areas of rapid tissue metabolism e.g. the brain, muscle and placenta.

Clinical features of sickle cell anaemia

Chronic haemolytic anaemia, abdominal pain/crises, jaundice, hand-foot syndrome, joint pains, bone pain, splenomegaly, hepatomegaly, pneumonias, chest pain due to lung infarct, chronic leg ulcers and pianism.

Radiological Features of Sickle Cell Anaemia

Musculoskeletal System

1. Hand – foot syndrome

This is sickle cell dactylitis occurring in infants aged 6 months – 2 years. Sickling of red blood cells (RBC) occludes blood vessels producing osteonecrosis and bone infarction, which appear as symmetrical:

    i.   Lytic areas or areas of radiolucency in the cortex (and medulla) of tubular bones of hands and feet.

    ii. Periosteal reaction which is often florid in the affected bone

    iii. Massive painful soft tissue swelling at the dorsum of hands and feet.

    iv. Sclerosis of the shaft of the affected tubular bones of hands and feet.

These findings are diagnostic of sickle cell anaemia

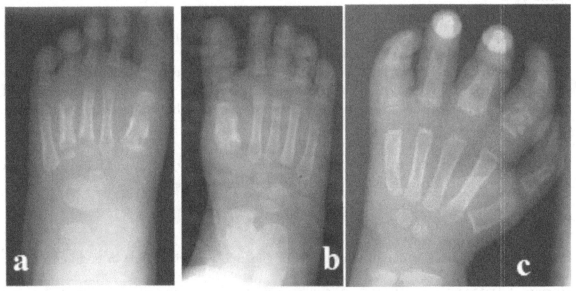

Figure 5.11: Hand-foot-syndrome in a 2-year old baby. The radiographs show multiple areas of oteolysis due to bone infarction affecting the metatarsal and the phalanges of the right and left foot (**a** and **b**) and the phalanges of the right hand (**c**). The left hand is similarly affected (not shown due to poor image quality).

Differential diagnosis of hand-foot syndrome

    1. Hypervitaminosis A

    2. Trauma with or without infection (osteomyelitis)

    3. Tuberculous dactylitis

    4. Infantile cortical hyperostosis

None is bilateral and symmetrical in both hands and feet

2. **Marrow hyperplasia**

   This is due to chronic anaemia. In general, it produces:
   i.   Widening of medullary cavity
   ii. Decrease in bone density (osteopaenia)
   iii. Cortical thinning due to endosteal bone resorption and osteopaenia
   iv. Coarse trabecular pattern

   a.   *In the skull it produces:*
        Widening of diplöe with sparing of inferior part of the occiput
        Ischaemia of the bones, causing headache
        Frontal bossing due to widening of the frontal sinus
        Hair-on-end appearance (5%)
        Thinning of outer table of skull
   b.   *The spine*
        Generalized osteopaenia /osteoporosis
        Coarse vertical striation/trabecular pattern
        Biconcave vertebrae or codfish vertebrae due to depression of central parts of the end-plates.
        Squared vertebrae
        Pathological fracture of vertebrae or collapse of one or more vertebrae
        Vanishing vertebra. One or more vertebra may dissolve and completely disappear.
   c.   *Tubular bones of hands and feet*
        Squared tubular bones, rectangular shaped tubular bones, and tri-radiate tubular bones with rectangular appearance.
        Increased medullary cavity with coarse trabecular pattern
   d.   *Enlarged vascular channels* with coarse trabecular pattern in small tubular bones of hands and feet.
        Rib notching due to enlarged vascular channels in the chest and ribs.
   e.   *Pathological fracture* due to porous bone produced by marrow hyperplasia with gross thinning of the tensile strength-providing cortex.

3. **Vascular occlusion**

   There is rouleaux formation or sickling of the red blood cells with blockage of vessels and osteonecrosis. This produces bone infarction, which is the hallmark of the disease.

   Long bones
   Diaphyseal bone infarction with osteolytic changes in early stages.
   Diaphyseal bone infarction with extensive sclerotic changes in late stages.
   Peg-in-hole appearance (central epiphyseal/metaphyseal bone defect or infarct). This is due to occlusion of nutrient artery to central part of metaphysis.
   Epiphyseal bone infarct in femoral head leads to:
   i.   Slipped femoral capital epiphysis (Type one Salter-Harris fracture)
   ii. Avascular necrosis of femoral head: This is observed in 12% of persons with sickle cell anaemia and 60% of those with HbSC disease
   Snow-cap sign of humeral head: This is dense sclerotic humeral head due to revascularisation of areas of avascular necrosis of humeral head.

Small tubular bones of hands and feet

Hand-foot syndrome (as discussed above)

H-shaped central metaphyseal defects in both ends of the small bones of hands and feet. This is due to occlusion of nutrient artery.

Vertebrae

H-shaped squared vertebrae: This is central metaphyseal or end-plate defect from infarction of the nutrient artery.

Fractures: Wedge-shaped or compression fracture of vertebrae or vertebra plana. There could also be multiple or single vertebral fracture.

Alignment deformities: Reduction in vertebral height from kyphosis and scoliosis, kyphoscoliosis and cod-fish vertebral deformities from generalised osteopaenia.

Skull bones

Bone infarction of the orbital wall, maxillary bone and skull base: This results from vaso-occlusion of the bone marrow: In bone infarction, CT demonstrates disruption of normal trabecular. Using T2-weighted and short inversion time inversion-recovery MR imaging, bone infarction with resulting marrow oedema are seen as areas of high signal intensity. In contrast MR imaging, areas of infarction demonstrate heterogeneous, rim-like enhancement and subperiosteal haemorrhage and adjacent fluid collections.

Subperiosteal haemorrhage and orbital compression syndrome: This arises from extravasation of blood due to necrosis of vessel wall, underlying bleeding abnormalities or minor trauma. Multiple focal lucencies that also could be due to infarct.

4. **Endosteal bone apposition**

There is internal cortical thickening with sclerosis.

There is also bone-in-bone appearance. This occurs when outer envelop of bone cortex is separated by a thin radiolucent zone from the inner cortex. This must be differentiated from infection.

There is narrowed or obliterated marrow cavity with diffuse or generalised increased density.

There is complete absence of endosteal apposition in axial skeleton due to persistent red marrow areas and this is diagnostic of sickle cell anaemia. All these lesions can also be found in the hands.

5. **Growth disturbances**

Retarded skeletal growth due to the following:
- Multiple Salter-Harris bone injuries or fractures
- Failure to thrive due to chronic anaemia

Premature epiphyseal fusion

Delayed closure of epiphysis

Reduction in height or stature due to:
- Cupped epiphysis due to osteopaenia and bone softening.
- Tibio-talar slant
- Reduced spinal vertebral height (kyphosis, scoliosis, kyphoscoliosis)
- Pseudo-Marfan's syndrome seen as long, slender long bones.

4. **Fractures**

Type 1 Salter – Harris fracture (slipped femoral capital epiphysis)
Vertebral collapse/fracture (single/multiple)
Fracture of long bones due to bone infarction or osteomyelitis
Compression fracture of femoral head resulting from avascular necrosis.
Cartilage fracture

5. **Osteomyelitis**

Long bones, small bones of the hand and feet, mandible and maxillary bones, Vertebrae (rare)
Salmonella organisms particularly *Salmonella typhinurium, Salmonella enteritidis, Salmonella choleraesuis,* and *Salmonella paratyphi* B are usually involved. *Staphylococcus aureus* may be involved. Chronic osteomyelitis heals rapidly with sequestrectomy and sensitive antibiotic therapy.

6. **Septic arthritis**

The offending organisms are Salmonella paratyphi group B and rarely *Staphylococcus aureus*

Extraskeletal Changes
The Chest
Acute chest syndrome: (It accounts for 25% of the deaths).

a. *This is an acute pulmonary illness* in which there are pulmonary consolidation, fever, chest pain and signs of chest compromise such as cough, dyspnoea or tachypnoea.

b. The causes of the acute chest syndrome are believed to be due to a combination of two or more of the following conditions: infection (bacterial or viral pneumonia), fat emboli from infarcting bone, pulmonary haemorrhage, pulmonary vascular occlusion; and pain from infarcting bones and lung preventing adequate ventilation.

Acute or adult respiratory distress syndrome
Pulmonary infarction (isolated).
Pulmonary fibrosis: This is called sickle cell chronic lung disease. There is interstitial fibrosis and high resolution CT shows scattered areas of lung scaring. These causes restrictive lung disease.
Sclerotic bones: Including ribs, scapulae, manubrum, spine and clavicle.
Chronic obstructive lung disease: This is rare occurring in less than 5% but can occur either alone or in combination with restrictive lung disease.
Asthma: There is slightly more incidence of asthma in sickle cell anaemia.
Pulmonary arterial hypertension: This is also more in sickle cell anaemia due to multiple small chronic pulmonary embolism.
Pulmonary embolism and pulmonary thromboembolism: This is also more common in patients with sickle cell anaemia and results from high viscousity of blood during vasoocclusive crises and problems with clothing mechanisms.

Extramedullary haemopoiesis
This gives rise to generalized or local enlargement of some organs and appearing as splenomegaly, hepatomegaly and as isolated masses in various organs (adrenal, skin, etc). Paravertebral masses may be seen in the thorax.

Herniation of medullary tissue into the paranasal cavities of maxillary, ethmoidal and sphenoidal sinuses due to underlying bone marrow hyperplasia leads to extramedullary haematopoiesis within the sinuses.

Liver

Cirrhosis: From dilatation of sinusoids and perisinusoidal fibrosis, ischaemia and necrosis. The causes of liver cirrhosis in patients with sickle cell anaemia could also be from hypoxic injury due to red blood cell sickling, hepatitis, gallstones, right heart failure, iron overload, and chronic use of other drug or chronic intake of alcohol.

Liver infarction: Resulting from ischaemia and necrosis.

Intrahepatic biliary duct stenosis.

Hepatitis: From repeated transfusion.

Sequestration syndrome: Less common than in the spleen.

Haemosiderosis: Evidence of iron overload from repeated transfusion in patients dependent on transfusion.

Gall bladder

Cholelithiasis: This is due to the release of iron pigments from accelerated destruction of erythrocytes. Jaundice is a major presenting symptom.

Spleen

What could be observed in the spleen includes:

i.   *Sequestration syndrome:* This results from rapid pooling of blood within a solid organ, usually the spleen in sickle cell anaemia. It could lead to sequestration crises and anaemia.

ii. *Splenic infarction:* This occurs from vascular occlusion and may progress to spontaneous splenic rupture.

iii. *Splenic rupture:* From splenic infarction.

iv. *Autosplenectomy*: Non-functioning spleen which could be removed from its bed and found elsewhere and could be completely calcified.

Heart

i.   *Cardiomegaly:* This results from anaemic heart failure with cardiac dilatation.

ii. *Congestive cardiac failure:* This is from increased anaemia. It could result to hyperdynamic cardiac failure.

iii. Vegetation could also be found in the heart.

iv. *Ischaemic heart disease*: Cardiac ischaemia, thrombus formation and myocardial infarction are also found.

Kidney

i.   Grossly enlarged smooth kidneys.

ii.   Nephritic syndrome

iii. Glomerulosclerosis

iv.   Renal papillary necrosis (15-36%)

v.   Renal failure (4-18%). Terminal in most cases of chronic renal failure.

vi.   Renal calculi

vii. Focal renal scarring and fibrosis

The Brain

Neurological complication is observed in about 25% of patients with sickle cell anaemia in their lifetime and over in 10% it occurs before the age of 20 years. These include:

Cerebrovascular accident/Stroke: This results in lifelong cognitive and functional impairment.

"Silent infarction" in 20% (asymptomatic). This is clinical ischaemic infarct and occurs in about 50% (symptomatic). The total rate of various degrees of infarction is about 70%. Infarction is also more common in patients that are less than 10 years.

Haemorrhagic cerebrovascular accident: This is intraparenchymal and results from aneurysms. It occurs in 20% of patients aged 20 – 30 years old.

Subarachnoid haemorrhage: It is more common in those aged 20 – 30 years.

Moyamoya disease: It is seen in 30% to 35% of patients with sickle cell anaemia. It has *"puff of smoke"* appearance in cerebral angiography and its combination with sickle cell anaemia results in moyamoya syndrome.

Atraumatic epidural haematoma: This results from skull bone infarction or orbital wall infarct with formation of sub-periosteal haematoma.

Multiple aneurysms: Particularly from the vertebrobasilar system.

Subdural haemorrhage: This could result from rupture of intracerebral aneurysms into the subdural space.

Sensory-neural hearing loss: This occurs in up to 3% to 4% of patients. It is due to recurrent vaso-occlusion of the labyrinthine blood vessels leading to labyrinthine haemorrhage. This stimulates a healing response that results to changes ranging from fibrosis to sclerosis and ultimately ossification of the inner ear structures.

The Eyes

Retinal haemorrhage: This is from occlusion of central retinal artery by retinal artery thrombosis causes. Retinal detachment, spontaneous vitreous haemorrhage and blindness also occur.

Proliferative retinopathy is increasingly reported.

Orbital compression syndrome: This is from infarct of osseous wall of the orbit with oedema formation and subperiosteal haematoma.

Proptosis: This is due to subperiosteal haemorrhage occurring as a result of vaso-occlusive crises.

Vascular involvement

According to imaging appearances, vascular involvement is classified as arterial *tortuosity, stenosis, occlusion, or aneurysm*, in line with imaging appearance.

Tortuosity of vessels: Tortuosity is diagnosed on the basis of the following features: *(i)* dilatation or ectasia of a vessel segment, *(ii)* abnormal increase in affected vessel segment length, and *(iii)* obvious bowing of affected artery.

In sufferers, arterial tortuosity is believed to be an adaptive response to chronic anaemia. And also, vessel tortuosity is a predictor of chronic brain hypoxia.

Stenosis, occlusion and aneurysm formation: It is thought that damage to the vessel intima leads to vascular stenosis and occlusion; and that endothelial damage leads to aneurysm formation.

Progressive bilateral nasal obstruction

There is expanded diploic space appearing grossly expanded and protruding into the sinus cavity. This may appear as soft-tissue mass within and filling the sinuses. This can lead to bilateral nasal obstruction.

Appendicitis
The occurrence of appendicitis is reduced in patients with sickle cell disease compared to the normal population. In sickle cell anaemia, this reduction is up to one third of the rate in normal population.

Skeletal muscle
There is infarction and calcification of skeletal muscles resulting in inability of the muscle to contract. Thus, the patient cannot bend the affected limbs. It results in severe movement disability with waddling gait.

Chronic leg ulcer
Ulcers, seen especially at soft tissue overlying bony prominences are common and are believed to result from venous stasis and tissue hypoxia and when there is vascular damage, they become difficult to treat leading to chronic changes and osteomyelitis as commensal organisms present on the skin invade them.

Hyperuricemia
Hyperuricemia results from increased cell turnover.

Dental abnormalities
Dental caries and necrosis of the dental pulp. This may result to mandibular osteomyelitis.

Lymphadenothy
Multiple lymph node enlargements, cervical and other regional lymphadenopathies occur in sickle cell anaemia as a result of recurrent infections, which the sufferers are predisposed to.

Malignancies
Haematologic malignancies such as lymphoma, multiple myelomas and hairy cell leukaemia are more common in patients with sickle cell anaemia.

(Adam & Dixon, 2008; Dahnert, 2011; Sutton, 1998 and 2003, Swischuk, 2004; Palmer & Reeder 2001).

References
1. Lagundoye SB. Radiological features of sickle cell anaemia and related haemoglobinopathies in Nigeria. Afr J Med Sci 1970; 1:315-342.
2. Longergan GJ, Cline DB, Abhondanzo SL. Sickle cell anaemia. Radiographics 2001;21:971-994.
3. Saito N, Nadgir RN, Flower EN, Sakai O. Clinical and radiologic manifestations of sickle cell disease in the head and neck. Radiographics 2010; 30:1021-34.
4. Williams OA, Lagundoye SB, Johson CL. Lamellation of the diploe in the skulls of patient with sickle cell anaemia. Archives of Disease in Childhood 1975: 50, 948-952.
5. Madani G, Papadopoulou AM, Holloway B, Robins A, Davis J, Murray D. The radiological manifestations of sickle cell disease. Clin Radiol 2007; 62:528-38.
6. Ozoh JO, Onuigbo MA, Nwankwo N, Ukabam SO, Umerah BC, Emeruwa CC. "Vanishing" of vertebra in a patient with sickle cell haemoglobinopathy. BMJ 1990 ;301:1368-9.
7. Akamaguna AI, Odita JC, Ugbodaga CI, Okafor LA. Cholelithiasis in sickle cell disease: a cholecystographic and ultrasonographic evaluation in Nigerians. Eur J Radiol 1985;5:271-2.

8. Babalola OE, Wambebe CO. Ocular morbidity from sickle cell disease in a Nigerian cohort. Niger Postgrad Med J 2005;12:241-4.

9. Ejindu VC, Hine AL, Mashayekhi M, Shorvon PJ, Misra RR. Musculoskeletal manifestations of sickle cell disease. Radiographics 2007; 27:1005-21.

10. Ogunseyinde AO, Obajimi MO, Fatunde OJ. Computed tomographic pattern of stroke in children with sickle cell anaemia in Ibadan. Afr J Med Med Sci 2005; 24: 115-118.

11. Emodi JI, Okoye IJ. Vertebral bone collapse in sickle cell disease: a report of two cases. East Afr Med J 2001;78:445-6.

5.2 RADIOLOGICAL FINDINGS IN HODGKIN'S LYMPHOMA

Definition
Hodgkin's lymphoma is a type of primary malignant neoplasm of the immune system (lymphoid tissues) characterised by the presence of Reed-Sternberg cells in the nucleus of lymphocytes. Hodgkin's lymphoma comprises 40% of all the lymphomas and it is a disease of the T-cells.

Epidemiology
In the UK, lymphomas comprise 4% of newly diagnosed malignancy. Hodgkin's disease comprises 25% of newly diagnosed lymphomas.

Lymphomas are the third most frequent malignancies in children after leukaemia and central nervous system neoplasia.

Hodgkin's disease accounts for 1% of all newly diagnosed malignancies.

Age distribution: Bimodal distribution.
1. 25 – 30 years
2. 70 – 74 years

Histology
Presence of Reed-Sternberg cells in the nucleus of lymphocytes is characteristic.

Pathological classification
1. **Nodular sclerosing type**

   It is the most common type, more common in females, shows mediastinal and supraclavicular lymphadenopathy and has good prognosis.

2. **Lymphocyte-predominant (LP) type**

   It is frequently localised, uncommon, shows strong host response, majority of patients are less than 35 years and it has excellent prognosis.

3. **Mixed cellularity type**

   It is more common than LP and LD, B-symptoms (B-symptoms means abdominal organ involvement) and has less favourable prognosis.

4. **Lymphocyte-depleted (LD) type**

   This is uncommon, shows very weak host response, occurs in older patient age, polysymptomatic, numerous Reed-Sternberg cells are seen, advanced disseminated disease at the time of initial diagnosis and is often rapidly fatal.

Radiological Features

The Chest
Anterior mediastinal lymphadenopathy
The anterior mediastinum is the focus of the disease. Lymph nodes involvement occur

Hilar lymphadenopathy

This is seen in 50 – 67% of cases. It is usually bilateral and asymmetrical (sarcoidosis is bilateral and symmetrical and also involves the anterior node).

Mediastinal widening

Asymmetrical widening of mediastinum from paratracheal, tracheobronchial and middle mediastinal lymph node enlargement. Carinal, unilateral or bilateral masses also involving the anterior mediastinum are shown.

Calcification of lymph node

This has **egg**-shell calcification. Calcification of lymph nodes may follow chemotherapy or radiotherapy. In radiotherapy-associated calcification, there is associated mediastinal fibrosis extending into the lungs with widening of mediastinum on both sides with characteristic vertical straight lines due to the treatment field.

Lobar consolidation

The involvement of the lung can appear as an area of lobar consolidation. Usually there is associated lymphadenopathy. The lung opacity often has air-bronchogram and shaggy borders. The lesions are most frequent at the bases.

Bronchopneumonia

Patchy areas of larger opacities which may be confluent involving one or more lobes may occur. They have shaggy borders.

Lung collapse

Involvement of the bronchial wall may lead to collapse of a lobe. The lymphadenopathy can also compress a bronchus and lead to collapse. There is consolidation of the contiguous lung close to the area of collapse.

Lung cavities

Both the lobar opacities and the more confluent opacities may cavitate. Usually they have thick walls but may occasionally have thin walls. Necrosis of an enlarged lymph node can also lead to cavitary appearance.

Lymphangitis carcinomatosa

Diffuse reticulonodular appearance due to the spread of the tumours along peribronchial connective tissue.

Pleural effusion

This is seen in about 30%. It is due to lymphatic obstruction and therefore benign. It consists of homogenous opacities with lateral meniscus sign.

Pleural plaques

Direct involvement of the pleura by the disease can lead to pleural plaques. Tumour masses adjacent to the pleura can be seen.

Miliary opacities

Multiple, varying size, pin-head opacities throughout the lung due to pulmonary infiltration by the disease. The appearance resembles miliary tuberculosis.

Solitary pulmonary nodule

Coin lesion or solitary pulmonary nodule may be seen. It can be subpleural or within the lung field and may suggest consolidation if it is small and round. Usually there is associated lymphadenopathy.

Multiple pulmonary nodules

They usually measure less than 1cm in diameter but are much larger than miliary opacities. Differentiation from metastasis is difficult.

Opportunistic infection

Other features which may suggest opportunistic infections are:
1. Consolidation with bulging fissure/border
2. Bilateral diffuse pneumonia due to pneumocystis jiroveci (carinii).
3. Multiple cavitations in rapid succession due to anaerobic organisms.
4. Multiple pulmonary nodules due to fungal infection especially aspergillosis.

The Vertebrae
Anterior erosion of vertebral bodies

This is almost diagnostic. Anterior erosion/scalloping may involve one or more vertebrae and it is caused by adjacent enlarged lymph nodes. There may be associated sclerosis. Aneurysms of abdominal aorta and Pott's disease with paravertebral abscess are other diseases that can cause the same appearance and therefore must be excluded.

Pseudoparavertebral abscess

Soft tissue mass, enlarged lymph nodes with some of its necrotic or cavitary component may simulate paravertebral abscess. TB must be excluded.

Vertebral collapse

Osteolytic destructive lesion from the bone or direct involvement of the vertebrae by the tumour may lead to collapse of one or more vertebrae. Intervertebral disc space and the density of the end-plates are spared helping to differentiate it from infection and infective discitis. Osteoporosis, TB, trauma, multiple myeloma and pyogenic spondylitis are other common differentials to exclude since they can cause one or more vertebral collapse.

Ivory vertebra/solitary dense vertebra

Well-preserved vertebral size with completely sclerotic appearance. This is almost pathognomonic of the disease especially when it occurs in the young adult.

Diffuse sclerosis of vertebrae

Diffuse increase in density of two or more vertebral bodies. The sizes of the vertebrae are preserved but there may be anterior erosion due to lymphadenopathy

Subcutaneous and spinal extension of the tumour. This may occur.

Rib Lesions
Osteolytic lesion which expands the affected rib. They are often observed in chest radiography.

Sternum
Osteolytic destructive lesion from direct invasion from the lung or mediastinum.
Mixed osteolytic and sclerotic lesion with bony spiculation. The affected area is usually expanded.
Retrosternal and presternal soft tissue masses/swelling are seen but only occasionally.

Pelvis
Mixed osteolytic and sclerotic lesion or purely sclerotic types are more commonly seen.
Increased density of medial part of inorminate bone.
Multiple diffuse small areas of non-specific osteolytic lesions are seen in the Ischium which may progress to the mixed pattern on serial examinations.

Long Bones
The metaphysis having persistent red bone marrow is affected in the femur and humerus. the features seen are as follows:

Small oval translucencies in the long axis of the bone
These may extend through a long length in the marrow cavity and may cause endosteal scalloping of the cortex. This can also be seen in leukaemia, non-Hodgkin's lymphoma and Gaucher's disease.

Endosteal scalloping of the cortex
This is seen as long-length osteolytic oval lesion within the bone marrow, oriented in the long axis of the bone.

Honey-comb appearance
Multiple small oval-shaped translucencies when close together produce honey-comb appearance. These translucencies are areas of lytic destruction. The remaining translucencies will appear coarse and will also simulate medullary change in Gaucher's disease.

Periosteal reaction
This can be seen occasionally and will differentiate HL from Gaucher's disease which does not have periosteal reaction or very rarely does it occur in exceptional cases.

Hypertrophic osteoarthropathy
Intrathoracic lesion may cause this appearance. There is bilateral fluffy periosteal reaction in some bones including the wrist and ankle.

Flat Bones (Clavicles, Skull, Scapulae)
They are occasionally affected.
1. Pathological fracture can occur.
2. Sclerotic type of lesion with absence of bony expansion which in the elderly differentiates it from Paget's disease.

CT and MRI in Hodgkin's diseases of the chest and abdomen

1. MRI is superior to CT in detection of lymph node enlargement in the hilum because of superior contrast resolution and the multiplanar capabilities of MRI.
2. MRI and CT have the same success rate in detection of mediastinal lymph node enlargement.
3. MRI can detect invasion of aorto–pulmonary window and subcarinal spaces better than CT.
4. CT scan detects abnormal lymph nodes as homogenous soft tissue mass with sharply defined and often lobulated margins. Lymph nodes enhance when intravenous contrast is given and decreased attenuation of the centre of lymph node is due to necrosis.
5. CT is useful in detecting diameter and patency of the airway especially in children who often show significant airway obstruction.

GIT (involved only in 10% of Hodgkin's lymphoma)

The Stomach

Multiple polyploid masses showing filling defects on barium meal and oral contrast-enhanced CT scan. Central ulceration of the lesions is shown.

Ulceration

This is often central. It is seen in double-contrast barium meal examination.

Bull's eye lesion

Target appearance due to central ulceration in polyploid masses. Barium collects within the central ulceration and this is seen contrasted against the filling defect of the mass. It may be single or multiple. Lymphoma is highly suggested but histology is needed to prove whether Hodgkin's or non-Hodgkin's.

Infiltrating lesion simulating gastric carcinoma

Filling defects on barium meal, thickening of stomach wall and narrowing of gastric lumen. Extensive infiltrating lesion which thickens the gastric mucosa suggests the diagnosis.

Giant cavitating lesion may occur and is almost characteristic.

Linitis plastic

Diffuse submucosal infiltrations which thicken the gastric wall, narrow and elongate the stomach.

Desmoplastic reaction

Only Hodgkin's lymphoma produces desmoplastic reaction reducing the distensibility of the stomach. Other lymphomas don't.

Narrowing of oesophago-gastric junction

Upwards spread of fundaly sited gastric lymphoma causes this appearance on barium swallow or barium meal examination.

CT features which suggest lymphoma rather than carcinoma of the stomach

a. Bulky tumour
b. Significant thickening of stomach wall
c. Transpyloric spread
d. Multicentricity

e. Widespread nodal disease
f. Splenic enlargement

The Duodenum

This is rare. Duodenal involvement is via spread from the stomach or jejunum as it contains only very little lymphoid tissue.

Small Intestine

Hodgkin's lymphoma is rare in the small intestine though there is relatively high incidence in patients with coeliac disease.

Nodular bowel lesion

Single or multiple round nodular filling defects are found which can be localised or extensively spread throughout the bowel.

Thickening of the mucosa

Ulceration

The nodules may erode into the bowels causing ulceration.

Intussusception

This is the invagination of one loop of bowel into the other causing intestinal obstruction. The nodules act as lead point.

Wide displacement of the bowel with separation of loops of bowel. This is caused by large tumours.

Lymphatic obstruction

This can cause ascites, oedema or thickening of the soft tissue.

Aphthoid ulcers

Multiple shallow ulcerations in the small intestines. This may simulate inflammatory aphthoid ulcers of Crohn's disease.

Widening of bowel loops with slow transit of barium

This is due to infiltration of nerve plexus with some degree of paralysis of intestinal muscles.

Fistulation

This can occur but very rare in Hodgkin's lymphoma. Large masses are also rare in Hodgkin's lymphoma.

The Colon

Hodgkin's lymphoma involvement of the colon is extremely rare.

SPLEEN
1. Splenic involvement may be so uniformly enlarged that no identifiable focal abnormality is seen in up to 50%.
2. Multiple focal low attenuating-lesions may be seen on CT scan.
3. On ultrasound scan, focal splenic deposits which are well-defined, round and poorly echogenic. Occasionally hyperechoic lesions may be seen.
4. Splenomegaly is seen in only 50% and if no focal lesion is seen, other diagnosis may be entertained.

Liver
1. This may appear as multiple, well-defined areas of nodular low-attenuating changes.
2. There is hepatomegaly
3. Necrosis within nodules may be seen if the nodules are very large.

Renal Lymphoma
Involvement of the kidney by Hodgkin's lymphoma is rare.
It may appear as renal enlargement which is often generalised.
It can also appear as solitary masses, multiple focal masses or diffuse infiltration.

Ultrasound in GIT lymphoma
1. This shows the presence of lymph node enlargement.
2. It will also show bowel thickening.
3. It will show infiltration of the spleen and liver which will appear as nodular masses.

CT Scan of GIT
1. **Sandwich sign**
   Enlarged gland may surround the superior mesenteric artery/or vein. The fat around the vessels seen in contrast with the enlarged lymph nodes gives this appearance/sign
2. Lymph node enlargement is accurately detected.
3. Presence of nodular masses/involvement of the spleen, kidney and liver by the disease.
4. Thick mucosal fold with slight bowel dilatation.
5. **Aneurysmal dilatation** of an end-exoenteric lesion can be seen.
6. **Retroperitoneal lymphadenopathy** can be accurately identified.

The Eye
Hodgkin's lymphoma of the eye is rare
Lymphoma in the eyes is almost always non-Hodgkin's type. Histology is essential for adequate categorization. It is often bilateral and there is female preponderance.

Proptosis
Involvement of the rectus muscle and lacrimal gland is seen and may extend posteriorly into the extra-conal space.

Venous congestion due to cavernous sinus thrombosis may result.

Orbital apex mass lesion with involvement of the ophthalmic vein may occur. This may cause confusion unless coronal CT/MRI is done.

The Neck

Clinical palpation is almost always diagnostic of enlarged lymph nodes. Histology is required to know the type, and for staging, while assessment of abdominal lesion is required to check for recurrence after treatment.

The Testes

Hodgkin's disease affects the testes less frequently than non-Hodgkin's disease. It occurs in the middle-aged and elderly men and about 25% are bilateral. It may spread to the lungs, regional inguinal and abdominal lymph nodes, neck and central nervous system.

Spinal Cord

1. This can occur as epidural, subdural or intra-medullary masses.
2. Transection of the cord at a particular level can occur.
3. Mass effect from destroyed vertebra/disc may impinge on the spinal cord.

The Brain

Solitary or multiple ring-enhancing lesions. These are often seen in HIV/AIDS and there is associated surrounding low-attenuating area.

AIDS–Related Lymphoma

Only rarely is this the Hodgkin's type.
1. There is hepatosplenomegaly
2. Enlarged abdominal lymph nodes
3. Bowel displacement due to abdominal lymphadenopathy
4. Direct involvement of stomach, rectum and distal ileum in patients with ileal disease.
5. On CT, bowel displacement is noted.
6. Bowel perforation may occur.

(Adam & Dixon, 2008; Dahnert, 2011; Sutton, 1998 and 2003, Palmer & Reeder 2001).

References

1. Leite NP, Kased N, Hanna RF, Brown MA, Pereira JM, Cunha R, Sirlin CB. Cross-sectional imaging of extranodal involvement in abdominopelvic lymphoproliferative malignancies. Radiographics 2007; 27:1613-34.
2. Ghai S, Pattison J, Ghai S, O'Malley ME, Khalili K, Stephens M. Primary gastrointestinal lymphoma: spectrum of imaging findings with pathologic correlation. Radiographics. 2007; 27:1371-88.
3. Toma P, Granata C, Rossi A, Garaventa A. Multimodality imaging of Hodgkin's disease and non-Hodgkin's lymphomas in children. Radiographics 2007; 27:1335-54.
4. Guermazi A, Brice P, Hennequin C, Sarfati E. Lymphography: an old technique retains its usefulness. Radiographics 2003; 23:1541-58.
5. Guermazi A, Brice P, de Kerviler E E, Fermé C, Hennequin C, Meignin V, Frija J. Extranodal Hodgkin's disease: spectrum of disease. Radiographics 2001;21:161-79.
6. Fishman EK, Kuhlman JE, Jones RJ. CT of lymphoma: spectrum of disease. Radiographics 1991; 11:647-69.
7. Gossmann A, Eich HT, Engert A, Josting A, Müller RP, Diehl V, Lackner KJ. CT and MR imaging in Hodgkin's disease--present and future. Eur J Haematol Suppl 2005; (66):83-9.

5.3 RADIOLOGICAL FINDINGS IN NON-HODGKIN'S LYMPHOMA

Definition
Non-Hodgkin's lymphoma is a malignant disease of mostly the B-cell lymphocytes. However, T-cell lymphocytes found in the skin and thymus (from peripheral T-cell) may rarely be involved and comprise 10% of the total lymphocytes involved in non-Hodgkin's lymphoma.

Incidence:
1. It is the third most common cancer in childhood (after leukaemia and CNS neoplasm)
2. It is four times more common than Hodgkin's disease
3. It is more common in the elderly.

Age affected: Median age is 55 years but all ages are affected

Sex ratio: M: F = 1: 1

Classification
A. According to grade of malignancy
   1. Low grade
   2. Intermediate grade
   3. High grade
B. According to lymph node involvement
   1. Low grade (nodular or follicular lymphoma)
   2. High grade (diffuse lymphoma)

Cell of origin
A. B-cells (nodal form within lymphoid follicles)
   a. Centrocytes (with irregular nuclei), cleaved cells.
   b. Centroblasts (with large round nuclei), non-cleaved cells.
   c. Mixture of A and B
   d. Histiocytes (monocytes lodged in body tissues (5%)).
B. B-cells which exist outside follicles (Diffuse form).

Predisposing factors
These present 40 – 100 times greater risk than in normal persons.
1. Congenital immunodeficiency syndrome
2. Patients with HIV/AIDS.
3. Patients with organ transplant.
4. Collagen vascular disease.

Clinical features
Painless enlarged lymph nodes, chest pain, shoulder pain, dyspnoea, dysphagia, limb/leg swelling, congestive cardiac failure, hypotension, superior vena caval obstruction, back ache, fever, weight loss, anorexia and enlarged lymph node in unusual sites (elbows, knees, ankle).

GIT symptoms
Nausea, vomiting, weight loss, diarrhoea, abdominal pain and melaena stool.

Region of involvement
A. Nodal involvement
1. Splenic hilar involvement 53%
2. Mediastinal involvement 51%
3. Para-aortic lymph node involvement 49%

B. Extranodal involvement
Spleen 41%, liver 14%, G.I.T. 12%, urogenital system 10%, skin   6%, (bone CNS, head and neck, and breast) 10%.

Radiological investigative modalities
1. Plain x-ray (Chest – PA, lateral, apical lordotic, penetrated view, Abdomen and Skull.
2. Ultrasound
3. CT scan
4. MRI
5. Barium studies
6. IVU
7. Lymphography

Radiological manifestations
Chest
Plain films
1. Single hilar lymph node enlargement
2. *Pulmonary lobar pneumonia*: Lung consolidation
3. Pulmonary infiltrates with bronchovascular involvement
4. *Metastatic spread* to the lung with lymphangitis carcinomatosa
5. *Pleural effusion:* This is due to pleural involvement and often precedes mediastinal involvement.
6. *Lymphangitis carcinomatosa* often associated with multiple lobar involvements.
7. *Lung collapse:* Due to endobronchial lymphoma and mediastinal adenopathy compressing the airway.
8. Miliary nodules/infiltrates with air-bronchogram.
9. *Cavitation:* This has thick or thin wall. Cavitation is often eccentric.
10. Soft tissue masses adjacent to rib deposits.
11. *Pericardial effusion*: Enlarged heart with palm-wine keg appearance and pencilled-in cardiac margins.

Mediastinum
The mediastinum is not commonly involved in non-Hodgkin's lymphoma and its involvement represents widespread disease.
1. Bilateral and asymmetrical widening of the superior part of the middle mediastinum
2. Enlargement of paratracheal and tracheobronchial lymph nodes
3. Splaying of the carina by subcarinal node involvement
4. Bilateral hilar mass
5. Unilateral hilar mass
6. Compression of oesophagus. Seen on barium swallow due to invasion of middle and distal oesophagus.

Oesophagus

1. Primary non-Hodgkin's lymphoma of the oesophagus resembles oesophageal carcinoma with short-segment narrowing, destruction of mucosal pattern, shouldering and apple-core deformity.
2. However it may also appear as diffuse nodularity of the whole length of the oesophagus seen as multiple polypoid filling defects on barium swallow
3. *Ulceration:* Submucosal nodules may ulcerate with ulcer craters seen on barium swallow
4. C T scan will identify oesophageal masses outside the lumen.
5. Achalasia-like appearance may occur with rat-tail narrowing and proximal dilatation if there is submucosal infiltration of the distal oesophagus.
6. Multiple serpiginous filling defects in the middle and distal oesophagus appearing like oesophageal varices may be seen. Repeated films to note whether there is change in position which is seen in varices is an important distinguishing feature.
7. Gastric lymphoma may spread upwards and involve the distal oesophagus with extensive filling defect, shouldering, irregular margins and destruction of mucosal pattern.

Stomach

1. The commonest site of development of GIT lymphoma, and 90% is non-Hodgkin's type.
2. Coeliac disease is a predisposing factor
3. Solitary polypoid tumour with filling defect on barium meal identical to features seen in benign polyp
4. Solitary polypoid, eccentric and infiltrative tumour with destruction of bowel wall and mucosal pattern similar to features seen in carcinoma.
5. Multiple polypoid tumour with central ulceration giving the "bull's eye" appearance or target lesion (characteristic)
6. Giant cavitating lesion
7. Extensive infiltrative lesion with great thickening of gastric mucosal fold.
8. Diffuse submucosal infiltration which also thickens gastric mucosal fold
9. *Linitis plastica:* Marked reduction of stomach capacity, stretching of stomach and narrowing due to tumour infiltration.
10. *Duodenal deformity:* This is due to spread of antral tumour.
11. *Filling-defect:* Filling-defect, shouldering, apple core deformity and mucosal irregularity due to antral tumour
12. Fundal tumour can spread to involve the distal oesophagus, cause lesion similar to Barrett's oesophagus or achalasia
13. Single or multiple ulcers with irregular margins
14. In CT scan and MRI lymph nodes larger than 1cm in diameter are enlarged.

CT Features that suggest lymphoma rather than carcinoma

1. Bulky tumour producing thickening of gastric wall
2. Significant growth outside the gastric wall
3. Transpyloric spread
4. Multicentricity
5. Widespread nodal involvement
6. Splenic enlargement
7. Duodena3l involvement is from gastric or jejunal spread since the duodenum contains very little lymphoid tissue.

Small intestines

Uncommon site, occurs only in 20% of GIT involvement, occurs in distal rather than proximal small intestines due to presence of Peyer's patches in the ileum. High incidence is seen in coeliac disease.

Features seen on Barium follow-through

1. Focal or extensive involvement throughout small intestine.
2. Single or multiple nodules causing filling-defects in the small intestine.
3. Thickening of mucosal fold. This is often associated.
4. Ulceration. Ulceration with ulcer crater are associated.
5. Intussusception. Nodules may act as lead point to intussusception causing intestinal obstruction.
6. On plain film, CT scan and barium follow-through, large tumour will cause bowel displacement to the contralateral side.
7. Bowel separation and obstruction (of lymphatics)
8. Aphthoid ulcers. Multiple small nodules undergoing ulceration simulate aphthoid ulcers.
9. Involvement or infiltration of nerve plexuses leads to widening of bowel loops and slow transit of barium.
10. Hepatomegaly (with finger clubbing).
11. Bowel perforation.
12. Fistula formation.
13. Malabsorption-like features in small bowel.
14. Annular long-segment or tubular constriction.
15. Aneurysmal dilatation with featureless bowel.

Colon

Almost always non-Hodgkin's type.

Mostly from secondary involvement from other primary sites, caecum and rectum are characteristically involved.

1. Bulky polypoid tumour is characteristic.
2. Long-segment narrowing or the entire segment may be involved.
3. Diffuse nodularity with filling defects.
4. Cavitations. The lesion may cavitate.
5. Short-segment narrowing with shouldering, apple-core deformity, and irregular mucosal pattern may occur.
6. Polypoid mass may induce intussusception or intestinal obstruction.
7. Constriction/tubular annular lesion.

Liver

1. Hepatomegaly
2. Lymphadenopathy at porta hepatis
3. Multiple polypoid nodular hypodensities in the liver

Spleen

1. Splenomegaly.
2. Lymphadenopathy at splenic hilum.

Eye and Orbital Lesions

Primary lymphomas of the orbit are often non-Hodgkin's type and represent 1% of lymphomas. They present with proptosis and pain in the eye.

Ultrasound, CT and MRI will show.

1. Poorly defined infiltrative mass
2. Hypodensity with marked contrast enhancement on CT scan
3. Hypoechogenicity or low reflective mass on USS
4. Marked contrast enhancement on MRI
5. May occasionally be bilateral and symmetrical
6. Lacrimal gland involvement is common
7. Bilateral proptosis can occur
8. Mass may be oval in shape affecting patients above 60 years.
9. Mass may be seen cupping the back of the globe
10. Ultrasound-guided biopsy is useful to histologically identify the lesion and to separate it from inflammatory conditions/intermediate group of lesions.
11. Orbital non-Hodgkin's lymphoma often disseminates systemically.

Neck

1. Multiple lymph node involvement affecting Waldeyer's ring.
2. Multiple round discrete masses with hypoechoic appearance on ultrasound.
3. Upper limb swelling may occur due to infiltration of venous drainage.
4. Superior vena caval obstruction can occur due to obstruction/infiltration of superior vena cava or jugular veins.
5. Involvement of lymph nodes of the neck is better appreciated clinically than radiologically.
6. Extra-nodal involvement of the neck has poor prognosis.

CNS

Primary non-Hodgkin's lymphoma represents 1% of primary brain tumours. Patients hardly develop systemic lymphoma.

The incidence is highest in:

1. Patients with HIV/AIDS.
2. Other immunocompromised patients.
3. Renal transplant patients.
4. Patients on long-term immunosuppression.

Features

1. Multiple pin-head-sized periventricular masses.
2. Multiple widespread pin-head-sized nodular masses throughout the brain
3. Marked contrast enhancement of sub-ependymal region due to tumour spread.
4. Solitary large spherical hyperdense lesion with mass effect on the basal ganglia with ring enhancement following contrast.
5. Occasionally, multiple hypodense lesions on CT with multiple ring enhancements.

Secondary CNS NHL

Occur especially in children.

Features

1. Up to 50% of patients develop cord compression.
2. Lymphomatous meningitis with nerve root lesion
3. Raised intra-cranial pressure with widening of sutures, sutural splitting, erosion of dorsum sellae due to obstruction of CSF absorption or diffusion
4. Often occurs from testicular, orbital and head and neck primary sites of lymphomas
5. Paravertebral masses
6. Anterior scalloping of vertebrae
7. Cord compression from paravertebral masses is common.

Retropharyngeal lymphadenopathy (Lymphographic appearance)

1. Enlarged lymph node with dense contrast uptake
2. Foamy internal appearance of lymph node
3. Non-filling of lymph nodes
4. Multiple-discrete filling defect in lymph nodes
5. Multiple micrometastases in lymph nodes of normal size (these lymph nodes have been erroneously confirmed normal in CT and MRI).
6. Surgery and histology are superior to lymphography CT and MRI in lymph node assessment.
7. CT demonstration of micrometastasis is possible in lymph nodes of the neck
8. Large amorphous mass with infiltration of tissue planes.

Testicular NHL

Occurs in middle-aged and elderly patients, up to 25% are bilateral. Aggressive, high-grade NHL. Metastasizes to the regional lymph nodes, lungs, brains, CNS and Waldeyer's ring in the neck. In ultrasound scan the lesion is hypoechoic

Soft tissue

1. Infiltration by the tumour into the muscle leads to increased bulk of muscle and distortion of muscle outline
2. Detection by CT is difficult because the density is the same as in normal muscle.

Bones

Mostly high-grade Non-Hodgkin's lymphoma. Rarer than Hodgkin's lymphoma in bone involvement. Male preponderance and age is 50 – 60 years.

Few children affected. Radiological characteristics of bone involvement are seen in 10 – 20%. More lesions are detected in post-mortem examination. Primary skeletal involvement is rare.

Radiological features

1. Osteolytic destructive lesion
2. Area of bone destruction is in red marrow area
3. Diffuse irregular margin and wide zone of transition
4. Scalloping of inner aspect of cortex
5. Solitary or multiple lesions with pathological fracture

6. Anterior scalloping of vertebrae due to paravertebral mass
7. Solitary or multiple wedge-shaped vertebral collapse
8. Femoral neck collapse/fracture
9. Humeral neck collapse/fracture
10. Multiple osteolytic round lucencies or moth-eaten appearance
11. Erosion of cortex associated with large soft tissue mass and little periosteal reaction.
12. Erosion occurs in areas already thinned or expanded by underlying pathology simulating Ewing's sarcoma.

Renal/kidneys

1. Unilateral or bilateral intrarenal masses especially in children.
2. Masses are hypoechoic on ultrasound scan
3. The masses fail to enhance on contrast CT scan.

(Adam & Dixon, 2008; Dahnert, 2011; Sutton, 1998 and 2003, Palmer & Reeder 2001).

References

1. Ghai S, Pattison J, Ghai S, O'Malley ME, Khalili K, Stephens M. Primary gastrointestinal lymphoma: spectrum of imaging findings with pathologic correlation. Radiographics 2007; 27:1371-88.
2. Toma P, Granata C, Rossi A, Garaventa A. Multimodality imaging of Hodgkin disease and non-Hodgkin lymphomas in children. Radiographics 2007; 27:1335-54.
3. Guermazi A, Brice P, Hennequin C, Sarfati E. Lymphography: an old technique retains its usefulness. Radiographics 2003; 23:1541-58.
4. Fishman EK, Kuhlman JE, Jones RJ. CT of lymphoma: spectrum of disease. Radiographics 1991; 11:647-69.

CHAPTER 6

HEAD AND CENTRAL
NERVOUS SYSTEM

6.1 RADIOLOGICAL DIFFERENTIAL DIAGNOSIS OF UNILATERAL PROPTOSIS

Definition

Unilateral proptosis is defined as the abnormal forward protrusion or displacement of one of the eye balls.

Differential diagnosis/causes

A. Dysthyroid diseases
1. Muscle enlargement (Grave's ophthalmopathy)
2. Increase in fat content

B. Intracranial lesions
1. Meningioma (sphenoid ridge meningioma)
   i. Meningioma en plaque
   ii. Meningioma of middle third of sphenoid ridge
   iii. Meningioma of clinoid process
   iv. Meningioma of planum sphenoidale
2. Subfrontal meningiomas
3. Intracranial (frontal lobe) abscess/haematoma

C. Lesions of Nasopharynx and paranasal sinuses

Juvenile nasopharyngeal angiofibroma, frontal sinus mucocoele, ethmoidal mucocoele, mucocoele of sphenoidal sinus, maxillary mucocoele, Wegener's granulomatosis, Stewart's granuloma, nasal polyps, carcinoma, fibrous dysplasia, ossifying fibroma, osteoma and malignant lymphoma.

D. Causes arising from the orbit
a. Vascular anomalies
   1. Haemangiomas
      i. Capillary haemangioma
      ii. Cavernous haemangioma
   2. Orbital varices

3. Arteriovenous malformations
4. Secondary varices (carotico – cavernous fistula)
5. Lymphangioma
6. Haemangiopericytoma

b. **Tumours of the orbit**
   1. Orbital meningioma
      i. Sheath meningioma
      ii. Extradural orbital nerve meningioma
   2. Optic nerve glioma
   3. Dermoids and epidermoids
   4. Secondary meningioma
   5. Neurofibromatosis
   6. Rhabdomyosarcoma
   7. Lymphoma
   8. Metastasis
   9. Lacrimal gland tumours
      i. Adenoma, carcinoma, adenocystic carcinoma, lymphoma, dermoids and epidermoids
   10. Retinoblastoma
   11. Granulomatous disease (sarcoidosis, histiocytosis and Wegener's granulomatosis).
   12. Ectopic lacrimal gland
   13. Sickle cell anaemia

c. **Inflammatory lesions**
   Acute bacterial infections (cellulitis/abscess), acute fungal infections, traumas, orbital pseudotumous, retro-orbital pseudotumours, haematoma from scurvy, orbital hydatid and Tolosa–Hunt syndrome

Radiological investigative modalities

1. Plain film
   Skull – PA, lateral, occipitomental (OM) view, Towne's view, Optic canal view.
   Neck – PA and lateral
   Chest – PA and lateral
   Others – abdomen, thoracolumbar, lumbosacral, extremities.
2. Ultrasound (3.5 MHz, 7.5 MHz frequency probe).
   Orbital ultrasound scan
   Cranial / Transfontanelle scan
   Abdominal scan
3. Colour Doppler ultrasound scan
4. CT scan (contrast, non-contrast), coronal and axial scan.
5. Helical CT scan
6. MRI
7. MRA (MR angiography)
8 Conventional tomography
9. Angiography
10. Venography

11. Radionuclide studies
12. Interventional studies

Important causes of differential diagnosis

Great majority of proptosis are caused by thyroid diseases, orbital infections/cellulitis, orbital and retroorbital pseudotumour, retinoblastoma and orbital varices/vascylar lesions.

Discussion

A. Dysthyroid Diseases

Muscle enlargement/Grave's ophthalmopathy

Dysthyroid diseases are the commonest cause of both unilateral and bilateral extraocular muscle enlargement and proptosis. It can occur in both hyperthyroid and euthyroid patient who was previously hyperthyroid. There is acute enlargement of the muscle in which the inferior, medial, superior and lateral rectus muscles are enlarged in that order. Enlargement is usually bilateral and symmetrical and is confined to the belly of the muscles sparing the tendinous origin and insertions.

On plain film of skull, there is characteristic indentation of medial wall of the orbit persisting even after regression of the enlargement.
Ultrasound scan will demonstrate a solid tumour mass. Sonography is also able to demonstrate muscle enlargement compared to the contralateral side.
On CT studies coronal section identifies enlarged muscle especially at apex of the orbit and differentiates it from tumour.
MRI   shows increased signal intensity of enlarged muscles. With its multiplanar capability MRI can differentiate enlarged muscle from tumour.

Increase in fat contents

In certain dysthyroid diseases, there is considerable increase in fat content with little or no muscle enlargement. CT scan will show no muscle enlargement. In addition, there is increase in interconal space or distance. There is also characteristic angulation of lateral rectus muscle where they are held by lateral check ligament. There is also characteristic angulation of lateral check ligament. Orbital CT studies will show forward displacement of one of the eyeballs.
On venography, there is characteristic downward displacement of second part of ophthalmic vein with exaggerated upwards concavity. This is caused by the combined increase in bulk of levator palpebrae and superior rectus muscles by lying immediately above that point of superior ophthalmic vein. Using CT number and FLAIR MRI studies, the increase in fat content is confirmed.

B. Intracranial Lesions

Sphenoid ridge meningioma

Meningiomas cause unilateral proptosis in only a small group of patients. Meningiomas are benign tumours of the meninges and arise from the arachnoid rest cells adjacent to the dura mater concentrated in the arachnoid villi which are more numerous in large dural sinuses, in smaller veins, along roots of sleeves of exiting cranial and spinal nerves and choroid plexus.

Sphenoid ridge meningiomas are the commonest intracranial tumours to cause proptosis.

Sphenoid ridge meningiomas comprise:

i. Hyperostotic meningioma en-plaque
ii. Meningioma arising from middle third of sphenoid ridge
iii. Meningioma arising from clinoid process.
iv. Meningioma arising from planum sphenoidale.

Plain films/CT scan

i. Hyperostosis of adjacent bone.
ii. Pneumosinus dilatans (enlargement of adjacent paranasal sinuses).
iii. Hyperostotic blistering of planum sphenoidale in CT with subfrontal and posterior growth into sella turcica and clivus.
iv. Bone changes consist of local expansion of diplöe.
v. Enlarged vascular grooves.
vi. Calcification in circular or radial pattern more common on CT scan.
vii. Sharply defined mass on CT scan.
viii. Marked contrast enhancement and early venous drainage are shown by CT, MRI and angiography. Meningioma en plaque shows poor vascularity and encasement of carotid and middle cerebral arteries in meningioma of the clinoid process.

Subfrontal meningiomas (secondary meningiomas)

These are meningiomas in the anterior and middle cranial fossae, purely benign but which cause proptosis by mass effect on the adjacent orbit and structures. Their radiological features are similar to other meningiomas.

Intracranial frontal subdural/epidural abscess/haematoma.

The presence of subdural or epidural abscess or haematoma in the cranial cavity adjacent to the orbit will result in proptosis of the involved orbit by mass effect.

CT scan will usually diagnose the concavo-convex lesion of subdural abscess/haematoma while the epidural lesion will appear biconvex.

C. Lesions in the Nasopharynx and Paranasal Sinuses

Juvenile nasopharyngeal angiofibroma

The mass arises in the nose close to the pterygoid lamina. It grows to a large size and invades the surrounding structures. It occurs at a mean age of 15 years, almost exclusively in males. Using plain films, the mass is solid with anterior bowing of posterior wall of the maxillary sinus. Also there is loss of scalloped margin of the sinus. If bone destruction is excessive the sinus will appear radiolucent. Bleeding into it or obstruction of drainage of secretion or infection may cause the sinus to have fluid-levels.

On computed tomography (CT) scan, there will be demonstration of upward, posterior and downward expansion of sinus, and CT is the best modality for this Air-fluid level may be demonstrated by CT.

CT number will show whether the mass is solid or cystic. Contrast CT will demostrate the vascularity of the tumour and rim-enhancement indicates infected mucocoele or pyocoele due to obstruction of sinus ostium.

Ethmoidal mucocoele 20 – 30%

Anterior and middle groups of ethmoidal air cells are most frequently involved. Diagnosis is often obvious clinically than radiologically. Plain films will show opaque ethmoidal sinus and there may also be expansion of ethmoidal sinus into the orbit laterally. CT scan is the best modality for demonstration of its expansion into the orbit.
Using CT scan, bony rim of ethmoidal air cells expanding into the orbit is shown.
Coronal and axial sections of CT studies show soft tissue component of the mass extending into the orbit

Maxillary sinus mucocoele, 10%

The sinus is opaque in plain radiography and there is expanded wall of sinus which is not breached. CT scan shows fluid content of the sinus and also the fact that the expanded wall is intact. MRI will establish the content to be fluid.

Sphenoidal sinus mucocoele (2 – 7%)

In plain films the sphenoid sinus will be opaque. There is expansion of sphenoidal sinus wall and this may appear late. There is also elevation and destruction of floor of pituitary fossa. Erosion of medial wall of optic canal which appears late and there may be elevation of planum sphenoidale. On CT scan there may be expansion of the sinus but with intact wall and CT number will shown that the content is fluid. MRI is optimal for demonstrating fluid content within the sphenoid sinus.

Frontal sinus mucocoele

The expansion of the sinus is palpable and obvious clinically. The eye is displaced forward and inferiorly by the mucocoele. It is well shown on simple x-ray.

Benign hypertrophy of mucosa of the nasal turbinate:

This is the cause of benign exophthalmos syndrome (BES). There is slow progressive onset of the exophthalmos, without any inflammatory and mass effect signs. This condition is associated in all cases with ipsilateral hypertrophy of the nasal mucosa providing a guide to a hypothetical mechanism for BES. According to this hypothesis, the therapy should be devoted to the nasal disease more than the orbital exophthalmos.

Wegener's granulomatosis

An autoimmune multisystemic disease characterised by necrotising granulation of upper and lower respiratory tract together with formation of glomerulonephritis and systemic vasculitis. M: F = 2: 1, mean age = 40 years. The lesions causing proptoses are sinusitis and mucocoele. There is sinus rhinorrhoea, pain and purulent discharge.
There is also ocular inflammation with proptosis and otitis media. The sinus lesion itself could lead to proptosis frequently.
Progressive destruction of nasal cartilage occurs in the nose
In the lungs there are lesions including solitary or multiple pulmonary nodules, pneumonia, haemorrhage, lymphadenopathies, and pulmonary cavities.

Focal areas of glomerulonephritis are seen in the kidneys. There is migratory polyarthropathy in the joints and cutaneous purpura in the skin.

Stewart's granuloma

This is a mid-facial destructive lesion causing bone necrosis and facial mutilation. On plain film, there is massive and aggressive bone destruction in the nose with little soft tissue component. Progressive proptosis is due to changes in the sinuses. All of the above features are also shown by CT scan

Nasal polyp

Ethmoidal air cell is the commonest site of origin, followed by maxillary sinus. They are pedunculated and often multiple and bilateral. Polyps can obstruct sinus drainage and cause mucocoele. Plain radiography will show opaque sinus with expansion and thinning of the walls. There may also be expansion and lateral displacement of the orbit with hypertelorism. CT scan will confirm the above features and shows solid content of the mass using CT number and tissue attenuation.

Osteoma

This is a benign tumour most commonly found in the frontal sinus. It is the commonest benign tumour in the sinuses. Large osteomas in the frontal or ethmoidal sinuses may cause proptosis by pressure effect on the orbital wall or obstruction of drainage of sinus causing mucocoele. On plain films osteomas are round with dense opacity of cortical bone density in the sinuses. There is expansion and loss of scalloped margin of sinus. There may be associated opacity of the whole of the sinus due to mucocoele.

Fibrous dysplasia

Here, normal bone is replaced by fibrous tissue and cysts containing blood, serous fluid and abnormal trabeculae. There is an osteolytic process with bony expansion and calcification or "ground-glass" appearance. In the maxilla it is located at the lateral wall of antrum and zygoma with dense bone encroaching into the nasal cavity, and proptosis. The lesion is diffuse, its growth ceases with skeletal maturity.

Ossifying fibroma

A localised form of fibrous dysplasia with presence of osteoid unlike fibrous dysplasia. The lesion is discrete, oval in shape, confined to one part of bone and encapsulated. They may enlarge after ceasation of growth and can be removed without recurrence.

Carcinoma

a. *Squamous cell carcinoma* is the commonest malignant tumour of the nose and paranasal sinuses. Most of them arise in the maxillary antrum and less in ethmoid. It is rare in frontal and sphenoidal sinuses.

b. *Adenocarcinoma*
    Seen mostly in wood workers. Arises in the naso-ethmoidal cells and may gain access to anterior cranial fossa through the fenestrations of the cribriform plate.
    Plain film in both lesions shows:
    Soft tissue mass with bony destruction especially at the roof of the orbit.
    Bowing of nasal cavity away from tumour.

Bone destruction with breach of adjacent sinus walls.

Other type of carcinomas
These tumours are not common. They originate from various tissues.
Origin from gland
Adenocarcinomas arises from seromucinous gland in the nose and sinuses

Connective tissue origin
This includes fibrosarcoma, osteosarcoma and chondrosarcoma

Muscle origin
This include leiomyosarcoma and rhadomyosarcoma

Neurogenic origin
This includes neuroblastoma and meningioma

Lymphoreticular origin
This includes lymphoma and plasmacytoma

The roles of imaging are:
i.   To make diagnosis because these tumours are inaccessible to clinical examination.
ii. To establish the full extent of the disease before treatment using CT and MRI. The aims are to show the best area of approach for biopsy, presence of bony destruction and the full extent of the outline of the mass both in the sinuses and in the adjacent structures.
iii. Post-operative follow up for recurrence of malignant lesion.

D. Causes arising from the Orbit

Vascular Anomalies
a. Ophthalmic vein aneurysm
This occurs most commonly at junction of the internal carotid and ophthalmic artery called carotico-ophthalmic aneurysm. Curvilinear calcification or arc-like calcification in the wall of the aneurysm may be seen on plain skull radiography. CT scan, MRI and angiography will clearly show the dilated aneurysmal vessel.

b. Arteriovenous malformation
This can be congenital or acquired. The congenital type is rare. The acquired type is due to fracture of bones around the orbit. The features include proptosis, audible bruit and pulsatile exophthalmos. Carotid angiography shows early filling of the veins without passing through the capillary phase. It will also show other nature of the lesion and its blood supply. Studies of both internal and external carotid vessels are needed to show the feeding vessels.

c. Haemangioma
This is common in women and consists of:
   i.   Capillary haemangioma (found in children)
   ii. Cavernous haemangioma (found in adults)

i. Capillary haemangioma

This presents with chemosis of the eye lid, injection of sclera, unilateral proptosis and may be associated with superficial naevus. It grows quickly and involutes spontaneously. They are associated with *von Hippel-Lindau syndrome*. It has no surrounding capsule and thus grows very large and infiltrate. There is remodelling of the orbit but no bone destruction.

ii. Cavernous haemangioma

This is the most common benign tumour of the orbit in adults. It grows slowly and is not always symptomatic. There is proptosis and visual loss if there is compression of the optic nerve by haemangioma located at the orbital apex. Plain film and conventional tomography show enlargement of the affected orbit. On CT scan, the mass appears sharply marginated due to a pseudocapsule. There is contrast pool and flow void in Gd–MRI. In Angiography, there is venous pool within the muscle cone in the capillary phase which may be fed by the external carotid artery.

Orbital Varices

Here, Valsalva manoeuvre or dependent head position or cough may lead to proptosis and when this is repeated may result in blindness. Classification:

i. Primary varices

  Congenital venous malformation

  Traumatic

  Varices associated with haemangioma

ii. Secondary varices

  Carotico-cavernous fistula

  Arteriovenous fistula

  – Intracranial arteriovenous fistula

  – Extracranial arteriovenous fistula

Congenital venous malformation

Increase of venous pressure in the head increases the proptosis which dates back to birth or childhood. Proptosis may be associated with Klippel-Trenaunay-Weber syndrome or venous malformation elsewhere in the body. Plain film may show phleboliths and prominent vascular markings on the same side as the lesion.

CT scan.	1.	This will show encasement of the orbit
	2.	Phleboliths in the orbit and adjacent structures
Venography	1.	Local saccular venous dilatation resembling aneurysm
	2.	Whole system of abnormal venous channel in the orbit.

MRI. This will show the above features better

Doppler studies. This will show absence of flow

Traumatic varices

Tear of superior ophthalmic vein at the superior orbital fissure due to rupture of pre-existing primary varices with extravasation of blood into the muscle cone. This may occur spontaneously.

Secondary varices
Carotico-cavernous syndrome
Skull base fracture and penetrating injury may injure the carotid artery and cavernous sinus resulting in their direct communication. Blood flow in the superior ophthalmic vein in reversed or arterialised. Arterial pulsation transmitted through the venous system results in pulsatile exophthalmos. Colour Doppler imaging is diagnostic and may be the only investigation required in mild cases. CT or MRI may show muscle enlargement. Carotid angiography is the diagnostic imaging modality of choice and will show early filling of cavernous sinus and internal jugular vein with dilated superior ophthalmic vein providing an important collateral channel to the external jugular vein.

Lymphangioma
There is proptosis which may be sudden or slowly progressive. They are hamartomas composed of primitive lymphatic tissue, fibrous tissue, dysplastic vessels and lymphoid tissue.
CT scan. Poorly defined, lobulated solid mass of mixed attenuation with variable enhancement. **MRI** shows heterogeneous mass with cystic and haemorrhagic areas and clearly delineates the boundaries. It shows minimal enhancement which is seen in areas that bleed.

Haemangiopericytoma
Occurs in adult and is composed of vascular encapsulated mass with homogenous density. They are similar to cavernous haemangioma. They may show bone destruction and muscle invasion. They may recur after incomplete excision and may rarely show distant metastasis. In **CT** there is homogenous density and marked contrast enhancement.
In **MRI** there is homogenous intensity with marked contrast enhancement.

2. Orbital Tumours
Orbital meningioma
Often seen in middle aged-women who present with visual loss, papilloedema and pallor of optic nerve head. This may be primary within the orbit or extension of growth originating in the anterior or middle cranial fossa. Primary intraorbital meningiomas are classified as:
1. **Extradural meningiomas:** Arising within the orbit remote from optic nerve.
2. **Sheath meningiomas:** Arise from clusters of arachnoid cap cells in the meningeal sheath covering the optic nerve. They are sub classified into:
   i. *Intracanalicular or foraminal tumours*
   ii. *Retrobulbar tumours (Retrobulbar part of optic nerve)*
Sheath meningioma originates from the optic nerve sheath and spreads circumferentially round the nerve. Proptosis is a frequent occurrence.
Plain film will show widening of optic canal. Hyperostosis of sphenoid wing is best shown by conventional tomography or computed tomography. Localised or generalised ocular enlargement may be demonstrated by CT scan. Plain film will also demonstrate calcification within tumour and pneumosinus dilatans.
CT and MRI will show sharply-defined tubular mass surrounding and paralleling the course of the optic nerve. Tram–track sign and marked contrast enhancement is also demonstrated using these imaging modalities.

Optic nerve glioma

This tumour is uncommon and is often associated with neurofibromatosis type 1, especially when bilateral. When the tumour occur in adult it often take its origin from the optic chiasma. Plain radiography will show asymmetrical widening of the optic canal and calcification is uncommon. CT scan will demonstrate dense homogenous optic nerve which is enlarged or expanded or fusiform. The optic canal is widened and asymmetrical. There is little or no contrast enhancement. MR studies will show homogenous intensity of nerve with uniform enhancement.

Dermoid and epidermoid cysts

Seen in the superolateral quadrant of the orbit close to the lacrimal fossa and produce cystic appearance. They may also occur in the medial part of orbital rim, greater wing of sphenoid and rarely inferior part of the orbit. They may arise in the diplöe and grow to expand both inner and outer tables. CT and MRI will demonstrate the fat content within these tumours which do not enhance with contrast. Kinking of optic nerve may be demonstrated.

Secondary meningioma

These are extension of meningioma arising from the middle and anterior cranial fossae. It also include meningioma en-plaque affecting the greater wing of sphenoid bone and to a lesser extent the lesser wing. They take origin from the pterion in most cases.

On CT or MRI there is encasement of optic nerve by a densely-enhanced tumour.

There is also extension through the optic canal into the orbit. Pneumosinus dilatans which is abnormal dilatation of a paranasal sinus as a result of meningioma close to it is shown.

Neurofibromatosis

Here, apart from the general form of the disease, the several nerves that pass through the orbit may be a site of neurofibroma.

The orbit is enlarged.

Bare orbit is produced by elevation of sphenoid ridge to the roof of the orbit.

Encephalocoele may occur due to bare orbit

Pulsatile proptosis may occur due to direct transmission of intracranial pulsating arteries. Other associated features include enlarged middle cranial fossa and enlarged optic canal and pituitary fossa.

Rhabdomyosarcoma

Occurs in children often below the age of 6 years. It is the most common cause of malignancy in the orbit and half are primary while half are metastatic. There is rapidly progressing proptosis.

On plain film, there is enlargement of the orbit with bone destruction. CT scan will show bone destruction due to the tumour and enhancement with contrast. MR imagng shows isointense tumour with respect to other normal extraocular muscles. Lesion enhancement with contrast is also demonstrated.

Lymphoma

Benign reactive hyperplasia is the benign type while the malignant type usually occurs in the elderly. CT scan shows a mass often palpable clinically, enveloping the orbit. Plain films are often normal. Even on CT scan the bones are preserved.

Metastasis

In adults, this is usually from the breast, prostate, bronchus, kidney and gastrointestinal tract. In children it is usually neuroblastomas and to a lesser extent Ewing's sarcoma, Wilm's tumour and leukaemia. Orbital invasion can occur from tumours in the adjacent paranasal sinuses. The features include rapid onset proptosis, and may occasionally be bilateral. Bone destruction may be seen both on CT and MRI. Prostate metastasis may show hyperostosis similar to what is seen on meningioma.

Lacrimal gland tumours

These include:

1. Benign tumours of which the most common is benign pleomorphic adenoma.
2. Lacrimal gland dermoid and epidermoid, simple cysts and abscess.
3. Chronic granulomatous sialadenitis (TB, sarcoidosis, actinomycosis).
4. Carcinomas including adenocarcinoma, adenocystic carcinoma, and undifferentiated type.
5. Lymphomas

There is local enlargement of the lacrimal fossa without bone destruction in benign lesion and 50% of malignant lesions. Radiological features of malignancy include bone destruction, bone invasion, sclerosis of adjacent bones, calcification within tumour and expansion of mass outside the gland area. CT scan will show the fat content of tumour in dermoid and epidermoid, calcification and bone destruction in malignant lesions.

Retinoblastoma

Childhood intraocular aggressive, malignant tumour of neuroectodermal origin. There is leukocoria, proptosis, strabismus, visual loss and other non-specific signs. Bilateral involvement occurs in a third of cases and rarely there is trilateral tumour when primitive neurectodermal tumour of pineal gland is also present. Ultrasound shows highly echogenic mass originating from the retina in the vitreous humour with posterior shadowing due to calcification. CT shows soft tissue solid mass with dense calcification originating from the retina. There is marked contrast enhancement of non-calcified soft tissue component on both CT and MRI.

Ectopic lacrimal gland

This occurs in the orbit. It is rare but it can cause proptosis and orbital wall destruction. It appears as a well-encapsulated mass on CT scan with extension to the subcutaneous tissue.

Sickle cell anaemia

Proptosis in sickle cell anaemia may be caused by orbital wall infarction with sub-periosteal haemorrhage. The resulting inflammatory response may compromise important structures, leading to orbital compression syndrome. Symptoms include pain of acute onset and swelling, with or without visual impairment. Proptosis, limited ocular motility, corneal hyperesthesia, and optic nerve dysfunction occur. There may be associated epidural haematoma. Lacrimal gland swelling or enlargement is a rare complication of sickle cell anaemia caused by vaso-occlusion of the vessels supplying the gland. The gland appears uniformly enlarged and homogeneously enhanced on contrast CT and MR images.

A. Inflammatory Conditions of the Orbit

Acute bacterial infections

Bacterial infections of paranasal sinuses, dental caries/abscess, haematogenous spread from valveless veins of the face are often the route of infection. Cellulitis, panophthalmitis or orbital cellulitis results.

Abscess formation occurs and this may appear as a mass. Plain film shows gas with or without air-fluid level. CT scan shows widening of extraconal space between ethmoidal and periorbital regions due to oedema. Focal rectus enlargement. Ring enhancement of abscess.

Fungal infection

This is seen in diabetes and immunocompromised patients. It presents with soft tissue mass due to abscess formation. There is marked aggressive bone destruction which may simulate malignant lesion. In both bacterial and fungal infections, there may be cavernous sinus thrombosis which is best demonstrated by MRI.

Trauma

Both blunt and penetrating trauma can injure the orbit directly or indirectly. Soft tissue oedema produces proptosis. Haematoma within the muscle cone, retrobulbar region or within other soft tissues appearing like mass also produce proptosis. CT scan may demonstrate bony fractures, foreign body or air. Clinical examination is often limited. MRI is useful in patients who have no metallic foreign body for better soft tissue delineation. Ultrasound scan in the absence of globe disruption when applied directly can show most lesions within the globe and surrounding structures. Retinal detachment, choroidal detachment, vitreous haemorrhage, optic nerve damage, dislocation of the lens, foreign body and rupture of the globe can be shown.

Haematoma from scurvy

Retro-orbital pseudotumour from haemorrhage or extradural haematoma in patients often an infant with scurvy may be so large as to cause proptosis. It is rewarding to recognise the scurvy for accurate treatment as patient can recover completely when treated. CT scan in axial and coronal plane will identify the haematoma using CT number.

Scurvy

This may develop from subperiosteal haemorrhage of ocular bones with the formation of pseudotumour. It can be difficult to diagnose and orbital tumour may be suggested or inflammatory pseudotumour but the pathology is essentially subperiosteal haematoma. Extradural haematoma can also occur from subperiosteal haemorrhage.

Orbital emphysema

This may follow sneezing or rupture of sinuses after nasal trauma or chronic sinus disease. Often there is a history of old periorbital trauma or surgery. Crepitant eyelid swelling, ptosis and mild unilateral proptosis may be elicited clinically. CT scan demonstrates the areas of emphysema within the orbit.

Hydatid disease of the orbit

Through the systemic circulation, any organ or tissue can be affected, but infestation of the orbit comprises far less than 1% of the total incidence of hydatid. The presenting symptoms are slowly progressive unilateral proptosis, with or without pain (80%), visual loss (48%), periorbital pain (24%), chemosis (16%), and headache (12%). Diagnosis of hydatid cyst can be made on the images obtained from ultrasonography, CT and/or MRI examinations. A well-circumscribed cystic mass is demonstrated in almost all the patients. Treatment involves total surgical removal without rupture. Blindness can occur if not well treated.

Orbital and retro-orbital pseudotumour

Idiopathic inflammatory pseudotumour is the most common cause of orbital mass in adult. Unilateral proptosis is the most common appearance although bilateral lesion can occur. All the components of the orbit may be affected in the diffuse form including lacrimal gland, muscle cone, optic nerve and sclera. Most of the patients present with proptosis and visual loss. Isolated lateral rectus muscle involvement from pseudotumour of lacrimal gland is also diagnostic. There is involvement of tendinous origin and insertion of the muscle as well as the belly of the muscle differentiating it from Graves' myositis where only the bellies of the muscles are involved. Plain film shows opaque sinus and enlarged optic canal. CT scan shows heterogenous poorly marginated mass. In MRI, discrete mass lesions, lacrimal gland enlargement and contrast enhancement of lesions are noted. On venography, there is displacement of the venous system. There is also venous block in the 2nd and 3rd part of the superior orbital vein.

Tolosa – Hunt Syndrome

Non-specific inflammatory process with presence of granulamatous tissue is seen in the superior orbital vein or cavernous sinus.

Other rare causes of unilateral proptosis

These include leukaemia, sarcoidosis, tuberculosis, amyloidosis, ipsilateral mucosal turbinate hypertrophy and solitary fibrous tumour of the orbit.

(Adam & Dixon, 2008; Dahnert, 2011; Sutton, 1998 and 2003, Swischuk, 2004; Palmer & Reeder 2001).

References

1. Calcaterra TC, Trapp TK. Unilateral proptosis. Otolaryngol Clin North Am 1988;21:53-63.
2. Bord SP, Linden J. Trauma to the globe and orbit. Emerg Med Clin North Am 2008;26:97-123.
3. Smith M, Castillo M. Imaging and differential diagnosis of the large eye. Radiographics 1994;14:721-8.
4. Scott IU, Siatkowski MR. Thyroid eye disease. Semin Ophthalmol 1999;14:52-61.
5. Fafowora OF, Cookey-gam AI, Obajimi MO. Radiological evaluation of orbital tumours in Ibadan, Nigeria. Afr J Med Med Sci 1996;25:361-4
6. Eze KC, Mazeli FO, Otoibhi EO, Okuonghae JT. Unilateral exophthalmos. A radiological differential diagnosis. Benin Journal of Postgraduate Medicine 2002; 6: 71-82.
7. Verma S, Sivanandan S, Aneesh MK, Gupta V, Seth R, Kabra S. Unilateral proptosis and extradural haematoma in a child with scurvy. Pediatr Radiol 2007; 37:937-9.
8. Eze KC, Enock ME, Eluehike SU. Ultrasonic evaluation of orbito-ocular trauma in Benin-City, Nigeria. Niger Postgrad Med J 2009 ;16:198-202.
9. Nzegwu CO, Nzegwu MA, Aligbe JU, Oghre E, Waziri-Erameh MJ. A review of 61 cases of ocular tumours seen over a 3-year period in Benin City, Nigeria: a 3-year descriptive retrospective study (1998-2000). Eur J Cancer Care (Engl) 2010;19:279-80.
10. Nzeh DA, Owoeye JF, Ademola-Popoola DS, Uyanne I. Sonographic evaluation of ocular trauma in Ilorin, Nigeria. Eur J Ophthalmol 2006;16:453-7.
11. Odebode TO, Ologe FE, Segun-Busari S, Nzeh DA. Recurrent bilateral fronto-ethmoidal mucocoele with intracranial extension: a case report. West Afr J Med 2005;24:268-71.

6.2 RADIOLOGY OF HEADACHE

Headache

Headache can be defined as pain in the head as a result of irritation of the meninges of the brain. The brain has no sensory receptors but the meninges have and its irritation from any cause frequently causes headache. Usually the pain originates from the head, neck or muscles of the shoulder.

Causes of headache

1. Inflammatory/infections
   a. Intracranial lesion
      i. Meningitis
      ii. Tuberculous meningitis, fungal, parasitic
      iii. Intracerebral/intracranial abscess
      iv. Intracranial infections/infestations
      v. Encephalitis
   b. Extracranial lesions
      i. Scalp infection
      ii. Osteomyelitis
      iii. Giant cell arteritis
   c. infections outside the head
      i. Bacterial infections, e.g. septicaemia
      ii. Viral infections, e.g. AIDS, Lassa fever
      iii. Parasitic infections, e.g. malaria
      iv. Infestatations, e.g. cysticercosis
2. Traction on arteries
   a. Raised intracranial pressure
      i. Aneurysms
      ii. Tumours – primary, secondary/developmental tumoral conditions
      iii. Hydrocephalus
      iv. Cystic space occupying lesion
      v. Cerebrovascular accident/stroke (subarachnoid, intracerebral haemorrhage)
      vi. Trauma (subdural, epidural haematoma, cerebral oedema, intracerebral haematoma).
3. Dilatations and traction on venous sinuses
   i. Post-lumbar puncture
   ii. Arachnoiditis
   iii. Venous sinus thrombosis
   iv. Venous thrombosis
   v. Carotico-cavernous fistula
   vi. Arteriovenous fistula
   vii. Dilatation of veins.
      i. Internal carotid artery aneurysm
      ii. Aneurysm of vein of Galen
   viii. Cerebral atrophy (focal, diffuse, pseudo-atrophy)
4. Arterial dilatations
   a. Intracranial lesion
      i. Systemic infections

        ii.   Hypertension

        iii. Intracranial arterial spasm

        iv. Anoxia (hangover headache)

        v.   Nitrates

        vi. Confusion/post-ictal state

   b. Extracerebral lesion

        i.   Migraine

        ii.   Arterial spasm in head and neck

        iii. Other systemic infections/infestations and conditions

5. Skeletal muscle contraction

   a. Tension headache

   b. Sternocleidomastoid spasm

   c. Spasm of scalp muscle due to tumour, infection, trauma, osteomyelitis

6. Referred pain from:

   a. Eyes diseases

        i.   Refractive error

        ii.   Orbital pseudotumour

        iii. Orbital cellulitis/infection/ophthalmitis

        iv. Orbital tumours (primary/secondary/retinoblastoma, melanoma)

        v.   Eye lid oedema

        vi. Orbital vascular anomalies

        vii. Thyroid ophthalmopathy

        viii.Retinal detachment

        ix. Orbital trauma/vitreous haemorrhage

   b. Ear

        i.   Otitis/ infection of mastoid

        ii.   Otitis media

        iii. Otosclerosis

        iv. Otitis externa

        v.   Other ear conditions/tinnitus

        vi. Tumours

   c. Sinuses/Nasopharynx

        i.   Sinusitis (Acute/chronic)

        ii.   Mucocoele/pyelocoele

        iii. Tumours (polyp, carcinoma, nasopharyngeal angiofibroma, osteoma)

        iv. Retropharyngeal abscess

   d. Dental origin

        i.   Dental pain

        ii.   Dental caries

        iii. Dental extraction

        iv. Dental and non-dental tumours

7. Trauma

   a. Skull fractures

   b. Leptomeningeal cyst

   c. Intracranial haematoma (subdural, epidural, intracerebral)

   d. Brain contusion/anoxic injury

    e.   Trauma to the eye, neck, teeth and mouth

    f.   Cerebral oedema

    g.   Lumbar puncture/low CSF pressure

    h.   Acute post traumatic headache

8. Conditions specific to females

    a.   Preganancy-induced hypertension (Pre-eclampsia)

    b.   Eclampsia

    c.   Migraine

9. Drugs

    a.   Fulcin, etc.

    b.   Acute or chronic substance abuse or withdrawal

10. Metabolic disorders

    i.   Hypoxia

    ii.   Hypercapnia

    iii.   Combined hypoxia and hypercapnia

    iv.   Hypoglycaemia

    v.   Renal dialysis

    vi.   Other metabolic abnormalities

Before radiological investigations

History is very important. History of presenting complaint, past medical history and family and social history are essential. This should be followed by adequate clinical examination if possible to determine the need and the order of radiological investigations. Not all patients with headache need radiological investigations. Most do not as history will exclude infections outside the head, metabolic disorders, drugs and substance abuse, female-specific conditions, muscle contractions, diseases of the ears, neck and eyes that do not require imaging.

Radiological investigative modalities

1. Plain film – skull, sinuses, face, abdomen

2. Ultrasound – transfontanelle, eye, abdomen

3. Echocardiography

4. CT scan –cranial, face, chest, abdomen

5. MRI

6. Angiography – before surgery

7. Radionuclide studies

8. PET/SPECT

9. Interventional Radiology – Embolisation of aneurysms, angiomatous malformations, tumours.

Radiological findings
Normal findings (great majority)

The bulk of the patients, indeed over 75% of the patients with headache, will show or have normal findings on radiological examination. This is because virtually no structural abnormality is found with these lesions, which could be elicited by radiological investigative modalities. The patients in this category are those with:

1. Migraine headache

2. Hypertension

3. Refractive error
4. Dental aches and early dental caries
5. Acute systemic infections and infestations
6. Acute otitis media
7. Tension headache due to skeletal muscle spasm
8. Arterial spasm in head and neck
9. Intracranial arterial spasm
10. Anoxia (hangover headache)
11. Post-lumbar puncture
12. Early stages of uncomplicated meningitis and encephalitis
13. Drugs, e.g. fulcin
14. Acute scalp infection
15. Dental extraction
16. Febrile illness

Infections and infestations
Purulent meningitis
CT scan and MRI of the brain are the preferred investigative modalities. In the pre-contrast CT, there may be increased density in the subarachnoid space due to increased vascularity. Cerebral oedema may cause effacement of the ventricles. In post-contrast scan of CT, there may be significant curvilinear or gyriform enhancement over the cerebral hemisphere and fissures with obliterations of the basal cisterns due to oedema from adjacent bleed and, subdural haematoma or effusion. Empyema, cerebral infarct, hydrocephalus, cerebral atrophy, cerebral abscess and cerebellar atrophy are also complications of meningitis which can be elicited by imaging studies.

Osteomyelitis of skull/facial bone
Areas of osteolytic lesion in skull or facial bones are seen with plain film. Rarely, button sequestrum is identified. There is often adjacent soft tissue swelling due to infection or trauma. History is very important.

Tuberculous meningitis
Plain film and CT scan may show calcification of meninges. Skull lucencies and spherical area of calcification may be due to tuberculoma. Communicating hydrocephalus results from inflammatory changes blocking the arachnoid villi leading to lack of absorption of CSF.

Intracerebral abscess
This may be pyogenic, tuberculous, fungal or parasitic (toxoplasmosis in AIDS). Plain films may not show any abnormal findings.

Pyogenic abscess
In pre-contrast CT scan, there is a hypodense wide area with small mass effect relative to the size of the hypodense area. Post-contrast scan will show a thin-walled regular ring enhancement of the capsule. The abscess itself is hypodense, and may be unilocular or multilocular. Hypodense area with CT number suggestive of air within the abscess cavity due to gas may be seen if there is communication with the exterior, or due to presence of gas-forming organism. Previous tapping or drainage can also introduce gas into an abscess cavity. MRI will show similar findings.

Tuberculous abscess

Pre-contrast CT scan will show small multiple isodense or hypodense lesions within the brain with some evidence of meningitis. Post-contrast scan will show multiple round areas with nodular enhancement. Multiple small dense ring enhancements are also seen. Occasionally the abscesses are large enough to simulate pyogenic abscess, cystic glioma, lymphoma, haemorrhagic cerebral infarct or parasitic abscess.

Encephalitis / viral infections

Different types of viral infections can manifest with headache. Such viral infections also include viral haemorrhagic fever like Lassa fever.

Cerebral Toxoplasmosis

This is seen in immunocompromised patients especially in HIV/AIDS. In CT scan, multiple or solitary low density subcortical, thalamic, or basal ganglia lesions are seen with small mass effect or localised oedema. Following contrast administration there is ring enhancement of the lesion. The patient will test positive to HIV I, II or both, and often, the CD4 count will be less than 200. MRI will show similar features as on CT scan.

Cerebral malaria

This presents with brain tissue swelling with effacement of the sulci on CT or MR imaging. The patient is usually living in the tropics of have recently migrated from there. Treatment with antimalarial drugs particularly intravenous quinine in titrated dose is life saving. Intravenous glucose infusion is necessary to avoid hypoglycaemia.

Trauma/ Skull Trauma/ Head Injury

In skull trauma with or without head injury, the following lesions may be seen.

Fractures

Plain films and CT scan will clearly show skull fractures as areas of breach in the continuity of the bone appearing as radiolucency or linear hypodensity. The fractures can be linear, depressed or stellate. Fractures of facial bones with or without Le Fort components may be seen. The mandible may also be fractured and all these will cause headache.

Leptomeningeal cyst

This results from escape of CSF from subarachnoid space forming a cyst beneath a fracture often in children. Pulsation of CSF may lead to widening of the fracture outline and by the time it is discovered the trauma leading to the fracture might have been forgotten. Plain film and CT scan will show extended or elongated radiolucent area with or without extension of fracture line to it.

Cerebral infarct

Interruption of cerebral blood supply leads to cerebral anoxia and death of the affected portion. There is a hypodense area within the area known to be supplied by major vessels. Marginal enhancement may occur in subacute and chronic cases.

Cerebral contusion

Both haemorrhagic and non-haemorrhagic cerebral contusions appear as focal areas of cerebral oedema. Non-haemorrhagic contusions are more focal with more marked mass effect and show contrast enhancement not seen in oedema. In haemorrhagic cerebral contusion, areas of haemorrhage are still seen in early stages (figure 6.21 a).

Epidural haematoma

The appearances are the same as with subdural haematoma except that the shape is biconvex. Adjacent skull fractures may also be shown.

Subdural haematoma

If old and calcified, plain film may show dense calcified concavo-convex lesion within the skull. However, CT scan is frequently used to show the lesion where in acute cases there is hyperdense concavo-convex lesion within the skull with mass effect. Adjacent skull fractures may be seen. In subacute cases, the lesion is isodense to brain in pre-contrast scan. Post-contrast scan will show it as hypodense lesion due to preferential enhancement of viable brain parenchyma. There may be curvilinear marginal enhancement due to disruption of blood-brain barrier. Chronic lesions are hypodense on precontrast scan with concavo-convex shape. Post-contrast scan may show marginal enhancement (figure 6.21 a, b and c).

Subarachnoid Haemorrhage

This causes very severe headache and CT scan is the most important investigative modality. Subarachnoid haemorrhage is often caused by aneurysms, angiomas, tumours which may be identified with CT scan (figure 6.21 b). Blood appearing hypodense may be identified within the subarachnoid space, basal cisterns, insula, sulci, and they are most commonly seen within the first 1 – 3 days of the haemorrhage. Associated intra-cerebral or intraventricular blood collection or haematoma may be seen. In the ventricles, the blood will gravitate to the dependent side with fluid-levels and blood in the ventricles has grave prognosis. Contrast injection is contraindicated in acute cases. Areas of cerebral infarction and post-haemorrhagic hydrocephalus may be seen in patients with subarachnoid haemorrhage.

Cerebrovascular Accident/Stroke

This can be thrombotic or ischaemic. Thrombotic cerebrovascular accidents are caused by hypertension, ruptured aneurysm, angiomas or haemorrhagic tumours. Ischaemic CVA is caused by vascular occlusion by embolism, atheromatous plaques, spasm, infection, tumour or arterial thrombosis/ embolus due to tumour, infection, trauma. Subdural haematoma, epidural haematoma, intracerebral haematoma, tumours, aneurysm or subarachnoid haemorrhage may be seen.

Intracerebral haemorrhage/haematoma

This can result from trauma or it may be spontaneous. The spontaneous causes are aneurysm, angioma, blood dyscrasias, hypertension, atheroma, tumours and amyloid angiopathy. Both CT and MRI are indicated. Pre-contrast CT scan in acute cases will show hyperdense area within the brain surrounded by low density area and contrast injection may show ring enhancement due to clot retraction and damage to blood brain barrier. Subarachnoid extension can occur. Subacute and chronic cases are isodense and hypodense respectively to brain with marginal enhancement due to damage to the blood-brain barrier.

Lesion of Sinuses and Nasopharynx

Sinusitis: This can be acute or chronic. In acute sinusitis plain film or CT scan will show opacity of affected sinus with or without air-fluid level. Chronic sinusitis will present with mucoperiosteal thickening of the sinus mucous membrane.

Mucocoele/pyocoele of sinuses: Opaque sinus with loss of internal scalloping or outward bulging of the sinus wall. Mucocoele is caused by blockage of the drainage ostium with accumulation of secretion. Infection of this will lead to pus formation or pyocoele. The maxillary and the frontal sinuses are commonly involved.

Polyp: Spherical radio-opacity of soft tissue density is found with plain film or CT scan. This can cause sinusitis and mucocoele.

Carcinoma: The antral carcinoma is the commonest. There is a solid lesion with destruction of adjacent bone, erosion of orbital floor and even the pterygoid lamina.

Nasopharyngeal tumours: Carcinomas, juvenile angiofibroma, chordoma, meningioma may grow at this region and involve the skull base.

Retropharyngeal abscess: Widening (> 0.6C4) of the prevertebral soft tissue with lucency within it due to gas. There is often straightening of the cervical spine. There may be associated meningitis, torticollis.

Adenoid and tonsilar hyperplasia and inflammation: These can cause headache. Round, nodular or curvilinear radio-opacity in the usual location of adenoid or tonsil is found on plain film of nasopharynx or CT scan. There may be narrowing of the nasopharyngeal airway.

Referred Pain from the Eye

Orbital pseudotumour
Orbital cellulitis/infection/ophthalmitis
Orbital tumours – primary/secondary (Retinoblastoma, metastasis)
Orbital vascular lesions including carotico-cavernous fistulas.

Thyroid ophthalmopathies

Many thyroid lesions can cause headache. Please see *unilateral proptosis* where they are well-discussed.

Tumours and Associated Lesions
Skull lucencies

Tumours will present with skull lucencies on plain films. This is caused by erosion of inner table of the skull. Such tumours include meningioma, glioma, dermoid and epidermoid cysts, and craniopharyngioma. Multiple myeloma causes multiple punched-out lesions or moth-eaten appearance in the skull. Metastatic neuroblastoma causes widening of the sutures usually seen in children. Metastasis from breast may cause multiple varied-sized radiolucent lesions or mixed sclerotic and osteolytic lesions. Skull defects may be seen in neurofibromatosis in the area of the lambdoid suture.

Intracranial calcification

This can occur in tumours e.g. meningiomas, craniopharyngiomas, chordomas, ependymomas, medulloblastomas; infections such as tuberculosis may show calcified tuberculous granuloma. Plain film will show round or irregular radio-opacity. Curvilinear calcification is seen in aneurysm. Biconvex bracket calcification is seen in agenesis of the corpus callosum.

Erosion of sella turcica

Erosion, widening or ballooning of sella turcica is caused by space-occupying lesion causing raised intracranial pressure. Hydrocephalus can also cause it. The sella turcica is the weakest part of the skull bone thus it becomes thinned and widened by increased intracranial pressure. Calcification or lucencies may be associated with erosion of sella due to tumour.
CT and MRI will clearly show the tumour mass.

Meningioma

Meningioma is an intracranial tumour, hyperdense on CT study, has a well-defined capsule and margin. It is vascular, frequently parasagittal in location and shows marked contrast enhancement.

Glioma

Gliomas often has irregular calcification and occasionally it may be cystic resembling abscess. Tumour masses are associated with surrounding hypodense lesions due to oedema causing mass effect. There is midline shift, and dilatation of contralateral ventricles.

Sturge-Weber syndrome

Gyriform calcification with areas of brain atrophy are seen in Sturge-Weber syndrome.

Tumours in the cerebellopontine angle

They can be associated with neurofibromatosis. In summary CT and MRI will identify tumour mass but biopsy and histology are required for accurate identification.

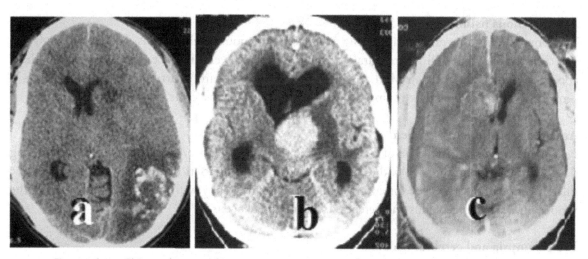

Figure 6.21. CT scan images of lesions causing headache. **a**. Angioma of the left occipital lobe demonstrated in contrast CT. **b**. Intracranial aneurysm with well-defined margin and mass-effect. **c**. Subacute right subdural haematoma demonstrated after contrast enhancement.

Arterial Lesions/Cystic Lesions
Hydrocephalus

Dilated ventricles can result from congenital lesions such as Dandy-Walker syndrome. Choroid plexus papilloma causing over-secretion of CSF will cause communicating hydrocephalus. This will be identified by CT and MRI.

Cerebral atrophy

There is dilatation of sulci, and only mild dilatation of the ventricles. Cystic space occupying lesions such as giant cisterna magna, arachnoid cyst, ependymal cyst, cyst of third ventricle, cyst of septum pellucidum. All these put traction on arteries and cause headache. They are all well identified by CT scan.

Arachnoid cysts

They are seen in the posterior fossa, more frequently in children. They can be intracranial and extracerebral with some hypoplasia of adjacent cerebral tissue. The cyst is posterior to the third ventricle and may cause obstructive hydrocephalus.

Aneurysm

These are seen on CT scan as high-density spherical lesions at the base of the brain. Contrast administration shows intense immediate post-contrast enhancement with fairly well-defined margins. Mass-effect on adjacent structures may be seen with compression and surrounding oedema (figure 6.21 b).

Angiomas

In pre-contrast CT scan, mottled appearance is seen with adjacent low-density areas due to cerebral infarction or haemorrhagic cyst. Post-contrast scan will show tortuous vascular hypendense areas with some of it superficial and others penetrating the brain like a wedge. Angiomas produce mass effect. Angiography will define the exact anatomy of the feeding vessels.

Arteriovenous fistulas

These may drain intracranially appearing as enlarged tortuous cerebral veins. More commonly the area is in the dura and drain extra-durally through superficial veins in the orbit, scalp or dura. These appear as signal void areas on MRI. Angiography of internal carotid artery or affected vessels will show early filling of the dilated veins. Arterial pulsation in dilated veins causes headache.

Aneurysm of the vein of Galen

Pear-shaped, grossly dilated vein of Galen found in the occipital lobe. Arteriovenous fistula occurring deep within the brain shunts blood to the vein of Galen leading to its dilatation. MRI will show the dilated vein without the need for contrast injection. Angiography will show the dilated vein in the venous phase. Hydrocephalus and cerebral ischaemia may occur.

Pre-eclampsia and cerebral oedema

There is swelling of cerebral tissues and parenchyma. The features are those of brain tissue oedema. CT and MRI will show effacement of sulci and widening of gyri. There will be reduction in the size of ventricles to slit-like appearance. It is best diagnosed retrospectively with improvement. Usually there is a history of recent delivery and that the patient is in the puerperal period or she may be pregnant. Headache peceeded by coitus has been described.

(Adam & Dixon, 2008; Dahnert, 2011; Sutton, 1998 and 2003, Palmer & Reeder 2001).

References

1. Medina LS, D'Souza B, Vasconcellos E. Adults and children with headache: evidence-based diagnostic evaluation. Neuroimaging Clin N Am 2003;13:225-35.
2. Provenzale JM. Imaging evaluation of the patient with worst headache of life--it's not all subarachnoid haemorrhage. Emerg Radiol 2010;17:403-12.
3. Dawson AJ, Rowland-Hill C, Atkin SL. A persistent headache. BMJ 2010;340:c2966.
4. Menon B. Symptomatic occipital epilepsy misdiagnosed as migraine. Headache 2007 ;47:287-9.
5. Onwuchekwa CR, Onwuchekwa AC. The role of computed tomography in the diagnostic work-up of headache patients in Nigeria. Headache 2010;50:1346-52.
6. Komolafe MA, Sunmonu TA, Oke O. Stroke-like syndrome in a middle aged Nigerian woman with metastatic brain cancer. West Afr J Med 2009;28:266-9.
7. Eze KC, Salami TA, Eze CU, Alikah SO. Computed tomography study of complicated bacterial meningitis. Niger J Clin Pract 2008;11:351-4.
8. Omoti AE, Waziri-Erameh MJ. Pattern of neuro-ophthalmic disorders in a tertiary eye centre in Nigeria. Niger J Clin Pract 2007;10:147-51.
9. Arogundade RA, Awosanya GO, Arigbabu SO. Role of computed tomography in the management of adult brain tumours. Niger Postgrad Med J 2006;13:123-7.
10. Harrison NE, Odunukwe NN, Ijoma CK, Mafe AG. Current clinical presentation of malaria in Enugu, Nigeria. Niger Postgrad Med J 2004;11:240-5.
11. Adinma JI, Agbai AO. Headache following parturition. J Obstet Gynaecol 2000;20:35-8.
12. Adinma JI. Acute puerperal coital headache and hypertension. Aust N Z J Obstet Gynaecol 1994;34:487-8.

6.3 RADIOLOGICAL FINDINGS IN RETINOBLASTOMAS

Definition
Retinoblastomas are highly malignant and aggressive primitive neuroectodermal tumours originating from the retina and they are the most common intraocular malignancies in childhood.

Aetiology
Some of them have autosomal dominant inheritance.
Some are congenital while others are non-inheritable

Presentation
They present with leucokoria (amaurotic cat eye) (abnormal light reflex), visual loss, strabismus, intraocular mass, intraocular calcification, retinal detachment, proptosis, phthisis bulbi, heterochromia iridis, neovascularization of iris, hyphaema and pain (secondary closed angle glaucoma).

Unilateral or bilateral
1. Initially presents in one eye
2. Bilateral in one third (⅓) of cases.

Incidence   1:20,000 live births

Sex Ratio: M:F = 1:1

Age at presentation
Mainly 6 months – 10 years but the age at diagnosis is mostly before 3 years.
Average age at diagnosis is 18 months.
Over 98% of tumours are detected at less than 5 years of age

Method of spread
Intra – orbital, Trans-scleral and Haematogenous spread.

Types of Retinoblastomas:
They are classified according to:
A. Inheritability (inheritable or non-inheritable)
B. Number of co-existing neuroectodermal tumours
C. Pathologic form/types

Classification according to inheritance
1. *Non-inheritable form* (66%)
    a. Sporadic post-zygotic mutation (unilateral disease with subsequent generations unaffected)
    b. Chromosomal anomaly.
2. *Inheritable form*
    a. Inheritable sporadic form (Bilateral Retinoblastomas) (up to 50% chance of occurrence in subsequent generations)
    b. *Familial retinoblastomas.* It is autosomal dominant with abnormality of band 14 in chromosome 13 (often have more than 2 tumours per eye and it is bilateral in up to 66% of cases).

Classification according to the number of tumours
a. *Unilateral tumour*
b. *Bilateral tumour* (Bilateral Retinoblastoma)

c. *Trilateral tumour* (rare): Bilateral Retinoblastoma with co-existing pinealoblastoma (Neuroectodermal pineal gland tumour).

d. *Quadrilateral retinoblastoma:* Trilateral retinoblastoma with a fourth tumour in the suprasellar cistern

Classification according to pathological types

a. *Exophytic form:* Haematogenous spread to subretinal space with retinal detachment

b. *Endophytic form:* Floating island of sharply demarcated tumour within the vitreous fluid due to centripetal invasion and calcification

c. *Diffuse form. En-plaque* thin lesion along retina with extension peripherally.

Histological origin

Tumour originates from cells derived from primitive embryonic retinal epithelium of the primary optic vesicle of early intra-uterine life.

Radiological features

Ultrasound

Echogenic soild mass within the globe: Highly echogenic mass within the globe originating posteriorly within the globe.

Heterogenous soild mass within the globe: Non-homogenous or heterogenous hyperechoic solid mass within the globe

Mushroom-shaped retina-based mass: Dome-shape, mushroom-shaped or irregular solid mass originating from the retina.

Cystic area within the tumour due to necrosis: Tumour necrosis may give the mass a cystic appearance

Calcification: Dense echogenic calcification within the mass with distal acoustic shadowing.

Retinal detachment: Secondary retinal detachment is very common appearing as v-shape, thin thread-like echogenic structure within the globe with apex of V at optic nerve head.

Vitreous haemorrhage: Echogenic area within the globe sometimes with fluid level due to gravitation of denser blood against the vitreous humour.

Normal ocular size at early stages: But later proptosis occurs with enlargement of the globe. Gross proptosis may make ultrasonography difficult if the eye lid does not cover the globe anymore.

Optic nerve infiltration: Optic nerve involvement with enlargement of optic nerve complex echo.

Sub-retinal exudates: There may be growth into the subretinal space and this may give features of sub-retinal exudates.

Orbital inflammatory changes: There may be features of inflammatory changes if the optic nerve is involved.

Doppler ultrasound scan

Increased blood flow is noted on Doppler imaging

Computed tomography scan

Retrolental solid mass: Smoothly marginated, lobulated, hyperdense solid retrolental mass.

Dense calcification: Dense calcification is seen in 75 – 95%. Retinoblastoma is the commonest cause of orbital calcification. Calcification on CT in paediatric patient is retinoblastoma until proven otherwise.

Vitreous haemorrhage: Dense vitreous humour (common) at late stages with proptosis. It may be normal-sized at early stages.

Changes in size of the globe with proptosis: Enlargement of the globe or macrophthalmia especially at late stages with proptosis. It may be normal-sized at early stages.

Intense contrast enhancement: Due to neovascularization there is contrast enhancement in post-contrast scan.

Extra-ocular extension: Extra-ocular extensions occur in up to one quarter (¼) of the cases. It is in the form of (a) Involvement with enlargement of the optic nerve, (b), Abnormal soft tissue mass in the orbit and (c), Intracranial extension.

Thickened wall of the globe: Thickening of outer wall of the globe.

Subarachnoid haemorrhage: CT scan detects subarachnoid haemorrhage due to metastasis to the meninges and subarachnoid space.

Pulmonary metastasis: Single or multiple pulmonary nodules, hilar enlargement and pleural effusion may occur due to metastasis to the chest.

Lymph node metastasis: Cervical, thoracic and intra-abdominal lymphadenopathy due to metastasis.

Hepatic metastasis: Multiple round hypodense lesion in the liver due to metastasis to the liver.

Multiple tumours: CT scan detects bilateral, trilateral and quadrilateral tumours.

Magnetic Resonance Imaging

Varied intensity in difference sequences: Mildly hyperintense lesion relative to the extra-ocular muscles on T_1WI and markedly hyperintense on T_2WI.

Calcification: Gradient echo shows hypointensity within mass due to calcification.

Enhancement of non-calcified component: Marked enhancement of non-calcified soft tissue component is seen in post-contrast MRI scan.

Sub-retinal exudates: Sub-retinal exudates are hyperintense on T_1WI.

Peri-retinal spread: MRI detects trans-scleral and periretinal spread better than CT scan.

Multiple tumours: Pineal gland tumour and quadrilateral tumour are detected by both CT and MRI but better by MRI.

Complementary to CT on calcific areas: MRI has poor detection of calcification and therefore both CT and MRI are complementary.

Multiplanar capability improves diagnosis: MRI detects metastasis in the liver and lymph nodes as well as lung and brain involvement in one session due to its multiplanar capability.

Sub-arachnoid haemorrhage: Sub-arachnoid haemorrhage, inflammation of meninges are seen due to metastasis.

Bone marrow metastasis: Metastasis can be detected within the bone marrow in sagittal and coronal section scans.

Plain films

Calcification: Calcification within the globe is seen in up to 50 – 75% of cases.

Metastasis to the lungs: Detects metastasis to the lungs
   a. Multiple/single pulmonary nodule
   b. Pleural effusion.
   c. Areas of consolidation due to exudative metastasis

Multiple congenital abnormalities: Microcephaly, finger and toe abnormalities associated with chromosomal anomalies in the non-inheritable form can be detected by plain films apart from clinical examination.

Others

Radiation-induced sarcomas: Radiation-induced sarcomatous changes can be detected by CT and MRI.

Other sarcomatous change: Other non-ocular malignancies which frequently have increased risk in familial retinoblastomas can be detected by CT and MRI. These non-ocular malignancies include osteosarcomas, fibrosarcoma, malignant fibrous histocytoma, chondrosarcoma. This is up to 20% in those aged 10 years and over 90% in 30 years.

Tumour recurrence: Both CT and MRI will detect recurrence of tumour. Tumour recurrence rates are high with recurrent enlargement of the orbit and an intra-orbital mass.

Prognosis

Retinoblastoma has the best prognosis of all childhood tumours with over 50% of survival records. Calcification denotes favourable prognosis. Contrast enhancement denotes poor prognosis. Non-involvement of optic nerve has mortality of less than 10%.

Optic nerve invasion, trans-scleral, haematogenous, subarachnoid and spread to vascular spaces of the orbit (choroidal invasion) denote very poor prognosis

If tumour is resected and margins of resection are not free from tumour, it also denotes very poor prognosis.

Complications

Metastasis, radiation-induced sarcomatous change and other non-ocular sarcomatous changes.

Differential diagnosis

1. Retinoma or retinocytoma (Benign variant).
2. Coat's disease (no calcification)
3. *Toxocara canis* infection (absence of calcification)
4. Persistent hyperplastic primary vitreous (hypoplastic globe, absence of calcification).

(Adam & Dixon, 2008; Dahnert, 2011; Sutton, 1998 and 2003, Palmer & Reeder 2001).

References

1. Apushkin MA, Apushkin MA, Shapiro MJ, Mafee MF. Retinoblastoma and simulating lesions: role of imaging. Neuroimaging Clin N Am 2005; 15:49-67.
2. Kivelä T, Tuppurainen K, Riikonen P, Vapalahti M. Retinoblastoma associated with chromosomal 13q14 deletion mosaicism. Ophthalmology 2003; 110:1983-8.
3. Saket RR, Mafee MF. Anterior-Segment Retinoblastoma Mimicking Pseudoinflammatory Angle-Closure Glaucoma: Review of the Literature and the Important Role of Imaging. AJNR Am J Neuroradiol 2009 Apr 15.
4. Sabourin SM, Jayashankar A, Mullins ME. AJR teaching file: lump on the head. AJR Am J Roentgenol 2008; 191:S31-3
5. Bekibele CO, Ayede AI, Asaolu OO, Brown BJ. Retinoblastoma: the challenges of management in Ibadan, Nigeria. J Pediatr Hematol Oncol 2009;31:552-5.

6. Chuka-Okosa CM, Uche NJ, Kizor-Akaraiwe NN. Orbito-ocular neoplasms in Enugu, South-Eastern, Nigeria. West Afr J Med 2008;27:144-7.

7. Ekenze SO, Ekwunife H, Eze BI, Ikefuna A, Amah CC, Emodi IJ. The burden of pediatric malignant solid tumours in a developing country. J Trop Pediatr 2010 ;56:111-4.

8. Agboola AO, Adekanmbi FA, Musa AA, Sotimehin AS, Deji-Agboola AM, Shonubi AM, Oyebadejo TY, Banjo AA. Pattern of childhood malignant tumours in a teaching hospital in south-western Nigeria. Med J Aust. 2009;190:12-4.

9. Eze KC, Enock ME, Eluehike SU. Ultrasonic evaluation of orbito-ocular trauma in Benin-City, Nigeria. Niger Postgrad Med J 2009;16(3):198-202.

10. Ukponmwan CU, Marchien TT. Ultrasonic diagnosis of orbito-ocular diseases in Benin City, Nigeria. Niger Postgrad Med J 2001;8(3):123-6.

11. Nzeh DA, Owoeye JF, Ademola-Popoola DS, Uyanne I. Sonographic evaluation of ocular trauma in Ilorin, Nigeria. Eur J Ophthalmol 2006;16(3):453-7.

6.4   RADIOLOGICAL FEATURES OF INTRACRANIAL MENINGIOMA

Definition
Meningioma is the commonest benign intracranial tumour arising from meninges of the brain. It is derived from arachnoid rest cell or meningeal rest cells, which are more numerous in the dura and are particularly concentrated in the arachnoid villi or granulations.

Age: 35 – 70 years, peak age is at about 45 years and it is rare below 20 years.
Sex ratio: Male to female ratios is 1:2

Table 6.41: Locations of meningioma	
Intracranial locations	**Ectopic locations**
Cerebral convexities	Extradural
Parasagittal Posterior fossa region	Outer table of skull
Sphenoid ridge	Scalp
	Paranasal sinus
Frontobasal region	Parapharyngeal space
Spine	Parotid
Intraventricular	Intra thoracic
Cerebellopontine angle	Mediastinum
Optic nerve sheath	Adrenal gland

Types of meningioma
1. **Globular meningioma:** Well defined compact spherical mass arising from the dura/falx, invaginating into the brain (commonest).
2. **Meningioma en-plaque:** Noted by extensive hyperostosis of adjacent bone especially around middle cranial fossa.
3. **Multicentric meningioma:** Rare. Associated with neurofibromatosis and many meningiomas discovered in some patients usually on one side of the head.

Radiological Features

Plain Films
Skull calcifications
Dense, amorphous or well marginated (appearing like football) due to the capsule f the tumour. They occur in the location of tumour as listed above. Less commonly, calcification may be nodular or speckled. Calcification can also be seen as homogenous when arising from psammoma bodies. Calcification is seen in 10 – 15%.

Skull lucencies
Erosion of inner table of the skull due to meningioma may present with areas of skull lucencies and there may be a mixture of osteolytic and osteoblastic lesion. Rarely angioblastic type of meningioma may leave areas of skull lucencies or a purely osteolytic response.

Falx calcification
Linear midline calcification, which can be dense, or multiple vertical strands in the region of the falx.

Local expansion of diplöe
This can also present as spotty appearance or lucency.

Hyperostosis
Areas of sclerosis, enostosis, exostosis or increased skull density due to thickening of the skull vault. It is often localised in meningioma. It initially affects the inner table, but it may later progress to involve the diplöe and outer table and may occasionally present a noticeable or palpable mass. Sun-burst or sunray spiculation may occur. There may be other features of meningioma like enlarged vascular groove or raised intracranial pressure.

Blistering
Meningioma sited at the anterior clinoid process, tuberculum sellae, jugum, planum sphenoidale or clivus (sphenoid wing meningioma) may show local bone expansion with pneumatization of the bone. The local bony expansion may also have increased density or hyperostosis. All these appearances when seen at characteristic sites are called *blistering*. They almost always signify meningioma en-plaque.

Enlarged vascular grooves
Meningioma is a highly vascular tumour and the meninges of the brain where it originates is in close proximity with the skull. The bulk of the blood supply to the meninges is from the middle meningeal branch of internal maxillary artery (a branch of external carotid artery). The grooves in the skull where these vessels pass are enlarged, widened, deepened, and become prominent. In addition, the enlarged vascular grooves tend to converge at the site of the tumour, which may be marked by calcification, lucencies or hyperostosis. Other minor vessels that may supply meningioma are also enlarged.

Enlarged foramina
Basal foramina where the vessels that supply the meninges involved in the tumour enter the cranium are enlarged. *Foramen spinosum* which *transmits middle meningeal artery* is widened in diameter compared to the contralateral side. Optic foramen may be enlarged in optic canal meningioma.

Pneumosinus dilatans
Enlargement, dilatation and widening of pneumatized paranasal sinuses.
There is increased pneumatization of sinuses adjacent to the meningioma. It is seen especially in ethmoidal and sphenoidal sinuses. The roofs of the sinuses are often thickened. This sign is a strong evidence of the existence of occult or not-yet-diagnosed meningioma or meningioma en-plaque close to the site (table 4.61).

Raised intracranial pressure
This may appear as erosion of dorsum sellae with sometimes thinning or depression of the bones of the sella turcica because the sella is the weakest and thinnest part of the cranial bone and it is the earliest to respond in cases of increased pressure within the inexpandible skull. Occasionally, there can be depression of bones of anterior cranial fossa due to tumour in this site causing raised intracranial pressure.

Proptosis

Meningioma of the sphenoid ridge will frequently cause proptosis which is forward protrusion of the eyeball. This can be identified clinically but imaging is frequently required to identify the underlying causes and CT and MRI are invaluable if the cause is within the cranial cavity.

Orbital changes

Narrowing of the optic canal due to hyperostosis in optic nerve sheath meningioma may occur. This can present with impairment of vision or blindness due to optic canal entrapment.

Calcification of optic nerve sheath meningioma may present with intra-orbital calcification. Optic canal enlargement can also occur by erosion from sheath meningioma.

Pressure changes

These include enlargement of superior orbital fissures, erosion of sella turcica, depression of anterior cranial fossa, erosion of petrous apex and orbital wall margins, depression of anterior cranial fossa and proptosis.

Sunray spiculation

This is seen in some parts of the skull in patients with meningioma. It is a pattern of calcification appearing to spread out from the tumour peripherially in a fan-like manner.

Computed Tomography Scan
Well-marginated tumour

Round well circumscribed sharply demarcated non infiltrative, high density tumour mass with homogenous density.

Broad–based attachment

The tumour has wide or broad-based attachment to the adjacent dura and inner table of skull.

Calcification

This in irregular, or radial and found in 16 – 20%. Calcification increases the pre-contrast density of the tumour.

En-plaque tumour

In bone window of CT scan the en-plaque type shows bone involvement with pronounced hyperostosis. This bone involvement is more difficult to see if the tumour is adjacent to the carvernous sinus or sphenoid ridge.

Cortical buckling of underlying brain

Compression of the adjacent brain with effacement of sulci and gyri.

Hypodense or Isodense mass lesion

This depends on the type of the tumour, tumour tissue necrosis, angioblastic component, and partial volume averaging. Psammomatous calcification increases the density.

No sign of infiltration
Characteristically the tumour is not infiltrative. It is well-circumscribed, well-defined and well-marginated with clearly defined and intact capsule. However the en-plaque variety is more infiltrative.

Intraosseous meningioma
Meningioma may permeate the bone with soft tissue component which can be intracerebral or extracerebral, intracranial or extracranial.

Hyperostosis
Increased thickening of adjacent skull bone and sclerosis are seen. These are more extensive in CT than are shown on plain film.

Cystic component/angioblastic meningioma
Areas of mass lesion with cystic components which are minor in about 15% and major in only 2%. They are caused by angioblastic meningioma. They may harbour areas of calcification/increased density.

Mild to moderate mass effect
Since the tumour is slow-growing, the shift of midline structures is strikingly small compared to the size of the tumour and the compression of adjacent ventricles is quite small.

Absent or mild surrounding oedema
The oedema elicited by even a large tumour mass is strikingly small and often only circumscribed. Only rarely is there extensive oedema or tail sign similar to malignant lesion.

Intraventricular meningioma
This comprises only about 2% of meningioma. Well-defined, high density, well marginated mass within the ventricle, usually within trigone of the lateral ventricle. It must be differentiated from papilloma of choroid plexus and ependymoma.

Falx meningioma
Meningioma arising from the falx in the parasagittal position will have tumour mass effect in both sides of the falx simulating a butterfly. Corpus callosum lipoma or cystic glioma must be excluded.

Intense and marked uniform enhancement
Absence of blood brain barrier leads to marked opacification of tumour by hypertrophied supplying blood vessels. This results in increased uniform density due to extensive contrast enhancement of tumour.

Magnetic Resonance Imaging
The tumour is hypointense/isointense on T1-weighted mgaes (T_1WI). It is isointense or hyperintense on T2-weeighted images (T_2WI). This is because the collagen element present in the tumour determines the tumour intensity/density.

Homogenous/heterogenous texture

High vascularity, cystic change and calcification in varied extent gives the tumour different texture and density.

Well-defined mass

The mass is well-defined and well marginated almost appearing like football.

Cortical buckling

There is cortical effacement of the sulci with arcuate bowing of white matter.

Low density tumour-brain interface

A low density linear area is seen between the tumour and the brain. However, cerebrospinal angle may show high intensity cleft on T_2WI.

High contrast enhancement

This is rapid and stays later as seen on CT scan. The enhancement is about 100 – 148% higher than normal brain parenchyma.

Dural tail sign

Broad-based attachment to the dura leads to curvilinear area of enhancement tapering off from tumour margin along dural surfaces in over 50% of cases.

Venous sinuse thrombosis

Superior and inferior sagittal sinuses and other venous sinuses are thrombosed due to tumour mass effect, compression of vessels and sluggish or stagnant blood.

Angiography
Mother-in-law phenomenom

Intense contrast enhancement which appears early in arterial phase and stays late into the venous phase.

Sun-burst enhancement pattern

This is also the same as sun-ray, spoke-wheel pattern of tumour enhancement or vascularity. The tumour has sun-burst or sun-ray or spoke-wheel pattern of vascularity which appears more marked with contrast enhancement showing this vascularity pattern more clearly. Occasionally this may appear cloud-like.

Early drainage vessels may rarely be seen especially in the angioblastic type. This is as opposed to the late drainage at the venous phase.

Thrombosis or occlusion of major sinuses

This occurs in the superior and inferior sagittal sinus or other major sinuses. They are also seen with MR imaging. MR angiography can show these lesions without the need for contrast administration.

Poor vascularity in meningioma en-plaque

This is characteristic. Without the use of CT scan to elicit hyperostosis or pneumosinus dilatans, the lesion may be missed.

Hypertrophied supplying vessels
1. *Middle meningeal artery – from internal maxillary artery, branch of external carotid artery:* This supplies the meninges of the brain and is thus almost always hypertrophied in most cases of meningioma.
2. *Posterior ethmoidal branch of ophthalmic artery* supplying suprasellar meningioma.
3. *Meningeal branch of meningohypophyseal artery,* branch of internal carotid artery supplying tentorial and suprasellar meningioma.
4. *Ascending pharyngeal artery and vertebral artery* supplying meningioma located in the clivus and the posterior fossa.
5. *Choroidal artery, branch of internal carotid artery* supplying intraventricular meningioma.
6. *Branches of external carotid artery* may supply scalp meningioma.

Other rare appearing meningiomas
1. Completely low-attenuating mass lesion. Due to tumour necrosis, old haemorrhage and cyst formation.
   a. Purely cystic meningioma is found in children.
   b. Lipoplastic meningioma. Metaplastic change of tumour cell origin to adipocytes. CT number will show density in the range of adipose tissue.
2. Ring enhancement/heterogeneous enhancement
   Necrosis and infarction of tumour may occur giving it ring enhancement in contrast CT scan. Ben0ign accumulation of fluid within tumour may rarely give it a cystic appearance.
3. Sarcomatous transformation. Rare. Following irradiation of tumour, sarcomatous change can also occur. There is invasion of cerebral hemisphere.

Interventional Studies
Tumour blood supply can be embolized during conventional angiographic studies using catheter technique to reduce the vascularity before neurosurgical intervention.

MENINGIOMA OF SPINE
Incidence: It comprises 12% of all meningiomas and 25 – 45% of all spinal tumours

Age: It occurs above 40 years (80%), is commoner in women and only 2 – 3% occur in children.

Location
More than 80% occur in the spinal canal and in the thoracic region.
About 50% – 90% is intradural extramedulary.
It is more common in the cervical spine especially at foramen magnum
More than 90% occur in the lateral aspect.
Extradural tumour suggests malignancy.

Radiological features
Plain films
1. Bone erosion
2. Scalloping of posterior aspects of vertebral bodies
3. Widening of interpedicular distances
4. Enlargement of intervertebral foramen on lateral view)

5. Partial calcification
6. Scoliosis/kyphosis

CT scan

1. Solid well-defined marginated mass
2. Density same as skeletal muscle
3. Marked contrast enhancement in contrast scan.
4. Intra-dural location is usual in CT myelography
5. Calcification is found within tumour
6. Broad-based dural attachment

MRI

1. Isointense to neural tissues especially the grey matter in both T_1WI and T_2WI.
2. Rapid, intense, marked contrast enhancement after Gd – DTPA.
3. MR myelography shows intradural location with obstruction or compression of spinal cord.
4. It has broad-based dural attachment.

(Adam & Dixon, 2008; Dahnert, 2011; Sutton, 2003)

References

1. Koeller KK, Sandberg GD. Cerebral intraventricular neoplasms: radiologic-pathologic correlation. Radiographics 2002;22:1473-505.
2. Buetow MP, Buetow PC, Smirniotopoulos JG. Typical, atypical, and misleading features in meningioma. Radiographics 1991;11:1087-106.
3. Siegelman ES, Mishkin MM, Taveras JM. Past, present, and future of radiology of meningioma. Radiographics 1991;11:899-910.
4. Eze KC, Mazeli FO, Otoibhi EO, Okuonghae JT. Unilateral exophthalmos: a radiological differential diagnosis. Benin journal of postgraduate medicine 2002; 6: 71-82.

6.5 RADIOLOGY OF TRAUMATIC BRAIN INJURY (HEAD INJURY)

Traumatic brain injury also called post-traumatic brain injury or head injury is a clinical condition caused by trauma to the head resulting in various degrees of alteration of sensorium or loss of consciousness. Head injury is said to occur when, following a trauma to the head, the Glasgow Coma Scale score is less than fifteen or when it is fifteen with a history of alteration of mental state or loss of consciousness as a result of the trauma. Post-traumatic brain injury is also defined as brain structural injury or disruption of brain function as a result of an external force. All the patients with head injuries need not undergo rigorous imaging with CT and MRI, but these should be based on clinical states of the patients and findings at plain radiography.

Causes of post-traumatic brain injury
Road traffic accidents, fall (children less than 4 years and elderly above 75 year), sports injury and recreation, assault, firearm-related injuries, and blasts injuries

The mechanism of brain injury in this condition is the transfer of energy from the external sources to body tissue to such an extent that the transferred energy becomes beyond the amount that can be absorbed by the body without dysfunction. The resulting brain dysfunction as a result of this excessive transferred energy in head injury manifests as intracranial lesion, loss, decreased, or altered level of consciousness, amnesia and neurologic deficit. Loss of input from the reticular activating system as a result of external force impairs consciousness.[1-3]

Indications for skull radiography
1. Abnormal neurological sign
2. Disturbance of consciousness
3. Loss of blood-stained or clear fluid from the nose or ear
4. Penetrating or suspected penetrating injury
5. Marked scalp bruising or swelling
6. Suspected skull fracture
7. Inability to assess neurological state because of influence of age–children and elderly, drugs, alcohol, uncooperativeness of patient, mental retardation, deafness, dumbness, foreign or unintelligible language.
8. *Medico-legal reasons:* This is for documentation of present extent of injury in the case of any subsequent injury to decide the insurance responsible for the cost since different insurances may operate in the same patients depending on where and when the injury occurs.

Indications for CT scan or MR imaging
1. Skull fracture
2. Abnormal neurological sign
3. Persistent confusion
4. Coma or drowsiness of moderate to severe degree
5. Persistent headache
6. Vomiting following head trauma

Radiological features on skull radiograph

1. *Fracture of skull:* Linear, stellate, depressed, open, e.t.c. skull fractures and best diagnosed using clinical examinations and plain radiographs.
2. Sutural diastasis. This is widening of the coronal or sagittal sutures by more than 3 mm in diameter.
3. Intracranial collection of air (pneumocephalus.) This occurs from fracture of the walls of the sinuses. The air appears translucent.
4. *Fluid in the paranasal sinuses or mastoid air cells:* This is due to haemorrhage. Fluid levels may be shown.
5. Foreign body in the cranial cavity or scalp.
6. Soft tissue emphysema
7. Fracture of facial bones

Imaging modalities
Plain films

Skull AP, Lateral, Waters view and Towne's view. It has poor diagnostic yield and correlation between fractures and intracranial injuries compared to CT and MRI. When CT and MRI are available, plain films add no additional information.

Computed tomography of the head

Scout film: lateral and AP which acts as digital radiography.

Non-contrast: 2.5-5 mm thickness slices from the base of the skull to the vertex in contiguous axial sections. Helical CT scan or helical multidetector scanning is preferred alternatives. CT is the *gold standard* for detecting intracranial haemorrhage and it can detect almost all the cerebral infarct 24 -48 hours in traumatic brain injury imaging. Its availability and short imaging time make it very versatile for imaging head injury. CT angiography can be done in the same session.

MR Imaging

When CT fails to detail the brain injury or fails to explain the clinical findings as correlated with the patient's condition, MRI is indicated.

MRI is also preferred in assessment of subacute or chronic brain injuries because of the tendency of the CT to fail to detect isodense lesions. In patients with small lesions, especially close to the skull, MRI is also preferred as partial volume averaging prevents the detection of these lesions by CT scan. Many protocols are used in MRI imaging in head injury and may be different for different centres.

Plain radiography of other parts of the body

1. Spinal radiography: Lateral cervical, anteroposterior cervical and open mouth odontoid view. Others such as oblique and swimmers of views cervical spine are also necessary to accurately assess the cervicothoracic junction. Plain radiography of thoracic and lumbosacral spine (AP and lateral views) are also necessary if injury to these regions are suspected.
2. Chest x-ray, plain abdominal x-ray may be necessary as frequently there are associated injuries to these organs.
3. Plain radiography of extremities if injuries to these areas are suspected, such as upper and lower limbs.

Other imaging modalities
Ultrasound of the abdomen, eyes and injuries soft tissue organs
CT scan or MRI of the neck chest, abdomen and pelvis for injuries to these organs.

Radiological features seen on CT scan
CT is the best imaging modality for assessment of head trauma and head injury. MR is contributory in some areas where CT scan has some drawbacks.
The findings in cranial CT scan include the following.

1. *Fractures:* Basal skull fractures which are difficult to demonstrate with clinical examination and plain radiography are usually very clearly shown by CT scanning (Figure 7.51).
2. *Scalp swelling:* There are many type including caput succedaneum, subgaleal haematoma, subgaleal cyst, and cephalohaematoma. The scalp swellings are differentiated.
3. *Fluid in paranasal sinuses* and mastoid air cells. Fluid in sphenoidal sinus indicates fracture of base of the skull
4. *Pneumocephalus:* Air in the ventricles, or subarachnoid space (Fracture of skull especially the cribriform plate)
5. *Cerebral contusion:* This is defined as patchy, ill-defined, nodular haemorrhages within the brain. It may appear as a mass of mixed density lesion and similar multifocal haemorrhage, more diffuse with widespread area of swelling. It is occurring close to the surface of the brain and can occur in both coup and contre-coup side of impact but haemorrhagic cerebral contusion is more common in contre coup side. It is often associated with subarachnoid haemorrhages and most frequent supratentorially. It is found mostly at anterior and inferior frontal and temporal lobes, and the gyra around Sylvian fissure.
6. *Intracerebral haematoma:* This appears as a well-circumscribed haemorrhage within the brain parenchyma often located within the deeper part of the brain. The frontal and temporal lobes of the brain are usually affected. When the intracerebral haematoma is due to trauma, it is usually multifocal, and associated with low density areas due to brain oedema, and there may be associated cortical contusions. This is as opposed to spontaneous haemorrhage. Involvement of the brain stem connotes poor prognosis. In acute stages, it is hyperdense with irregular margins and depending on the size may compress the ipsilateral ventricle with associated compensatory dilatation of the contralateral ventricle. The falx may be shifted to the contralateral size. Skull fracture and scalp oedema may be seen. *Intracerebral haematoma is* irregular in shape (table 6.51, Figure 6.51 b).
7. *Sub-arachnoid haemorrhage:* This appears as hyperdense areas around the falx, Sylvian fissues, basal cistern and sulci (Figure 6.51 a). Its commonest manifestation is along the posterior falx. It may result from superficial cerebral contusion with leakage of blood into the subarachnoid space; or direct initial injury to the leptomeninges or intraventricular bleed with reflux through the foramina of fourth ventricular into the subarachnoid space. Its presence denotes possible secondary effects such as vasospasm and ischaemia, or a marker of more serious brain injury. Sub-arachnoid haemorrhage may be associated with intracerebral or intraventricular haemorrhage (table 6.51, Figure 6.51 b).

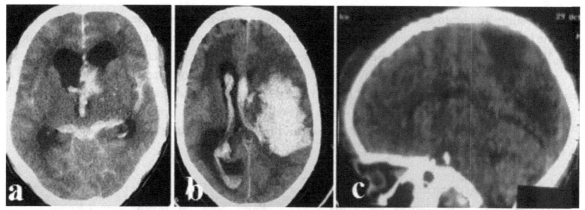

Figure 6.51: Non-enhanced CT scan studies in traumatic brain injury. Subarachnoid haemorrhage with fresh blood in Sylvian fissures and subarachnoid spaces (**a**). Irregular hyperdense area in the left temporal lobe due to actute intracerenral haematoma with surrounding hypodense area due to oedema with compression of left lateral ventricle; also note blood in the right lateral ventricle due to intreventricle extension (**b**). Irregular hypodense area in the occipito-parietal region with multiple linear hypodense areas within the brain due to brain infarction in child with non-accidental injury (**c**).

8. *Intraventricular haemorrhage:* Pure and isolated intraventricular haemorrhage is uncommon in head injury but it may be associated with intracerebral or subarachnoid haemorrhages. It results from tearing of the ependymal veins which line the ventricular cavities. The commonest occurrences are the ventral surface of corpus callosum, along the falx and the septum pellucidum. Intraventricular haemorrhage may be due to reflux of subarachnoid haemorrhage through the fourth ventricular foramina or extension from intracerebral haemorrhage. It denotes poor prognosis but associated injuries that cause it may be more important (tables 6.51, 6.52 and 6.53, Figure 6.51 b).

9. *Subdural haematoma/bleed:* Acute subdural haematoma (within 48 hours) is crescent- or concavo-convex-shaped spreading over the adjacent skull in the cerebral hemisphere. The haematoma is hyperdense and often located in fronto-parietal region or middle cranial fossa. There is associated hypodense surrounding areas of the brain due to brain oedema. Sudural haematoma is hyperdense in 0-7 days-2 weeks, isodense in 2-3 weeks and hypodense from above three weeks until it approaches the density of CSF after 4 weeks (table 6.52, 6.53).

10. *Epidural haematoma/bleed:* Acute epidural haematoma is biconvex-shaped and sited adjacent to the skull within the cranial cavity. The haematoma is hyperdense and often associated with skull fracture (table 6.52, 6.53).

11. *Leptomeningeal cyst* (late effect, due to unrecognised skull fracture in children). There is dural tear with herniation of pia and arachnoid layers of the meninges containing arachnoid fluid through it. CSF pulsation leads to increasing erosion of bones forming the fracture margins and leading to its widening. It occurs in children usually less than 5 years and noticed clinically as a soft tissue cystic swelling in the scalp. Repair of the dura after excision of the cyst is the treatment.

12. *Intraventricular bleed* (poor prognosis). Hyperdense lesions are seen within the ventricles with CSF-blood levels appearing as fluid level. In chronic stages, it can lead to hydrocephalus due to fibrotic obliteration of the aqueduct and ventricular foramina (Figure 6.51 b).

13. *Cerebral oedema:* There is obliteration of sulci and widening of gyri confirmed by repeat CT scan. Repeat scan and seeing the sulci wider than the previous scan appearance confirms the diagnosis.

14. *Haemorrhagic contusion:* This may appear as an area with mixed low and high densities similar to intracerebral haemorrhage. Frontal and temporal lobes are frequently affected though the

cerebellum and brain stem may also be involved. There is often a window period of 24 hours when the haemorrhagic area may not be seen apart from areas of low densities due to brain swelling.

15. *Non-haemorrhagic contusion*: Brain swelling with areas of mass effect is seen. Mass effect or compression of the ventricles. This is due to epidural, subdural and intracerebral haemorrhage

16. *Cerebral infarction without atrophy*: Both cerebral contusion and intracerebral haematoma could lead to cerebral infarction. At early stages this will appaear as an irregular or linear hypodense area. There is often no cavitation or shift of midline brain structures at the early stages (Figure 6.51 c).

Table 6.51: Imaging characteristics of intracranial haemorrhage using MRI and CT Scan.[1-5]

Parameter/ Haemorrhage type	Hyperacute haemorrhage	Acute haemorrhage	Early subacute haemorrhage	Late subacute haemorrhage	Chronic haemorrhage
Time duration	1-6 hours/ less than 12 hours	12 – 24–48 hours	2– 4 – 7 days	7 days – 4 weeks	4 weeks to one year and beyond
Event	Extravasation of blood	Formation of deoxy-Hb	Clot retraction and formation of met Deoxy-Hb	Cell lysis	Clot digestion by macrophages
Signal intensity on T1WI	Iso- or hypointense	Iso- or hypointense	Hyperintense	Hyperintense	Iso or hypointense
Signal intensity on T2WI	Hyperintense	Hypointense T2 PRE	Hypointense T2 PRE	Hyperintense	Hypointense T2 PRE
Non-enhanced CT	Hyperdense	Hyperdense with ill -defined hypodense margins	Isodense	Iso-or Slightly hypodense	Hypodense
Enhance CT	Contraindicated	Contraindicated	Isodence with marginal ring enhancement	Hypodense with marginal ring- enhancement	Hypodense area with ill-defined marginal ring enhancement.

(MR signal intensity is relative to brain gray matter)

17. *Cerebral atrophy*: This may be associated with subdural or epidural haemorrhage where there may be expansion or thinning of the skull vault.

18. *Infection of haematoma*: This may be seen as air loculation within the haematoma, increased density of the haematoma and by significant enhancement of the capsule of the haematoma cavity.

19. *Cerebral hygroma*: CT can detect subdural or epidural fluid collection due to neurosurgery. The fluid is clear but will be crescent-shaped in subdural and biconvex-shaped in epidural collection.

20. *Calcifications*: When there is epidural or subdural haematoma without infection, the capsule can calcify over a long period of time. The haematoma itself may calcify over a very long time and be visualized using CT scan.
21. *Diffuse brain injury*: This is identified in very severe and in fatal head injuries. These present as multiple petechial haemorrhages and hypoxic brain damage (Figure 6.51 c).
22. *Retrobulbar or subperiosteal haemorrhage:* It appears as high-density mass lesion close to the bone and within the orbits. Retrobulbar mass must be differentiated if head injury is not confirmed by history.
23. *Non-haemorrhagic cerebral contusion:* It appears similar to cerebral oedema however, these enhances with contrast administration unlike cerebral oedema. Similar areas are affected.

Useful signs to diagnose isodense haematoma[1-5]
a. *Shift of midline structures* to contralateral side e.g. falx cerebri, pineal gland (tables 6.52).
b. *Compression of the ventricle* on the affected side and its dilatation on the unaffected side.
c. Effacement of the sulci on the affected side. This sign is unreliable in bilateral haematoma since comparison with the contralateral side will be unhelpful.
d. *Rabbit's ear" appearance in bilateral haematoma*. The two frontal horns of the lateral ventricles are squeezed together by bilateral subdural haematoma.
e. *Effacement of the basal cisterns* in bilateral subdural haematoma.
f. *Marginal enhancement*: Contrast administration will show enhancement of the margins of the haematoma. If increased dose of the contrast is used, there will be enhancement of the normal brain making the haematoma more obvious.
g. *Subdural haematoma* of mixed density indicates fresh bleeding into a subacute or chronic haematoma. The fresh bleeding tends to gravitate to the dependent side.
6. *Epidural or extradural haematoma/bleed:* Fresh haematoma is hyperdense, biconvex in shape, seen close to the skull vault and is more common in the fronto-parietal regions. It can also occur in the posterior fossa where they are often missed by CT scanning due to partial volume averaging. Recurrent epidural haematoma after surgery often loses the classical shape (tables 6.51 and 6.52).
12. *Local oedema*: Due to fracture, subdural, epidural or intracerebral haemorrhage or bleed.
13. Foreign body within the cranial cavity or scalp.

Raised intracranial hypertension
When brain swelling is severe or when there is large space occupying lesion within the cranium such as large haematoma, the brain tissues may be displaced. When the pressure in one dural compartment increases beyond the level that can be accommodated by the normal physiological compensatory mechanisms, raised intracranial pressure occurs. There then develops displacement of brain, CSF, shift of midline structures such as falx from one compartment to the other and cerebral herniations.

Cerebral herniations[1,2,3]
Tonsillar herniation: The cerebral tonsil is displaced inferiorly through the foramen magnum. It is most often caused by a posterior fossa mass or mass-effect from a supra-tentorial lesion. At imaging, there is noted, a downward displacement of cerebellar tonsils below the level of foramen magnum with obliteration of cistern magna. Posterior inferior cerebellar artery may be infarcted due to its compression by the displaced tonsil.
Ascending transtentorial herniations: Through the tentorial insusura, the vermis is displaced superiorly. It is caused by a large posterior fossa mass or haematoma. At neuroimaging, there is obliteration of

the fourth ventricle, and effacement of the superior cerebellar and quadri-geminal cisterns. There may be associated cerebellar infarction due to compression of superior cerebellar artery.

External brain tissue herniations: This is the external extrusion of brain tissues through a skull defect. It is caused by raised intracranial pressure associated with traumatic or surgical skull defect. At imaging, there is an area of bone defect observed in CT with external displacement of brain tissue. Venous infarction with high tendency for haemorrhage may result from venous obstruction caused by the brain tissue herniations.

Other types of cerebral herniations:

Subfalcine herniation or midline shift: These include displacement of cingulate gyrus under the free edge of the falx celebri.

Uncal herniation:

This is seen when the medial temporal lobe herniates through the tentorial incisura and compresses the ipsilateral suprasellar cistern. The oculomotor nerve is compressed leading to loss of normal papillary reflex.

Downward shift of diecephalon, mesecephalon and the midbrain may occur in head trauma and head injury.

Table 6.52: Consensus-based classification (Department of Defence and Veteran Affairs) of closed traumatic brain injury (TBI) severity[1-5]

Criteria	Traumatic brain injury severity		
	Mild	Moderate	Severe
Structural imaging	Normal	Normal or abnormal	Normal or abnormal
Loss of consciousness	0-30 minutes	Above 30 minutes to 24 hours	Above 24 hours
Alteration of consciousness/ mental states	Less than 24 hours	More than 24 hours	More than 24 hour plus other criteria
Post-traumatic amnesia	0-1 day	More than 1 to 7 days	More than 7 days
Glasgow coma scale (done within 24 hours)	13-15	9-12	Less than 9

Cerebral oedema

This co-exists with raised intracranial pressure and tends to become very severe at about 24 to 48 hours following trauma. The dangerous effect of cerebral oedema is ischaemia or under-perfusion of oedematous brain due to compression of the vessels within the brain. In long standing and severe cases there could be herniation of the brain through the foramen magnum or other characteristic sites causing compression of the brain stem with compromise of breathing and cardiac functions which may then lead to death.

Facial bone fractures

There can be fractures of the facial bones including the classical Le forte I, II and II fracture. Fracture of the zygomatic arch, mandibles and asymmetrical Le Forte and blow out fracture also occur and are common.

MR imaging

1. It shows all of the above features but has increased sensitivity to blood collection especially around middle or posterior cranial fossa where partial volume effect reduces CT sensitivity.
2. *Contusion:* MRI can show contusion not seen with CT scan.
3. *Vascular injury:* MRI can assess the vascular system for injuries without the need for contrast administration.
4. *Extra-cerebral fluid collection:* This is better demonstrated by MRI

Advantages of MR imaging over CT in imaging traumatic brain injury

1. MRI is superior to CT at demonstrating extra-cerebral fluid collection such as epidural and subdural chronic haemorrhages and hygroma. This is because of their fluid contents which make them to be more hyperintense at the MRI compared to the surrounding brain.
2. MRI is better at demonstrating cerebral oedema (brain swelling) evidenced by obliteration of the cisterns around the brainstem on T1-weighted spin echo images.
3. MR images are better at showing injuries in the hidden areas of the brain and skull, viz: cerebral sulci, dural sinuses, orbits and globe, cavernous sinuses, clivus, Meckel's cave, brain stem and base of the skull. Beam hardening artifacts and partial volume effect prevent CT from detecting the exact nature of small injuries in these regions.
4. MRI can show brain subacute subdural and intracerebral haematoma and small collections which CT scan failed to show.
5. MRI has the highest sensitivity in detecting intra-parenchymal lesion.
6. MRI is best at detecting diffuse axonal injury due to shearing stress and cortical contusions occurring close to the skull. Over 80% of diffuse axonal injuries shown normal findings on CT because they are non-haemorrhagic and thus undetected by CT. MRI can detect both haemorrhagic and non-haemorrhagic diffuse axonal injuries. The findings of retraction balls and spheroids at histology with or without beta amyloid precursor protein (βAPP) detection is the hallmark of diffuse axonal injury.
7. In patient with acute subdural haematoma who also has severe anaemia or in patients with chronic subdural haematoma co-existing with acute bleed, or in those in which CSF from arachnoids tear is admixed with acute haemorrhage, the imaging finding in CT may be normal as the lesions may appear isodense. MRI can differentiate and detect these lesions accurately.

The limitations of MRI are its inability to detect cortical bone fracture, small bone fragments and subarachnoid haemorrhage.

Cerebral infarction and ischaemia

Cerebral ischaemia and infarction are seen in about 2% of patients imaged with CT for head injury. *Mechanical compression:* Ischaemia is caused by mechanical compression of a blood vessel from cerebral herniation across the falx cerebri and/or tentorium. Infarctions result from mechanical shift usually seen affecting the anterior cerebral artery following acute subfalcine herniation or the affecting the posterior cerebral artery area following acute uncal herniation. Infarction of callosomarginal branch of the anterior cerebral artery is caused by its compression against the free edge of the falx when there is subfalcine herniation. In uncal herniation, the displaced medial temporal lobe can compress the posterior communicating artery, resulting in infarction; or constrict the anterior choroidal artery, leading to infarction of the posterior limb of the internal capsule.

Table 6.53: Probability of Mortality in Patients with Traumatic Brain Injury (Rotterdam Score)[1,3,4,5]

Predictor	Score
Basal cisterns	
Normal	*0*
Compressed	*1*
Absent	*2*
Midline shift	
No shift or shift of ≤ 5 mm	*0*
Shift more than 5 mm	*1*
Epidural/subdural mass lesion	
Absent	*0*
Present	*1*
Intraventricular or subarachnoid bleed	
Absent	*0*
Present	*1*
Sum of score#	+1

# The sum of score predicts 6 months mortality as shown below.
1 = 0% mortality; 2 = 7%; 3 = 16%; 4 = 26%, 5 = 53%; 6 = 61% mortality.

Vasospasm: This is another important cause of ischaemia and infarction. Extra-axial hematomas that apply a significant mass effect on the adjacent cortex may compress cortical veins and end up with venous infarction.

Direct vascular injury: Direct vascular injury, such as dissection, occlusion, or pseudoaneurysm from a skull base fracture, can also result in ischaemia.

Prediction of severity of traumatic brain injury using imaging[1-5]

1. Subarachnoid haemorrhage due to trauma seen at CT is associated with a twofold increase in mortality.
2. Intracranial haemorrhage has an approximately 80% positive predictive value for poor functional outcome, and the prognosis worsens as the hematoma volume increases in size
3. Haemorrhage in the basilar cisterns has a 70% positive predictive value for poor prognosis and outcome.
4. Compression or absent basilar cisterns at CT imaging indicate a threefold higher risk of raised intracerebral pressure and are associated with a two- to threefold increase in mortality
5. Midline shift at CT imaging indicates raised intracranial pressure and is also associated with a poor clinical outcome, although this association is to some extent complicated by the fact that midline shift is caused by intracranial haemorrhage that also negatively impacts on outcome.
6. Observed mortality is higher in patients with acute subdural hematomas compared with those with epidural hematomas (table 6.53).

Table 6.54: Predicting accidental versus non-accidental injury using brain CT finding[1,3,4,5]

Parameter	Accidental injury	Non-accidental injury
Injury duration type	Acute or chronic	Combination of chronic and acute injury
Skull fracture	Common	Rare
Type of skull fracture	Single	Multiple or cross suture line
Epidural haematoma	Common	Rare
Intraparenchymal haemorrhage	Common	Rare
Subdural haematoma	Rare	Common
Outcome	Better	Worse

Trauma to the brain in neonates and children

This can be from (a) Birth injury (normal delivery with cephalo-pelvic disproportion, traumatic delivery, vacuum delivery, breach delivery (table 6.54)), (b) Battered Baby (child) Syndrome, (c). Other accidental injuries such as fall from height, road traffic injury, sports and recreational activities.

(a) *Birth injury*: Scalp injuries, intracerebral haemorrhage, subdural effusion or periventricular leukomalacia.

(b) *Battered baby syndrome*: Scalp injuries, intraventricular, intracerebral haemorrhage, subdural haemorrhage or effusion or periventricular leukomalacia may occur. Slit-like cavities at gray/white matter interface representing shearing injuries are pathognomonic.

(c). *Other traumas:* These could be fall from height, domestic accident, road traffic injuries and other trauma from recreation or civilian blast injuries. Scalp injuries, intraventricular, intracerebral haemorrhage, epidural haemorrhage/effusion or periventricular leukomalacia may occur.

Cerebral oedema may be the only sign of head injury in children following head trauma or non-accidental head injury (table 6.54).

Transfontanelle ultrasonography

This is useful in neonates. Ultrasound of neonatal or infant brain through the patent fontanelles or thin skull bone.

Technique: 5 – 15 MHz probe (curvilinear, sector or linear and rectangular small head preferred).

Radiological features identified

1. *Normal findings.* There may be no injury elicited.
2. *Cerebral oedema*: The brain is hypoechoic due to increased water content with obliteration of the ventricles and sulci. It is better diagnosed in a repeat scan after the brain oedema has subsided.
3. *Intracerebral haemorrhage*: This hyperechoic and can be in the germinal matrix in premature infants vascular choroid in term infants or it may be white matter haemorrhage in both term and preterm infants.
4. *Periventricular leukomalacia:* Associated with haemorrhage occurring in germinal matrix in pre-term infants. Ultrasound shows periventricular hyperechoic areas with multiple cystic spaces formed.

5. *Diffuse intraparenchymal haemorrhage* and petechiae form in cortical areas seen in term neonates.
6. *Subarachnoid haemorrhage* (difficult and unreliably demonstrated).
7. *Intraventricular haemorrhage:* This is intraparenchymal or subarachnoid haemorrhage which ruptures into ventricles. It is hyperechoic with fluid levels. It may lead to:
   a. Enlargement of ventricles
   b. Brain atrophy
   c. Hydrocephalus due to obstruction of CSF flow
   d. All of the above may occur and monitoring is required.
8. *Subdural haemorrhage:* Crescent or concavo-convex lesion separating the brain and skull. It is often hypoechoic.
9. *Other accidental injuries*
   a. The findings will very much simulate the findings in adult and in children of older age.
   b. Leptomeningeal cyst (late effect due to unrecognised skull fracture in children).

Post-traumatic sequelae

1. *Cerebral infarction:* This leads to macrocystic encephalomalacia appearing as cavitations due to loss of brain tissue in area of cerebral injury.
2. *Cerebral atrophy:* This is diffuse non-focal enlargement of the ventricular CSF spaces within the brain with widening of gyrae and sulci. This also includes poroencephalic cysts.
3. *Hydrocephalus:* This may be due to decreased CSF absorption due adhesive subarachnoid haemorrhage.

Table 6.55: Scalp lesions in the newborn following head trauma[4,5,6]

Type of lesion	Caput succedaneum	Subgaleal haematoma	Subgaleal hygroma/cyst	Cephalohaematoma
Nature of lesion	Scalp oedema	Extracranial subdural haematoma	Cyst containing cerebrospinal fluid	Extracranial epidural haematoma
Location	Scalp, superficial to galeal aponeurosis	Scalp, beneath the galeal aponeurosis	Scalp, beneath the galeal aponeurosis	Subperiosteal in flat skull bone
Composition	Oedema with minimal bleed	Venous blood clot	CSF	Subperiosteal bleed/clot
Skull fracture	No	Yes/no	Yes	yes
Crosses suture line	Yes	Yes	Yes	Yes
Clinical presentation	Pitting oedema immediately after birth (usually normal deliver)	Distributed firm fluctuant mass	Localised, well-defined fluctuant mass	Localised, well-defined firm mass
Occurrence	After normal vaginal delivery	After birth injury or head trauma	Birth trauma (usually following forceps delivery)	Birth trauma (when there is skull fracture)

4. *Aerocoele or pneumocephalus:* This is the presence on intracranial air bubbles and is an ominous sign in the presence of CSF leakage or fistula.

5. *CSF fistula:* This is more common in penetrating injuries. In the fracture of the floor of anterior cranial fossa, CSF would leak into the paranasal sinuses and nasal cavity. In the fracture of bones of the middle cranial fossa, the CSF would leak into the middle ear.

6. *Infection: Meningitis* may follow open fracture, or iatrogenic skull defect It may progress to diffuse cerebral inflammation, cerebral abscess formation and ventriculitis. Hydrocephalus may develop when inflammation leads to adhesive obliteration of arachnoid villi, foramina and aquaduct. *Subdural abscess* results from infection of the liquifarcted subdural haematoma. *Empyema* is due to pus collection.

7. *Carotico-caverneous fistula:* This is a communication between the high pressure carotid artery and the low pressure carverneous sinus. It is caused by a defect in the wall of intracaverneous portion of the internal carotid artery. There is gross dilatation of the superior ophthalmic vein cuased by intressed pressure of the sinus. CT and MRi shows widening of the affected sinus. MRA will show dilated superior ophthalmic vein.

8. *Encephalomalacia:* This is intra-parenchymal brain tissue loss surrounded by area of gliosis. It is a direct result of cerebral contusion and haematoma caused by trauma. On CT scan there may be one or more area of brain tissue loss associated with focal dilatation of ventricle nearest to the traumatic lesion. It is hyperintense on T2WI. Frank cavitations may occur.

9. *Post-traumatic stress disorder:* This occurs when a person experienced, witnessed, or was confronted with an event or events that involved actual or threatened death or serious injury or a threat to the physical preservation of self or others; and the person's reaction involved intense fear, helplessness, or horror and the person seems to relive this trauma in the form of unintentional recollections which are vivid and long-lasting. This has been described as a 'signature injury' of blast traumatic brain injury. On MRI, there is reduction in anterior cingulate cortex and hippocampal volumes. There is also persistence of headache.

10. *Post traumatic aneurysm* and *traumatic vascular dissection.*

11. *Leptomeningeal cyst:* (see above).

(Adam & Dixon, 2008; Dahnert, 2011; Sutton, 1998 and 2003, Swischuk, 2004).

Reference

1. Brenner LA. Neuropsychological and neuroimaging findings in traumatic brain injury and post-traumatic stress disorder. Dialogues Clin Neurosci 2011;13(3):311-23.

2. Blyth BJ, Bazarian JJ. Traumatic alterations in consciousness: traumatic brain injury. Emerg Med Clin North Am 2010;28(3):571-94.

3. Van Boven RW, Harrington GS, Hackney DB, Ebel A, Gauger G, Bremner JD, D'Esposito M, et al. Advances in neuroimaging of traumatic brain injury and posttraumatic stress disorder. J Rehabil Res Dev 2009;46(6):717-57

4. Suskauer SJ, Huisman TA. Neuroimaging in pediatric traumatic brain injury:current and future predictors of functional outcome. Dev Disabil Res Rev 2009;15(2):117-23.

5. Parizel PM, Philip CD. Neuroradiological diagnosis of craniocerebral trauma:current concepts. In: Holder J, von Schulthess GK, Zollikoffer ChL. Diseases of the brain, head and neck, spine: Diagnostic imaging and interventional technique (syllabus IDKD 2008). Springer-Verlag Italia, Milan 2008(syllabus IDKD 2008).

6. Prabhu SP, Young-Poussaint T. Pediatric central nervous system emergencies. Neuroimaging Clin N Am 2010 ;20:663-83.

7. Giannatempo GM, Scarabino T, Simeone A, Casillo A, Maggialetti A, Armillotta M. Head injuries. In: Scarabino T, Salvolini U, Jinkins JR (Eds). Emergency neuroradiology, Springer Berlin Heidelberg, Germany 2006: 142-167.

8. Erly WK, Ashdown BC, Lucio RW 2nd, Carmody RF, Seeger JF, Alcala JN. Evaluation of emergency CT scans of the head: is there a community standard? AJR Am J Roentgenol 2003; 180:1727-30.

9. Murshid WR. Management of Minor Head Injuries: Admission Criteria, Radiological Evaluation and Treatment of Complications. Acta Neurochir (Wien) 1998; 140: 56 – 64.

10. Thanni LO. Evaluation of Guidelines for Skull Radiography in Head Injury. Niger Postgrad Med J 2003; 10: 231 –233.

11. Burke CJ, Thomas RH, Owens E, Howlett D. The role of plain films in imaging major trauma. Br J Hosp Med (Lond) 2010;71:612-3.

12. Ogunseyinde AO, Obajimi MO, Ogundare SM. Radiological Evaluation of Head Trauma by Computed Tomography in Ibadan. West Afr J Med 1999; 18: 33 – 38.

13. Agunloye AM, Adeyinka AO, Obajimi MO, Malomo A, Shokumbi MT. Computerised Tomography of Intracranial Subdural Haematoma in Ibadan. Afr J Med Med Sci 2003; 32: 235 –23 8.

14. Irabor PF, Akhigbe AO. Leptomeningeal cyst in a child after head trauma: a case report. West Afr J Med 2010;29:44-6.

15. Gean AD, Fischbein NJ. Head trauma. Neuroimaging Clin N Am 2010;20:527-56.

16. Prabhu SP. The role of neuroimaging in sport-related concussion. Clin Sports Med 2011;30:103-14.

17. Odita JC, Hebi S. CT and MRI characteristics of intracranial hemorrhage complicating breech and vacuum delivery. Pediatr Radiol. 1996;26:782-5.

18. Eze KC, Mazeli FO. Computed tomography of patients with head trauma following road traffic accidents in Benin City, Nigeria. West African Journal of Medicine 2011;30(6):404-407.

19. Adeyekun AA, Obi-Egbedi-Ejakpovi EB. Computerised tomographic patterns in patients with head injury at the university of Benin teaching hospital. Niger J Clin Pract 2013;16(1):19-22.

20. Mezue WC, Ndubuisi CA, Chikani MC, Achebe DS, Ohaegbulam SC. Traumatic extradural hematoma in Enugu, Nigeria. Niger J Surg 2012;18(2):80-4.

21. Abiodun A, Atinuke A, Yvonne O. Computerized tomography assessment of cranial and mid-facial fractures in patients following road traffic accident in South-West Nigeria. Ann Afr Med 2012;11(3):131-8.

22. Ohaegbulam SC, Mezue WC, Ndubuisi CA, Erechukwu UA, Ani CO. Cranial computed tomography scan findings in head trauma patients in Enugu, Nigeria. Surg Neurol Int 2011;2:182.

23. Mezue WC, Ndubuisi CA, Erechukwu UA, Ohaegbulam SC. Chest injuries associated with head injury. Niger J Surg 2012;18(1):8-12.

24. Udoh DO, Adeyemo AA. Traumatic brain injuries in children: A hospital-based study in Nigeria. Afr J Paediatr Surg 2013;10(2):154-9.

6.6 RADIOLOGY OF CYSTIC LESIONS OF THE JAW BONES (JAW TUMOURS)

Causes of Cystic Lesions of the Jaw

Cystic lesion of the jaw on plain film may be due to:

1. **Cysts of dental origin**
   a. Developmental cysts
      i. Primordial cysts (odontogenic Keratocyst)
      ii. Dentigerous cyst / Follicular cyst
   b. Post inflammatory cyst.
      i. Radicular or apical or periodontal cyst

2. **Non-Dental cysts**
   a. Developmental (Fissural) cysts
      i. Medial mandibular cyst
      ii. Medial maxillary cyst
      iii. Nasopalatine cyst
   b. **Non-epithelial bone cysts**
      i. Simple bone cyst
      ii. Aneurysmal bone cyst
   c. **Neoplasms**

Benign

1. Giant cell tumour/ osteoclastoma
2. Ameloblastoma
3. Osteoma
4. Enchondroma
5. Osteochondroma
6. Haemangioma
7. Brown tumour of hyperparathyroidism
8. Langerhans cell histiocytosis

Malignant

1. Osteosarcoma.
2. Ewing's sarcoma.
3. Multiple myeloma.
4. Burkitt's lymphoma.
5. Metastases

Discussion on the Tumours

Primordial cyst

This is more common in young men but can be seen in all ages. Slow-growing, but may reach very large size. Seen in ascending or posterior ramus of mandible and is unilocular. There is a cystic mass with expansion and thinning of the cortex. Expansion is common in the buccal lingual plane. If secondarily infected there may be discharge of pus. Primordial cyst results from cystic degeneration of the enamel organ before the tooth is actually formed so that in most cases the cyst replaces the tooth. They have also been said to arise from ectopic odontogenic epithelium. If normal complement of the teeth is present, the cyst is practically assumed to replace a supernumerary tooth. The cyst is keratinized. Long-term follow up is necessary because recurrence is very common unless the cyst is completely removed. If they grow large and reach an unrelated unerupted tooth, they may simulate dentigerous cyst though their location may help in differentiation from each other.

Dentigerous cyst

Here the cyst results from cystic degeneration of the enamel organ after the tooth is formed but before it erupts. The cyst that is formed is adjacent or related to the crown of unerupted tooth. The tooth may be prevented from erupting and become displaced for some distance, although part of the crown is always in contact with the cyst. The cyst may be unilocular or multilocular and well–defined. When located in the maxilla it may extend into the maxillary antra or nose. Multiple cysts are often associated with *Gorlin's syndrome (Multiple basal naevi, rib anomalies, lamellar falx calcification and the inheritance is by autosomal dominance)*. They are usually seen related to the permanent third molar and maxillary canine teeth. Adolescents and young adults are often affected.

Radicular cyst

This is also called apical cyst. Cysts of the jaw are frequently radicular. This is post-inflammatory and usually follows inflammation of the pulp and apex bone of the tooth. Chronic inflammation could lead to formation of granulomas which are epithelialised. The cyst measures about 1–1.5 cm and may be multiple especially when there are chronic and extensive carious changes in the teeth. Dental extraction and curettage is the treatment. Persistent cyst after dental extraction is known as *residual cyst*.

Non-dental cyst

1. Medial mandibular cyst
   The cyst is located in the mandible close to the midline.
2. Medial maxillary cyst or Nasolabial cyst.
   The cyst is located in the soft tissue with resorption of the adjacent maxilla close to the midline
3. Nasopalatine duct/ incisive canal cyst.
   The cyst is small, asymptomatic and close to the anterior palatine papilla. It occurs in 40 – 60 year age group.
4. Globulomaxillary cyst
   This is a small cyst between the lateral incisor and canine. It looks like an inverted pear with the roots of the teeth appearing divergent.

b. Non-Epithelial Cysts
i. Simple bone cyst

They are also known as traumatic cysts because they may follow trauma. They are spherical and well-defined. The margins are thin with dense sclerosis. The lesion is likely to extend upwards between the teeth and alveolar margin. Occurs in 5 – 15 years age group. Well-defined lucency with sclerotic margin. They are central in location. There is a thin cortex with slight expansion. There may be thin internal septations.

ii. Aneurysmal bone cyst

Not common in the jaw. Well-defined expansile lucency is seen displacing the adjacent teeth. Occurs in 10 – 30 years age group, up to 70% are before 18 years.

The well-defined expansile lucency thins the cortex with a balooning appearance. The internal septa or strands may be noted. There may be new bone in the angle between the original cortex and the expanded part simulating Codman's triangle.

Fluid level is noted on CT and MRI. It may be secondary to other tumours. Histology is usually necessary for specific diagnosis.

Neoplasms
Giant cell tumour/ osteoclastoma
There is a central soft tissue mass replacing the bone with cystic appearance. The margin may be well-defined or irregular and not well-defined. The cyst is seen displacing developing or erupting teeth. The bone is expanded. The cyst arises in the tooth-bearing part of the jaw. It is common. It may have internal septa with multiloculated appearance. It is seen in the young between 7 – 20 years, only rarely does it occur after 20 years. True osteoclastoma is rare

Ameloblastoma
This is a benign tumour that is locally aggressive. It accounts for about 10% of jaw tumours and seen mostly in persons aged 30-50 years. Over 75% of the cases are found in the molar region or ramus of the mandible. It is typically multilocular with multiple internal septations giving a 'soap bubble' appearance. The tumour is expansile, with well-defined with corticated and scalloped margins. The tumour also typically produces sharp margins of adjacent teeth due their resorption. Irregularities of tumour margin on pain radiography or CT may denote a rare malignant variety. This may have lung metastasis. In some occasions, ameloblastoma may be associated with the crown of an unerupted tooth. An uncommon unilocular type is noted in younger age group.

Osteoma
A dense, well-defined lobulated mass may be seen with surrounding cystic lesion. Osteomas may also be seen in Gardner's syndrome. Occasionally old trauma or sepsis may present as a cystic lesion with sclerosis.

Enchondroma
These are well-defined lucency with sclerotic margins occurring within the medulla of the mandible or maxilla. It expands the cortex and thins it. The margin is sclerotic. There is usually ground glass appearance in which there may be associated calcification. They are not common in the jaw but do occur. They are more common in the hand and wrist located at the diaphysis or metadiaphysis. In long bones, they may be multiloculated. The usually affected age group is 10 – 50 years and over 50% are seen in the hand and wrist.

Osteochondroma
Osteochondroma or cartilage-capped exostosis may grow in the jaw bone. The exostosis may occasionally have cystic appearance and therefore resemble a cyst. There is always some calcification or evidence of ossification within the cystic exostotic lesion. The cortical margin of the mass merges with the underlying bone and the trabecullar pattern merges with that of the parent bone. The cartilage cap is more clearly defined on CT and MRI than on plain film. It usually occurs before epiphyseal closure and may occasionally regress without treatment.

Haemangioma
This is possible because all the tissues that make up the jaw bone are capable of undergoing neoplastic changes. A lytic lesion with sun burst or sunray appearance or radial spiculation is seen. The spiculation is usually seen within a central lucency. The vertebrae and skull are often more affected but occasionally the jaw bones are involved and it may be confused with osteosarcoma. The age affected is 10 – 50 years. The dorsolumbar vertebrae and the skull are most frequently affected. There are multiple coarse vertical striations mostly affecting the body of the vertebra only. The appendages of the vertebra are usually spared but only rarely are they affected.

Fibrous Dysplasia
This causes localised areas of osteolysis and frequently ossifies with time.
There are three types of fibrous tissue dysplasia that affect the jaw
1. Fibrous dysplasia
2. Cherubism
3. Cementomas

Fibrous dysplasias
Here medullary bone is replaced by fibrous tissue. It is usually seen in 10 – 30 years age group. Diagnosis is made because of the bony deformity and often at 3 – 15 years. The mandible is frequently affected in the jaw. It may be monostotic or polyostotic. Polyostotic cases are often unilateral but rarely may be bilateral, in which case it is usually asymmetrical. In younger ages, polyostotic disease is more frequent.

The radiological features include:
1. Lytic expansile lesion almost appearing cystic with thinned intact cortex and endosteal scalloping.
2. There is often ground glass appearance of the internal aspect of the lesion with multiple calcifications and sclerotic areas.
3. There is usually a thick sclerotic border looking like orange rind.
4. Periosteal reaction is remarkable by its absence.
5. The lesion is medullary, expanding down the cortex with a front of osteolytic lesion, and with rather small cortical expansion compared to the extent of the lesion.
6. The lesion is diametaphyseal rather than metaphyseal
7. Lesion is often multiloculated
8. It leads to accelerated bony maturation.
9. Involvement of bones of the skull leads to leontiasis ossea. This is sclerosis with bony expansion and asymmetry affecting the facial bones.
10. There may be expansion of the paranasal sinuses making the face appear mask – like.
11. Other bony deformities include growth disparity, shepherd's crook deformity of the proximal femur.
12. Other bones frequently affected include the pelvis, femur, skull, and ribs

Cherubism
This is also called hereditary fibrous dysplasia of the jaw. This is because the disease is histologically identical and indistinguishable from fibrous dysplasia and has obvious familial incidence. The disease occurs only in maxillary tuberosity.

Features
1. Lytic expansile or cystic lesion in the mandible with prominent jaw line.
2. Dental agenesis or unerupted separated or widely displaced teeth if the teeth ever erupt.
3. Bony changes start about one year and stop or start to regress after puberty.
4. At the time of maximal appearance the affected children resemble cherubs with chubby faces.
5. It is an autosomal dominant disorder more severe in males.

Cementoma
This affects the apex of the tooth especially in the mandible. There is a radiolucent lesion due to fibrous outgrowth of the periodontal membrane space. The teeth are normal. However, there are multiple apical lucencies with destruction of the lamina dura.

Brown Tumour *(Brown tumour of hyperparathyroidism)*
This is a lytic expansile lesion with occasional cortical destruction and endosteal scalloping. It is well-defined and multiloculated. The site of the lesion is eccentric and cortical and it is usually solitary. There may be pathological fracture. There is a classical appearance of destruction of mid portion of distal phalanges with telescoping. This is more frequent in primary hyperparathyroidism and only rarely does it occur in secondary hyperparathyroidism. These lesions result from a locally destructive severe osteoclastic activity occurring rapidly and stimulated by parathyroid hormone. The bone is replaced by vascularised fibrous tissue with an abundance of giant cells. Necrosis and liquefaction make the lesion appear cystic. Common sites of involvement include the jaw, pelvis, ribs, facial bones, axial skeleton and the metaphyses of the long bones especially the femur.

Langerhans cell histiocytosis *(Eosinophilic granuloma)*
The lesion is due to influx of eosinophilic leucocytes, resembling inflammation and the true cause is unknown. It occurs in 1 – 4 years of age and male-to-female ratio is 1:1. In Hand-Schuller-Christian disease the mandible may be involved with cystic lesion making the teeth appear floating due to loss of the anchoring substance. (Floating teeth). In eosinophilic granuloma there is gingival swelling including its surrounding soft tissue with cystic lesion of the mandible and 'floating teeth'. Occasionally fracture may occur. There may be the appearance of multiple well-defined cystic lesions in the mandible.

Malignant tumours
Osteosarcoma
The age affected in the jaw is the older age group than in classical osteosarcoma. It occurs in 30-40 years of age. The prognosis is however better than for classical osteosarcoma.
Osteosarcoma due to irradiation of the jaw: The features are those of osteosarcomas elsewhere.

Ewing's sarcoma
Poor prognosis. Mostly lytic. The lesion in the jaw is same as elsewhere.

Multiple myeloma
Multiple round well-defined lucencies in the mandible are more likely to be multiple myeloma than metastases. Multiple myelomatous lesion of the mandible is however less common than of the skull. The appearance is the same as the features of multiple myeloma elsewhere in the skeleton.

Burkitt's lymphoma

It is more common in Africa but can occur elsewhere. It accounts for about 50 % of all childhood mitotic diseases. There is the occurrence of massive tumour with involvement of the jaw. The tumour may present as destructive bone lesion with exfoliation of the teeth.

Features

1. Large osteolytic rapidly destructive lesion with large soft tissue component.
2. Resorption of lamina dura of teeth when the jaw is affected.
3. Multiple lytic foci which may later coalesce.
4. Multiple radiating spiculations with sun burst or sunray appearance.
5. Associated with Epstein – Barr virus.
6. Also associated with malaria.
7. Regression may follow when cytotoxic drug is used.

Metastases

The incidence of secondaries to the jaw is low. This is because the mandible has low marrow content. The blood-borne secondaries are trapped in the red marrow-rich areas of the skeleton. Detection of secondaries in the mandible is also low because the secondaries appear much earlier in the skull and axial skeleton and metaphyses of the long bones before appearing in the mandible. The appearance is that of secondaries elsewhere in the skeleton. They are multiple, varied-sized, well-defined lesions in the background of a normal bone. Involvement of the inferior dental nerve may lead to anaesthesia of the lip.

(Adam & Dixon, 2008; Dahnert, 2011; Sutton, 2003; Swischuk, 2004; Palmer & Reeder, 2001).

References

1. Dunfee BL, Sakai O, Pistey R, Gohel A. Radiologic and pathologic characteristics of benign and malignant lesions of the mandible. Radiographics 2006;26:1751-68.
2. Onuigbo WIB. Jaw tumours in Nigerian Igbos. British Journal of Oral Surgery 1978;15:223-226.
3. 3. Scholl RJ, Kellett HM, Neumann DP, Lurie AG. Cysts and cystic lesions of the mandible: clinical and radiologic-histopathologic review. Radiographics 1999;19:1107-24.
4. Lagundoye SB, Akinosi JO, Obisesan AA, Oluwasanmi O. Radiologic features of ameloblastoma in Nigerians. Oral Surg Oral Med Oral Pathol 1975; 39:967-75.
5. Yoshiura K, Weber AL, Runnels S, Scrivani SJ. Cystic lesions of the mandible and maxilla. Neuroimaging Clin N Am 2003;13:485-94.
6. Olasoji HO, Nggada HA, Tahir A. Recurrence of multicystic ameloblastoma in soft tissue. Trop Doct 2004;34: 112-114.
7. Nzeh DA. Importance of Jaw Radiography in the diagnosis of Burkitt's lymphoma. Clin Radiol 1987;18: 411-412.
8. Nzegwu MA, Uguru C, Okafor OC, Ifeoma O, Olusina D. Patterns of oral and jaw tumours seen in eastern Nigeria: a review of sixty cases seen over a 5-year period--1 January 2000 to 31 December 2004. Eur J Cancer Care (Engl) 2008;17:532-4.
9. Macdonald-Jankowski DS. Glandular odontogenic cyst: systematic review. Dentomaxillofac Radiol 2010;39:127-39.
10. Scully C, Langdon J, Evans J. Marathon of eponyms: 7 Gorlin-Goltz syndrome (Naevoid basal-cell carcinoma syndrome). Oral Dis 2010;16:117-8.

6.7 RADIOLOGY OF STROKE

Definition
Stroke, also known as cerebrovascular accident, is defined as a sudden central nervous system injury of vascular origin that leaves a lasting neurological damage.

Incidence
It is the third leading cause of death in United States after heart disease and cancer. It is also the second leading cause of death due to cardiovascular disease in U.S. It is the second leading cause of death in patients aged over 75 years of age. It is the leading cause of death in Asia.

Affected age
Mostly those aged above 55 years
But about 12% occurs in young adults

Sex ratio
M:F = 2:1

Risk factors
Heredity, hypertension, smoking, atherosclerosis, excessive alcohol consumption, diabetes (15%), obesity, angiomatous malformation, intracranial aneurysm(accounts for one third of intracranial bleed), congestive heart failure, familial hypercholesterolemia, myocardial infarction, atrial fibrillation, substance abuse, oral contraceptives, pregnancy, high anxiety, stress, sickle cell anaemia.

Aetiology:
A. Nonvascular (5%): eg, tumour, hypoxia.

B. Vascular (95%)
1. Brain infarction or ischemic stroke
    (a) Occlusive atheromatous disease of extracranial arteries
    (b) Small vessel disease of penetrating arteries
    (c) Cardiogenic emboli
    (d) Hypercoagulability states

2. Haemorrhagic stroke
    (a) Primary intracerebral haemorrhage
    (b) Nontraumatic subarachnoid haemorrhage causing vasospasm
    (c) Veno-occlusive disease such as sinus thrombosis

In developed countries, ischaemic stroke is observed in 80% of cases and haemorrhagic stroke is seen in 20% while in developing and emerging nations, there is increased incidence of haemorrhagic stroke.

Hotspots
Hypodensity involving more than 50% of the territory of middle cerebral artery has a fatal outcome in over 80% (figure 6.71 A).

Clinical diagnosis is inaccurate in 10-20%. Haemorrhagic stroke affect younger aged patients and has more mortality than ischaemic stroke. Most cases of haemorrhagic strokes are caused by hypertension and risky lifestyle such as physical inactivity, obesity, unhealthy diet, excess alcohol consumption, and smoking most of which are preventable.

Roles of imaging
1. To confirm the clinical diagnosis
2. To identify any primary intracerebral haemorrhage
3. To detect any structural lesions mimicking stroke such as tumour, vascular malformation, subdural haematoma.
4. To detect early complications of stroke such as cerebral herniation and hemorrhagic transformation.
5. To quickly detect patients with severe strokes due to occlusions of large cerebral arteries such as the distal internal carotid artery (ICA), proximal middle cerebral artery (MCA) and basilar artery (BA) and institute appropriate catheter-based intervention therapy to convert such major strokes to minor strokes.
6. More recently, to identify penumbra and monitor the effect of an instituted appropriate therapy to salvage the tissue at risk (figures 6.71 A and B).

What are the problems of stroke?
1. Only a small fraction of patients are eligible for acute stroke therapy with reversal of occlusion in ischaemic stroke.
2. There is increasing prevalence of hypertension especially in developing countries leading to more stroke incidence.
3. A majority of stroke survivors live with profound neurological deficits, resulting to significant loss in quality of life, economic productivity and substantial caregiver burden.
4. The problem is deteriorating in the developed world, due to increase in senior citizens brought about by improvement in medicine, environment and quality of life.
5. Stroke is a major cause of poverty among families as its sudden death approach may leave the family in financial disarray as the affected person may be the bread winner, custodian of family finances, business, inheritance, even investments and some types of social security.

Radiological imaging of stroke
Preparedness for imaging a patient with stroke
'Time is brain' in acute stroke and ideally, everything should be made ready before the patient arrives the radiology unit.[1] These include:
1. There should be a stroke code which its activation leads to stopping of other work at the emergency department CT scanner.
2. The CT power injector has to be loaded with 125 mlL of low osmolar nonionic contrast material with iodine concentration of 300 mg per milliliter and 50 mL of saline solution.
3. There should be a peripheral intravenous access line with an 18–20-gauge cannula to support the 4 mL/sec injection rate needed for perfusion CT.
4. Metallic hardware or ferromagnetic material or clothing, including dental and hair prostheses, should be removed from the patient before arriving the department incase the patient requires MR imaging.[2-5]

The main questions to be asked in imaging stroke are:[2,3]

1. *Parenchyma*: Is the stroke ischaemic or haemorrhagic? If haemorrhagic start with non-enhanced CT and avoid intravenous contrast injection.
2. *Pipes*: Is there a flow obstruction in a major vessel? If this is yes do CT angiography.
3. *Perfusion*: Which tissue is already infarcted?
4. *Penumbra:* Which tissue is still salvageable? Perfusion CT and CT angiography will answer the last two questions.

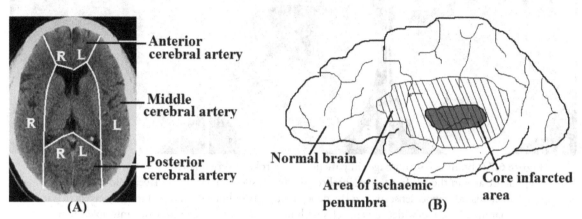

Figure 6.71: Areas of brain haemorrhage or infarction in stroke according to the blood supply (A), and a diagram of brain changes in hyperacute ischaemic stroke (B).

Radiological features of Haemorrhagic Stroke seen on CT scan

CT is the best imaging modality for assessment of haemorrhagic stroke. However, MR is contributory in showing lesions of the posterior fossa and in differentiating minor bleed due to partial volume effect of CT. The findings in brain CT scan in haemorrhagic stroke include the following.

1. *Intracerebral haematoma:* This appears as a well-circumscribed hyperdense area in acute stages and the temporal lobes of the brain are usually affected due to the involvement of middle cerebral artery. It is usually a solitary area in spontaneous haemorrhage as opposed to trauma which is usually multifocal. Involvement of the brain stem connotes poor prognosis. In acute stages, it is hyperdense with irregular margins and depending on the size may compress the ipsilateral ventricle with associated compensatory dilatation of the contralateral ventricle (Fig. 6.51 b). The falx may be shifted to the contralateral side. There may be signs of old brain infarct due to previous episode of small ischaemic or haemorrhagic stroke. Cerebral oedema is less marked in spontaneous haemorrhage compared to traumatic ones (table 6.71).
2. *Subdural haematoma/bleed:* Acute subdural haematoma (within 48 hours) is crescent- or concavo-convex-shaped spreading over the adjacent skull in the cerebral hemisphere. The haematoma is often located in fronto-parietal region or middle cranial fossa. There is associated hypodense surrounding areas of the brain due to brain oedema (Fig. 6.72 c)
3. *Sub-arachnoid haemorrhage*: This appears as hyperdense areas around the falx, Sylvian fissures, basal cistern and sulci in the acute stage. Its commonest manifestation is along the posterior falx. Sub-arachnoid haemorrhage may be associated with intracerebral or intraventricular haemorrhage (Fig. 6.51 a)
   In MRI subarachnoid clot shows as a relatively higher signal than the low signal of CSF in the late acute stage. MRI reliability at detecting subarachnoid or intraventricular clot decreases markedly after 10-14 days due to liquefaction of the clot as xanthochromia. On the whole MRI

is less sensitive than CT in detecting subarachnoid haemorrhage even within the first few days of its maximum sensitivity (table 6.71).

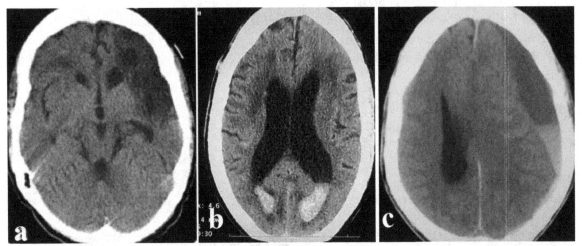

Figure 6.72: Brain CT scan images in patients with stroke. Non-enhanced CT scan study showing hypodense area in the left fronto-pariental region due to silent infarct in a 24-year old patient with sickle anaemia (**a**). Hyperdense area in the dependent parts of both vebtricles due to intraventriclear haematoma; note also widened ventricles with prominent sulci due to previous multiple small infarcts due to chronic (**b**). A cresent area in the left hemisphere close to the skull with hydepense area in the inferior part showing fluid level due to acute on chronic subdural harmorrhage (**c**).

4. *Intraventricular bleed* (poor prognosis). Hyperdense lesion are seen within the ventricle with CSF-blood levels appearing as fluid levels. Its presence indicates spontaneous haemorrhage as a more likely cause than trauma. In chronic stages it can lead to hydrocephalus due to fibrotic obliteration of the aqueduct and ventricular foramina (Fig. 6.51 b).

5. *Cerebral atrophy*: It may be caused by minor chronic cerebral anoxia or ischaemia due to vasocclusive diseases. This may be associated with subdural or epidural haemorrhage where there may be expansion or thinning of the skull vault (Fig.6.72 b).

6. *Epidural haematoma/bleed:* Acute epidural haematoma is biconvex-shaped adjacent to the skull within the cranial cavity. It is very rare in spontaneous haemorrhage (table 6.71).

7. *Calcifications*: Aneurysms, arteriovenous malformations and angiomatous malformations which could precipitate spontaneous haemorrhage could show curvilinear marginal calcifications or calcifications of chronic intravascular thrombus.

Radiological features of Ischaemic stroke
Definition of terms
Cerebral perfusion: Perfusion is defined as nutritive delivery of arterial blood to a capillary bed in the tissue of an organ. This blood delivery is responsible for delivery of glucose, oxygen and clearance of carbon dioxide and removal of heat.

Mean transit time (MTT): Cerebral vascular mean transit time (MTT), is defined as the ratio of cerebral blood volume to cerebral blood flow (CBV/CBF). It is a valuable indicator of the cerebral circulation and the most sensitive indicator of stroke.

Cerebral blood flow (CBF): Cerebral blood flow is the blood supply to the brain in a given time. In an adult, the brain weighs 1400 g or 2% of the total body weight but CBF is normally 750 millilitres per minute or 15% of the cardiac output. This equates to 50 millilitres of blood per 100 grams of brain tissue per minute. Since cerebral blood flow delivers oxygen and glucose to the brain tissue, it varies with the level of neural activity. It is affected by cerebral perfusion pressure and the radius of cerebral blood vessels. Within the brain CBF ranges from 20 ml/100g/min in white matter to 70 ml/100g/min in grey matter. Normal value is 50-80% ml/100g/min depending on the extent of metabolic activity and energy requirement. The mathematical relation is CBF = CBV/MTT

Table 6.71: CT and MRI appearances of various types of intracranial haematoma[2,3]					
Stage	**Time**	**Non-enhanced CT**	**Enhanced CT**	**T1WI MRI**	**T2WI**
Hyperacute	0–12 hours	Hyperdense (50-90 HU) (increasing in volume)	Contraindicated	Iso or hypointense	Hyperintense
Acute	12 hours – 7 day	Hyperdense with ill-defined hypodense margin.	Contraindicated	Iso or hypointense	hypointense
Subacute	7 – 28 days	Isodense or slight low density.	Isodense with marginal ring enhancement	Hyperintense	Hyperintense
Chronic	Over 1 month	Hypodense area	Hypodense area with ill-defined ring enhancement barrier.	Iso- or hypointense	Markedly hyperintense

Cerebral blood volume (CBV): Cerebral blood volume (CBV) is defined as the fraction of tissue volume occupied by blood vessels, and in the brain this fraction is approximately 0.04 or 4%. Both CBF and CBV are more specific indicator for distinguishing ischaemia from infarction. Its value is obtained by dividing the areas under curve in the parenchymal pixel by the area under curve in the arterial pixel in perfusion studies. It is also obtained from the equation CBF X MTT = CBV.

Cerebral ischaemia: This is defined as a condition in which there is too little blood flow to the brain; below 18 to 20 ml per 100 g per minute, and tissue death occurs when the flow decreases to below 8 to 10 ml per 100 g per minute.

Cerebral metabolic rate for oxygen (CMRO2): This is defined as the oxygen consumption of the brain which is 3.3ml/100g/min (50ml/min in total) amounting to 20% of the total body consumption. Since it parallels the cortical electrical activity it is higher in the cortical grey matter.

Cerebral Perfusion Pressure (CPP): Cerebral perfusion pressure is defined as the difference between the mean arterial blood pressure (MAP) which is usually 90 mmHg and the mean cerebral venous pressure. Mean cerebral venous pressure is approximately equal to the intracranial pressure (ICP) which is usually about 10 mmHg. CPP = MAP – ICP = 80 mmHg.

The concept of stroke penumbra in ischaemic stroke

Stroke penumbra is defined as a peripheral area of ischaemic but salvageable brain tissue surrounding a core area of irreversibly infarcted tissue in acute ischaemic stroke. The penumbra contains metabolically challenged but reversibly injured neural tissues surrounding a region of dead infarcted tissue. It is also called ischaemic stroke penumbra or tissue at risk in acute ischaemic stroke.

Penumbra is characterized by:

1. Increased activity and cerebral metabolic rate of oxygen ($CMRO_2$) on PET studies, with:
    a. Reduced cerebral blood flow (CBF) in the 12-20 ml/100 g/min range.
    b. Cerebral blood flow in the infarct core is less than 12 ml/100g/min
    c. Cerebral blood flow in the irreversibly dead or already dead tissue in the core is less than 10 ml/100g/min however established infarct core has CBF value of less than 2.0 ml/100g/min
2. Although neurons in the penumbra may be viable, they exhibit loss of function or function in a suboptimal manner.
3. Neurologic symptoms indistinguishable from those produced by infarcted tissue are produced by the non-functional or reduced functional neurons in penumbra.
4. Neurons in the penumbra may be potentially salvageable through neuroprotective or thrombolytic therapy when made within a narrow time limit.

Pathology of ischaemic infarct and penumbra in ischaemic stroke[1-4]

Normal neuronal tissue blood flow is above 50 ml/100g/minute. Brain tissue has negligible neuronal energy store and is therefore greatly sensitive to infarction. Available energy can maintain neuronal viability for only about 2-3 minutes. This narrow range of time of energy store in the brain has led to the time-tested truth slogan that "Time is brain" depicting that any response for beneficial therapy in stroke must be timely. Approximately 1.8 million neurons and 12 km of axonal fibres are lost for every minute that appropriate effective therapy is not instituted in a major stroke event according to Jeffery Saver.

Decrease in cerebral perfusion leads to cessation of neuronal protein synthesis and loss of membrane transport and synaptic activity.

Further reduction in perfusion pressure leads to irreversible infarction.

However, ischaemia is almost always incomplete in acute stroke because the injured area receives collateral supply from uninjured arteries and from leptomeningeal territories.

The central area of complete irreversibly infarcted tissue forms the core while the periphery surrounding the core with incomplete ischaemia forms the penumbra. The aim of radiology is to quickly re-establish blood flow by vessel recanalization with catheter-based or thrombolytic therapy so that penumbra is completely salvaged and any area of infarct core that is not completely dead could also be salvaged and in essence reduce further spread of irreversible infarcted area apart from what occurred in the initial stroke event.

In summary, three zones are recognized in the area affected by acute stroke (figure 6.71B).

1. **Core:** A central area with tissue that is dead or will inevitably die.
2. **Stroke penumbra:** An area with reduction of blood flow below 20 ml/100g/min leading to impaired function but preserved tissue integrity. The tissue in time may die or survive depending on intervention and is called tissue at risk (penumbra).

3. **Oligaemic area:** An area with blood flow of 20 ml/100g/min to 50 ml/100g/minute is oligaemic but it still has normal function, cellular and tissue integrity and will, in principle, survive. This area which surrounds the immediate vicinity of penumbra and is area of potential spread of penumbra. It is sometimes called normal brain because neuronal function is intact and preserved.

Radiology of penumbra

1. Conventional CT and T2-weighted MR imaging and similar techniques such as FLAIR are unable to differentiate penumbra because of the similarities of its water states to those of the unaffected normal brain.
2. In hyperacute ishaemic stroke CT may show brain swelling at the area of the penumbra.
3. In the hyperacute stroke setting, a region that shows both diffusion and perfusion abnormalities is thought to represent irreversibly infarcted tissue, while a region that shows only perfusion abnormalities and has normal diffusion likely represents viable ischemic tissue, or a penumbra.
4. In CT angiography, intravascular thrombi causing the ischaemia can be diagnosed and if appropriately trained personnel are available, lysis of the thrombus or its extraction with re-establishment of flow is feasible and advocated.
5. In CT perfusion images, penumbra shows:
   a. Increased mean transit cerebral blood volume (70-100% or higher) secondary to time with moderately deceased cerebral blood flow (>60%) and normal or increased autoregulation mechanism.
   b. Increased *mean transit time* (MTT) (>145%) with markedly reduced cerebral blood flow (>30%) and moderately reduced blood volume (>60%) whereas infarcted tissues shows severely decreased cerebral blood flow (<30%) and blood volume (<40%) with mean transit time.

Significance

1. Penumbra can help in selection of appropriate therapy. Intravenous thrombolytic therapy can benefit carefully selected patients according to CT perfusion and diffusion mismatch or penumbra at MR imaging if instituted within the first three to four and half hours following the onset of stroke.
2. Presence of penumbra can help in predicting clinical outcome as the aim of stroke therapy in hyperaacute stages is to improve the blood supply in the area of penumbra to the extent that the tissue will surely survive.
3. The cells in penumbra have ceased to function or have sub-optimal function but are potentially salvageable with early recanalization following therapy.
4. Without early recanalization the infarction within the core gradually expands to include the penumbra. This is because within the infarct core, there is no more autoregulation and cerebral blood volume (CBV) is decreased.
5. The penumbra is a dynamic entity that exists within a narrow range of perfusion pressures and the duration of delay in recanalization is inversely related to the size of the penumbra and survival of the brain tissue.
6. The concept of penumbra and possible salvageable brain tissue in imaging studies has driven the development of functional imaging techniques such as brain perfusion imaging and diffusion weighted MR studies.

Table 6.72: CT appearances in hyperacute ischaemic stroke[3-5]

	Non-enhanced CT	Perfusion CT studies		
		Mean transit time (MTT)	**Cerebral blood flow (CBF)**	**Cerebral blood volume (CBV)**
Normal parenchyma	Normal attenuation (Gray matter 36-46 HU White matter 22-32 HU)	Normal (4 s)	54-70 mL/100 gmin^{-1}	4–5 mL/100 g
Penumbra	Normal findings or cerebral oedema	Increased (> 6 s or >145%)	Reduced (0-10 mL/100g/min	Normal or mildly elevated due to autoregulation.
Infarcted core area	Hypoattenuating	Increased	Markedly reduced	Markedly reduced (<2.0 mL x 100 g-^{1})

Non-contrast enhanced CT features of hyperacute ischaemic stroke

1. *Normal findings:* This is observed in about 10-50% and could be more when the studies are done by inexperienced performers/observers.
2. Reduced gray matter density with brain swelling evidenced by effacement of sulci. This is most likely from abnormal perfusion.
3. Loss of distinction between gray and white matter.
4. *Insula ribbon sign:* A decrease and later loss in the clarity of the boundaries of the lentiform nucleus and cortex, characteristically in the insula denoting early middle cerebral artery infarct.
5. On early CT studies in hyperacute ischaemic stroke, any hypodensity affecting more than 30 – 50 per cent of the territory supplied by middle cerebral artery is a significant sign of a major infarct and is associated with a high mortality rate.
6. *Disappearing basal ganglia sign:* Reduction and loss of distinction between the gray and white matter in the basal ganglia.
7. *Hyperdense middle cerebral artery sign:* This is relative hyperdensity of the middle cerebral artery due to acute intraluminal thrombus in which the serum content has been extruded making it appear markedly hyperdense as a result of clot retraction.
8. *Middle cerebral artery dot sign:* This is seen as a nodular focus of hyperattenuation within the sylvian fissure caused by thromboembolus.
   Pattern of contrast enhancement

Advantages of MR imaging over CT in patients with stroke

1. MRI is superior to CT at demonstrating extra-cerebral fluid collection such as epidural and subdural chronic haemorrhage and hygroma. This is because of their fluid contents which make them to be more hyperintense at the MRI compared to the surrounding brain.

2. MRI is better at demonstrating cerebral oedema (brain swelling) evidenced by obliteration of the cisterns around the brainstem on T1-weighted spin echo images.

3. MR images are better at showing small bleed or clots or fluid in the hidden areas of the brain and adjacent to the skull, viz: cerebral sulci, dural sinuses, orbits and globe, cavernous sinuses, clivus, Meckel's cave, brain stem and base of the skull. Beam hardening artifacts and partial volume effect prevent CT from detecting the exact nature of fluid or blood collections in these regions.

4. MRI can show small subacute, subdural and intracerebral haematoma and small collections which CT scan failed to show.

5. MRI has the highest sensitivity in detecting intra-parenchymal lesion and can detect very small haemorrhage and very small infarct which CT may fail to show.

6. In patient with acute subdural haematoma who also has severe anaemia or in patient with chronic subdural haematoma co-existing with acute bleed, or in those in which CSF from arachnoid tear is admixed with acute haemorrhage, the imaging finding in CT may be normal as the lesions may appear isodense. MRI can differentiate and detect these lesions accurately.

Table 6.73: CT and MRI appearances of various types of ischaemic stroke[4-5]

Stage/parameter	Time	Non-enhanced CT	Enhanced CT*	T1WI	T2WI
Hyperacute	0–12 hours	Isodense	Contraindicated	Iso or hypointense	Isointense
Acute	12 hours – 7 day	Slightly hypodense	Slightly hypodense with marginal enhancement	Iso or mildly hypointense	Iso or mildly hyperintense
Subacute	7 – 28 days	Isodensity or slight low density.	Isodense with marginal ring enhancement	Hyperintense	Hyperintense
Chronic	Over 1 month	Hypodense with loss of volume	Hypodense area with ill-defined marginal enhancement.	Hypointense	Markedly hyperintense with loss of volume
*Contrast enhnacement can be variable					

Radiological findings of functional MR images in hyperacute ischaemic stroke:

1. In perfusion (perfusion weighted images PWI) and diffusion (diffusion weighted images DWI) MR images there is a mismatch between diffusion and perfusion parameters in favour of diffusion (tables 6.72 and 6.73).

2. MR imaging techniques in penumbra offer great potential for an early predictor of therapeutic outcome of thrombolytic drugs and recanalization procedures and a guide to choice of therapeutic modality.

3. In MR images the infarct core is characterized by reduction of CBF and CBV on perfusion MR images, 40%-50% reduction of apparent diffusion coefficient (ADC) on diffusion MR images, and reduced metabolism on PET scans. The area of reduced CBV is hypothesized to be a marker of final infarct size in ischaemic stroke (table 6.72).

4. PWI (perfusion studies) sometimes overestimates the tissue at risk and DWI in diffusion studies does not represent irreversible injury and DWI abnormalities can include the core and penumbra

Transient ischaemic attack

This is defined as an occurrence of transient focal neurological deficit due to cerebral ischaemia lasting less than 24 hours with a return to pre-attack state. The causes are cerebral embolic events generally from ulcerative plaque at cervical carotid artery, and haemodynamic events from fall in cerebral perfusion pressure distal to a severe arterial occlusion. Predisposing factors are the same for stroke. The symptoms include transient motor *or* sensory dysfunction in the hand, face, sensory organs, upper and lower extremities. Diffusion weighted images (DWI) correctly diagnoses TIA by showing an abnormality in the presence of a motor deficit, aphasia or an event lasting more than one hour. The abnormality confirms cerebrovascular lesion and indicates the location and the vascular territory. CT scan is often normal. Diffuse rather than non-specific ischaemic changes may sometimes be shown by CT. Patients with significant arterial occlusion of more than 70-90 percent using Doppler carotid scan may require endarterectomy surgery. Reversal flow demonstrated in any of the vertebral arteries signifies occlusion, severe stenosis or subclavian steal syndrome. CT- and MR-angiography are diagnostic of the causative lesions of TIA but conventional angiography of carotid artery is required when surgery or angioplasty/catheter dilatation is contemplated.

Prognosis:
Coma due to stroke is observed in about 30% of emergency admissions.
Death during hospitalization is observed in a quarter of cases
Survival with varying degrees of neurologic deficit is observed in about 75% of cases
There is good functional recovery in about 40% of cases

(Adam & Dixon, 2008; Dahnert, 2011; Sutton, 1998 and 2003, Swischuk, 2004).

References

1. Saver JL. Time is brain--quantified. Stroke 2006; 37:263-266.
2. Srinivasan A, Goyal M, Al Azri F, Lum C. State-of-the-art imaging of acute stroke. Radiographics. 2006 Oct;26 Suppl 1:S75-95.
3. Ahmed M, Masaryk TJ. Imaging of acute stroke: state of the art. Semin Vasc Surg 2004;17(2):181-205.
4. Beauchamp NJ Jr, Barker PB, Wang PY, vanZijl PC. Imaging of acute cerebral ischaemia. Radiology 1999;212(2):307-24.
5. Alves JE, Carneiro Â, Xavier J. Reliability of CT perfusion in the evaluation of the ischaemic penumbra. Neuroradiol J 2014;27(1):91-5.

CHAPTER 7

MAJOR MULTISYSTEMIC DISEASES

7.1   RADIOLOGY OF NEUROFIBROMATOSIS

Introduction

Neurofibromatosis is one of the diseases collectively referred to as phakomatoses or neuroectodermal dysplasias or neurocutaneous syndrome / tumours. They are characterised by

1. Lesions of the skin
2. Lesions of the retina
3. Lesions of nervous system
4. They are developmental lesions.

There is the development of benign tumours and malformations in organs of ectodermal origin. Increased propensity of tumour formation is due to defective tumour – suppressor genes.

Other members of the groups are

1. Tuberous sclerosis
2. Sturge-Weber syndrome
3. von Hippel-Lindau syndrome
4. Ataxia telangiectasis

Definition

Neurofibromatosis is an autosomal dorminant inherited disorder considered to be of neural crest origin affecting all three germ layers and capable of involving many or any organ or system, or structure in the body.

Types of neurofibromatosis

Type 1 is known as peripheral neurofibromatosis. It is also called von Recklinghausen's disease and accounts for 90% of the disease. There is a defect in long arm of chromosome 17. It has an automosal dominant inheritance and 50% occur by spontaneous mutation. The incidence is 1:4000 of population and Male to Female ratio is 1:1.

Diagnostic criteria for NF – 1

This is diagnosed if two or more of the following are present:

1. *Six or more Café-au-lait spots*
    a. 5 mm in diameter in prepubertal persons
    b. 15 mm in diameter in post pubertal persons
2. *Two or more neurofibromas* of any type
3. *One plexiform neurofibroma*
4. *Axillary or inguinal frecklings*
5. *Optic nerve glioma*
6. *Two or more Lisch nodules* (pigmented hamartoma of the iris)
7. *Typical bone lesions*
    a. Sphenoid dysplasia
    b. Pseudoarthrosis of tibia
8. *One or more first degree relatives with NF – 1*
    It may be associated with MEN IIb.
    MEN II b is syndrome recognized by a combination of pheochromocytoma, medullary carcinoma of thyroid, multiple neuromas, congenital heart disease (10-fold increase). The congenital heart disease includes pulmonary valve stenosis, ventricular septal defect and atrial septal defect.

Table 7.11: Radiological Investigative Modalities	
Plain film, Skull (PA/lateral), chest x-ray, lumbosacral spine, radiograph of extremities	Myelography; conventional, CT- and MR-Myelography
Ultrasound	Angiography and MRA
Tomography (conventional)	Radionuclide studies
Computed tomography, helical CT, CT angiography	Barium swallow, meal and follow through and enema
Magnetic Resonance Imaging, MR angiography	Intravenous urography, CT and MR urography

Neurofibromatosis type 2 (NF – 2)

Also called central neurofibromatosis. It is rare.

It is characterised by:

1. *Autosomal dominant inheritance*
2. *Propensity for developing multiple schwannomas*, meningiomas and gliomas of ependymal derivations.
3. *Eighth (VIII) cranial nerve tumours*
4. *Rare in childhood*, symptomatic in $2^{nd} – 3^{rd}$ decades of life
    The incidence is 1:50,000. There is deletion of long arm of chromosome 22 and it accounts for 10% of all neurofibromatosis.

Diagnostic criteria of NF-2

Neurofibromatosis type 2 is diagnosed if one of the following is present:

1. *Bilateral cranial nerve VIII tumours*
2. *Unilateral cranial nerve VIII tumour* in association with any of the following:
    i. Meningioma
    ii. Neurofibroma
    iii. Schwannoma
    iv. Juvenile posterior subcapsular cataract
3. *Unilateral cranial nerve VIII tumour* with other spinal or brain tumour as above in a first degree relative.

Note that in central neurofibromatosis (type 2).
    i. There is no Lisch nodules, skeletal dysplasias, optic pathway gliomas, vascular dysplasias and learning disability.
    ii. Café – au – lait spots (< 50%), pale, < 5 in number.
    iii. Cutaneous neurofibroma is minimal in size and number or absent.

Radiological features

Orbital bone defect

Dysplastic change in sphenoid bone: 'Bare orbit' of sphenoid bone, partial or total absence of greater or lesser wing of sphenoid bone and / or orbital plate of frontal bone. This presents as bare orbit of neurofibromatosis. Lucency of the affected orbit is seen in comparison with contralateral side. Ultrasound scan will demonstrate ability to see brain structures through the orbit since no bone is present and the globe of the affected orbit acting as acoustic window. CT scan and MRI will clearly demonstrate absence of the bones (table 7.11).

Absent posterolateral wall of the orbit: This may lead to herniation of meninges containing the CSF and transmission of the CSF pulse into the orbit leading to pulsatile proptosis. Ultrasound scan (USS) will demonstrate transonic fluid posterior to the orbit. CT scan and MRI will clearly show absence of the bone and demonstrate the herniated content to be fluid of CSF density.

Encephalocoele: Defect in the sphenoid bone may lead to extension of content of middle cranial fossa (temporal lobe of the brain) into the orbit.

Ultrasound will demonstrate the herniated tissue to be brain with gyri and sulci. CT scan is optimal for demonstrating bone defect. MRI will identify the bone defects, the brain tissue and CSF herniation. The bone changes are due to failure in development of membranous bone.

Concentric enlargement of orbital foramen: This will be seen using optic foramen view in plain film of the skull. CT scan will demonstrate the asymmetrical enlargement of the optic canal and optic foremen. The enlargement is caused by optic nerve glioma. The glioma may be appreciated using CT as hypodense lesion in the optic nerve with or without calcification. Bony erosions causing widening of the foramen will be appreciated by CT.

Hyperostosis with optic nerve narrowing: Sclerosis or hyperostosis with narrowing of optic canal and optic foramen: Hyperostosis is caused by optic nerve sheath meningioma. Optic canal view of the skull will show the area of increased density. However CT scan is optimal for showing the increased density and it may be more than what is demonstrated by plain film.

Enlargement of orbital margins and superior orbital fissure: This is caused by plexiform neurofibroma of peripheral nerve and sympathetic nerve within the orbit. Optic nerve glioma may be involved. PA view of the skull will show asymmetrical widening of affected orbit but this is best demonstrated with coronal section CT scan. MRI is optimal for demonstrating soft tissue tumour mass.

Deformity of ethmoidal and maxillary sinuses: Deformity and decrease in size of the ipsilateral ethmoid and maxillary sinus

The Skull

Lytic defect or congenital bone defect in the skull: Spherical defect in lambdoid suture is the commonest. A defect adjacent to squamo- temporal suture also common on plain film and CT scan. These will appear as skull lucencies or holes in the skull. The characteristic sites help in the diagnosis.

Mandibular abnormalities:

a. Enlarged hemimandible
b. Erosion of mandible from pressure effect of superficial neurofibroma
c. Widened nerve canal and its opening. This is by intra-osseous enlargement of inferior dental nerve which has intraosseous course through the mandible (type 2).

Skull calcifications: Psammoma bodies / calcifications. The calcification is of choroid plexus in the lateral (temporal horn) and third ventricles.

J-shaped sella: This is due to sphenoid bone dysplasia.

Enlarged internal auditory meati caused by:

• Dural ectasia without acoustic neurofibroma
• Acoustic neuroma

Macrocranium or macrocephaly

Cranial asymmetry: Cranial asymmetry with hypoplasia of one side or macrocranium of the other side

Erosion of tuberculum sellae

• Optic nerve glioma will enlarge optic foramen
• Optic chiasma involvement will lead to erosion of tuberculum sellae and posterior and superior displacement of third ventricle

Widening of internal auditory meatus: Enlargement or erosion of internal auditory meatus due to acoustic neuroma (type 2).

Pneumoecephalography: Caused by bilateral cerebellopontine angle tumour (type 2).

Enlargement of foramen ovale: Due to neurofibroma of trigeminal nerve (type 2)

Crania bifidum: Varing degrees of lucent defects of the skull may be seen which may progress to the extreme of cranial bifidum although extremely rare.

Pneumosinus dilatans: Pneumosinus dilatans of ethmoidal and frontal sinuses occur and are caused by intra – orbital meningioma in NF type 2.

The Brain

Macrocephaly

Optic pathway glioma: This may be isolated to a single optic nerve with extension to other optic nerves, chiasma, or optic tract. Optic nerve is an embryonal part of hypothalamus and develops glioma instead of schwannoma. Ten percent of optic nerve gliomas are associated with neurofibroma.

Cerebral and brain stem astrocytoma: This is associated with anomalies of migration resulting in various types of dysplasia and heterotopia of white matter: Gliomatosis cerebri – unusual confluence of astrocytes

Hydrocephalus: Obstruction of aqueduct of Sylvius is caused by

- Benign aqueduct stenosis
- Glioma of tectum
- Glioma of tegmentum of mesencephaon

Schwannoma of cranial nerves V and VIII

Craniofacial plexiform neurofibroma

Common in orbital apex and superior – orbital fissure. Tortous cord of schwann cells neurons and collagens progressing along the nerve of origin and the nerve often unidentified or inseparable from the mass.

CNS harmatoma: Intracerebral and intracerebellar harmatomas with no mass effect. Located in cerebellum, cerebral peduncles pons, basal ganglia (globus pallidus is the commonest). It appears as high signal intensity on T_2WI MRI studies ("*unidentified bright objects*"). There is no enhancement with contrast injection.

Brain atrophy: Focal or generalised brain atrophy may be diagnosed with CT or MRI. They are associated with mental retardation.

Arachnoid cysts

Vascular dysplasias: Occlusion or stenosis of

- Distal internal carotid artery
- Proximal middle cerebral artery
- Anterior cerebral artery

Meningioma: Intraventricular, and arises from choroid plexus of lateral ventricle (type 2).

Moyamoya syndrome: Multiple progressive stenosis or occlusion of intracranial arteries especially in children. Multiple tiny basal collaterals develop. On angiography, the vessels appear as a meshwork or a mass of sponge. It was first diagnosed in Japanese but now found in other races.

The Spines

Scoliosis: It is typically acute angle, thoracic region and short segment.

Kyphoscoliosis: This is due to abnormal development of vertebral bodies. Found in lower thoracic and lumbar spines.

Widened interpedicular distance

Vertebral body erosion: This is due to erosion of vertebral bodies by asymptomatic neurofibroma.

Dysplastic pedicle: Absence or hypoplasia of a pedicle, transverse or spinous process. The position of the pedicle is filled with fat. Benign neurofibroma may lead to erosion of a pedicle.

Dumb-bell tumour

Paravertebral soft tissue mass projecting through enlarged foramina. This is caused by dural ectasia existing through enlarged foramina as lateral meningocoele. Usually asymptomatic but may cause pain. It is often diagnosed as an incidental finding. MRI and CT will demonstrate it, and filling defect is seen in myelography.

Dural ectasia: This causes CSF pulsation to be transmitted directly to the vertebral bodies causing posterior scalloping.

Posterior scalloping of vertebral bodies (r Marfans).

Enlarged spinal neural foramina

Paravertebral plexiform neurofibroma: Localised infiltrative mass lesion along nerve bundle on MRI

Spondylolisthesis: Due to defects in bony development of the vertebrae

Sub-arachnoid haemorrhage: Spinal neurofibroma may rarely present with subarachnoid haemorrhage. Intradural extramedullary mass on myelography.

Raised intracranial pressure: Due to mass lesions blocking CSF flow and absorption.

Paraspinal neurofibroma: Arising from posterior nerve root. $^2/_3$ intradural while others are either entirely extradural or have extradural component. They may cause bone erosions and occasionally are very large. They may displace spinal cord to one side.

Syringomyelia: Frequently associated with neurofibroma.

Paraplegia: This is due to kyphoscoliosis, subluxation, dislocation, vertebral deformity or intraspinal tumours e.g. neurosarcoma, neurofibroma, meningioma.

The Chest

Twisted-ribbon rib: This is seen in the upper thoracic segment with or without Kyphoscoliosis. Associated with abnormal tubular splaying or localised widening of one or several ribs including posterior rib due to neurogenic tumour

Localised cortical rib notching: Not found at 4th – 8th ribs as in coarctation. The depression is in the inferior margin of ribs.

Neurogenic mediastinal mass: Round or oval soft tissue mass with well-defined outline in paravertebral gutter usually project over one side of posterior mediastinum. Bony destruction, pleural effusion or rapid increase in size suggests malignant change. It may rarely occur in middle or anterior mediastinum. Neurofibroma of the vagus nerve is associated with neurofibromatosis in 50% of the cases.

Intrathoracic meningocoele: MRI and CT myelography can diagnose the meningocoele.

Pulmonary neurofibromas: These will appear as single or multiple pulmonary nodules.

Pulmonary fibrosis: Occurs in 10% of patients.

Honey-comb lung: Multiple recticular shadowing with lace-like appearance. Bullae may be seen in upper and middle lung zones. Bullae may appear as ring shadows in children.

Pulmonary haematoma or haemothorax: Due to rupture of aneurysm.

Lung collapse: Huge neurofibroma in the thorax can cause lung collapse.

Cardiovascular system

Congenital heart disease (10-fold increase)

a. Pulmonary valve stenosis
b. Ventricular septal defect
c. Coarctation of aorta
d. Atrial septal defect
e. Complete heart block
f. Idiopathic hypertrophic subaortic stenosis

Renal artery stenosis with post stenotic dilatation

Renal artery aneurysm without stenosis

Narrowing of abdominal aorta

Stenosis of mesenteric, coeliac, iliac and pulmonary arteries occurs but are rare.

Stenosis of supraclinoid portion of internal carotid artery

Moyamoya disease

Cerebrovascular accident due to haemorrhage from tumour, ischaemia from stenosed vessel or haemorrhage from hypertension as a result of renal artery stenosis or phaeochromocytoma.

Coronary artery aneurysm, stenosis and ectasia.

Hepatic artery aneurysm, ectasia and stenosis

Appendicular skeleton

Focal gigantism: Overgrowth of long bone with increase in length of the bones and soft tissue usually unilateral e.g. the lower limb, the upper limb.

Marked enlargement of a digit: In the hand or foot. This is diagnosed clinically. The bones are also enlarged.

Undergrowth of long bones: This may very rarely be observed. Poliomyelitis is a major differential diagnosis when the lower limb is involved.

Overtubulation/ undertubulation of bone: Overtubulation or undertubulation of bone the later being due to cortical thickening. Other causes of cortical thickening and defective modelling with enlargement of the bone are the major differential diagnosis.

Anterior and lateral tibia bowing: Anterior and lateral bowing of tibia with irregular periosteal thickening frequently progressing to pseudoarthrosis.

Pseudoarthrosis: Marked absorption of fracture margins so that they become pointed. Most commonly seen in tibia followed by radius and clavicle.

Intra-osseous lucency: Due to intra-osseous neurofibroma presenting as subperiosteal cortical lucency with smooth expanded outer margin.

Pressure resorption of cortical bone: Cortical bone pressure resorption from adjacent soft tissue neurofibroma.

Fibrous cortical bone defect: May be due to dysplastic periosteum

Single or multiple cystic lesion within the bone: Probably due to deossification or association of non-ossifying fibroma with neurofibromatosis.

Subcutaneous haematoma: Massive, fast, life threatening and frequently at the back due to NF – type 1.

Decreased bone mineral density

Decreased muscle bulk

Rhabdomyosarcoma

Breast cancer, peripheral nerve sheath tumour.

GIT manifestation, 10 – 25%

Constipation: Constipation or obstruction of intestines simulating Hirschsprung's disease caused by plexiform neurofibroma of the colon. It may be associated with pain and bleeding. Plexiform neurofibroma may be located in jejunum, stomach, ileum or duodenum in that order.

Carcinoid tumour and other GIT stromal tumours: The increased prevalence of carcinoid tumour in neurofibromatosis is due to presence of plexiform neurofibromas in GI tract.

Solitary subserosal or submucosal filling-defects: This is due to solitary polypoid neurofibroma, neuroma or ganglioneuroma, schwannoma (mucosal ganglioneurofibromatosis). The subserosal lesions lie in antimesenteric border anywhere in GIT from oesophagus to rectum.

Intussusception: Submucosal lesions may act as lead point and cause intussusception. Bleeding from the mass presents as melaena stool.

Plexiform neurofibroma: Regional enlargement of nerve root causing:

1. Mass-effect on adjacent barium-filled loops of bowels
2. Multiple eccentric polypoid filling defects
3. Mesenteric fat trapped within enlarged network (15 – 30 HU on CT), characteristic
4. Multiple leiomyomas with or without ulcers

Steatorrhoea: This is secondary to obstruction of pancreatic duct.

Dysphagia: Neurofibroma in subcutaneous adipose tissue of posterior neck.

Renal and urogenital tract

Retroperitoneal neurofibroma: This may displace and obstruct the ureter.

Neurofibroma of the bladder: This causes frequency and urgency of urination

Intra-renal vessel aneurysm (rare).

Urinary retention: Neurofibroma of lumbar spinal root compressing the urinary bladder and ureter retroperitoneally.

Ocular manifestations

Pulsatile proptosis: Unilateral pulsatile exophthlamos (proptosis). This is due to herniation of sub-arachnoid space into the orbit through defect in the sphenoid bone.

Congenital glaucoma: Aberrant mesodermal tissue obstructing the canal of Schlemm (scleral venous sinus).

Lisch nodules: Pigmented iris harmatoma, < 2 mm. Bilateral and first appear in childhood.

Optic nerve glioma: 12% of patients, 4% bilateral and 75% in the first decade.

Choroidal haematoma (in up to 50%)

Perioptic meningioma (causes pneumosinus dilatans of ethmoidal and frontal sinuses).

Plexiform neurofibroma (Found in up to 90% of cases)

Neural crest tumours (endocrine tumours)

Phaeochromocytoma: Found in 1% of patients with neurofibromatosis. 5% of cases of phaeochromocytoma are associated with neurofibromatosis.

Parathyroid adenomas: Associated with hyperparathyroidism (MEN II).

Sipple syndrome: This consists of neurofibromatosis, bilateral phaeochromocytoma and medullary carcinoma of thyroid and parathyroid adenoma.

Small bowel carcinoids: Carcinoid tumour of small bowel and multiple endocrine abnormalities.

Precocious sexual development

Somatostatinoma (NF – type 1)

Ampullary carcinoid tumour presenting as pancreatitis

Skin manifestations

Café-au-lait spots: Have smooth outline, may cause misdiagnosis of pulmonary nodule when found in the chest.

Cutaneous neurofibroma: this comprises of elephantiasis neuromatosa. It is due to partial or local gigantism. This may be secondary to increased blood supply to a digit or a limb. It may also be caused by plexiform neurofibromatosis.

Massive soft tissue haematoma: Involvement of periosteum leads to its loose attachment to the bone and may lead to massive subperiosteal haemorrhage after mild bruising similar to scurvy.

Periosteal cloaking: Calcified extensive massive haemorrhage may appear as cyst and cloak the bone. It leads to increase cortical thickening with defective modelling when incorporated into the bone.

Specific features of neurofibromatosis type 2
Intracranial
Bilateral acoustic neuroma (sine qua non)

Schwannoma of other cranial nerves (olfactory and optic nerve excluded because they don't have Schwann cells).

Multiple meningiomas

Meningiomatosis: Innumerable small meningiomas studded in the dura.

Glioma of ependymal derivatives

Spine
Bone abnormalities are absent

Large bilateral neurofibromas may be seen sometimes at every level of the spine

Spinal cord meningioma

Ependymoma of the cord and filum terminalae

Others
Pre-eclampsia and eclampsia. When any of these develops recently in a pregnant woman, it may be from neurofibromatosis. Adverse foetal and maternal outcome may occur.

Whole body MR imaging can estimate the tumour burden in NF-1 and 2.

(Adam & Dixon, 2008; Dahnert, 2011; Sutton, 1998 and 2003).

References
1. Klatte EC, Franken EA, Smith JA. The radiologic spectrum in neurofibromatosis. Semin Roentgenol 1976; 11: 17-23.
2. Gutmann DH, Aylsworth A, Carey JC, Korf B, Marks J, Pyeritz RE, Rubenstein A, Viskochil D. The diagnostic evaluation and multidisciplinary management of neurofibromatosis 1 and neurofibromatosis 2. JAMA 1997;278:51-7.
3. Cai W, Kassarijian A, Bredella MA, et al. Tumour burden in patients with neurofibromatosis types 1 and 2 and schwannomatosis: Determination on whole body MR images. Radiology 2009; 250:665-673.
4. Restrepo CS, Riascos RF, Hatta AA, Rojas R. Neurofibromatosis type 1: spinal manifestations of a systemic disease. J Comput Assist Tomogr 2005; 29:532-9.
5. Czyzyk E, Jóźwiak S, Roszkowski M, Schwartz RA. Optic pathway gliomas in children with and without neurofibromatosis 1. J Child Neurol 2003;18:471-8.
6. Jacquemin C, Bosley TM, Svedberg H. Orbit deformities in craniofacial neurofibromatosis type 1. AJNR Am J Neuroradiol 2003 ;24:1678-82.

7. de Andrade GC, Braga OP, Hisatugo MK, de Paiva Neto MA, Succi E, Braga FM. Giant intrathoracic meningoceles associated with cutaneous neurofibromatosis type I: case report. Arq Neuropsiquiatr 2003;61:677-81.

8. Zisis C, Dountsis A, Dahabreh J. Multiple bilateral recurrent neurofibromas of the lungs. Eur J Cardiothorac Surg 2003; 24:826.

9. Agarwal U, Dahiya P, Sangwan K. Recent onset neurofibromatosis complicating eclampsia with maternal death: a case report. Arch Gynecol Obstet 2003;268:241-2.

7.2 RADIOLOGY OF SCHISTOSOMIASIS

Definition

Schistosomiasis is a disease caused by infestation by a parasitic worm of a specie of trematodes of the genus known as Schistosoma. It is also called Bilharziasis or Biharziosis There are many types:

1. *Schistosoma haematobium*
   Found in Africa, South East Asia, Mediterranean regions
2. *Schistosoma mansoni*
   Found in Africa (affects over 70 million), Caribbean, Arabian Peninsula and northern part of America
3. *Schistosoma japonicum*
   Found in China, Japan, Philippines and other Asian countries.
4. *Schistosoma intercalatum*
5. *Schistosoma mekongi*

It is worldwide in distribution
Male:Female   = 9:1

Radiological Features

Radiological features are found in the urogenital system, chest and lungs, gastrointestinal tract, liver, spinal cord, brain and meninges and the pulmonary circulation

Genitourinary system

Plain Film
Kidneys
Renal calculi: Polypoid granulomatous tissue calcification.
Calcified auto-nephrectomised kidney (unilateral)

Ureters
Calcification starts at distal ureter: It may be unilateral or bilateral
Cow-horn calcification of distal ureter: Dilated calcified distal ureters appearing as cow horns.
Ureteric calculus: Confirmed by excretory urography.
Dilated calcified entire ureter in continuity.

Bladder
Pencil-like linear bladder wall calcification: This appears parallel to the base of the bladder.
Eggshell calcification of the bladder wall peripherially. Necrotic dead ova in the fibrous tissues are what calcify.
Punctate, polypoid or nodular bladder wall calcification due to clusters of encasements of eggs in moulds of polypoid granulomatous tissue.
Very dense calcification of bladder wall
There may occur vesical calculus that is different from calcification.
Flat-shaped or flat-topped bladder: Fibrotic urinary bladder with thickened wall appearing almost box-like especially at the top.

Excretory urography (EU)
Kidney
Increased calyceal cupping with calyceal dilatation
Hydronephrosis with or without hydroureters
Non-functioning kidney: This is unilateral as bilateral occurrence is incompartible with life.

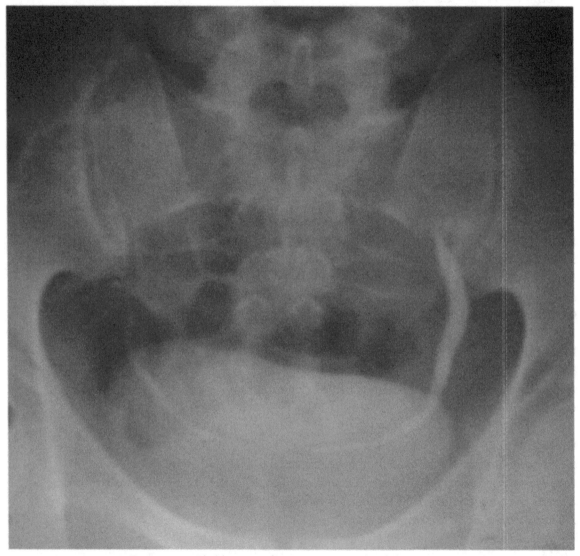

Figure 7.21: Bladder view of excretory urography showing cow-
horn appearance of distal ureters in schistosomiasis.

Ureter
Polypoid filling-defects in the ureters
Ureteric narrowing and stricture: Ureters tapering distally to a point.
Cow-horn dilatation of distal ureter. This is demonstrable in bladder view of IVU showing cow-horn
appearance of distal ureters (figure 7.21).
Hydroureters with columnization of ureters.
Aneurysmal dilatation of ureters. Grossly dilated ureters may have aneurysmal configuration.

Cobra-head ureter due to pseudo-ureterocoele formation.
Ureteric reflux with dilatation and columnization.
Aperistaltic ureter on fluoroscopy
Fistulations: Ureteroperineal fistulas may be seen.

Bladder (cystography)
Normal bladder contractility: Calcification does not affect the bladder distensibility and the bladder has normal filling and emptying.
Bladder ulcers: They occur in early carcinoma and may cause haemorrhage.
Bladder carcinoma: Mass of malignant tissue with irregular margin and filling- defect seen in the bladder in cystography.

Ultrasound, CT scan and MRI
The lesions that are demonstrated by the modalities include polypoid bladder masses, bladder calculus, bladder carcinoma and bladder calcification.

Others
Calcification in various organs: Calcification in the prostate, calcification in the posterior urethra, calcified seminal vesicles appearing as honey comb, calcification in the testes, calcification in the cervix, calcification in the vagina and calcification in the uterus

Renography
Renographic (131 – Hippuran studies) abnormalities are seen and may persist after water load and are commonly found in infected children. The renographic abnormalities are reversible following treatment.

Computed tomography
CT scan identifies bladder calculus, calcification in the bladder, ureter and kidneys better than plain films. Ureteral calculus and nephrolithiasis are better identified by plain films.

Magnetic resonance imaging
This can identify lesions similar to those identified by CT scan.
CT or MR urography: New methods with reconstruction can show changes in the genitourinary system without the use of conventional IVU.

The Lung (Plain film features)
Katayama syndrome: Acute pneumonia-like appearance from direct antigenic and indirect circulating antibody reaction from liver worms and dead eggs respectively. There is an inhomogenous opacity similar to pneumonia. There are also areas of patchy opacities similar to bronchopneumonia. Liver worms can also produce focal granulomatous reaction which is acute stages resembles pneumonia.
Miliary opacities: These are caused by small granulomas and eosinophilia. The opacities are small, pinhead in size and widespread in both lungs and result when eggs lodge in pulmonary arteries of less than 100 mm. Miliary TB and sarcoidosis are differentials.
Lung calcification: Calcified solitary or multiple pulmonary nodules. The areas that have undergone granulomatous reactions can have the granulomas calcify.
Lung fibrosis: Fibrotic scarring can also result from granulomatous reaction. This leads to relative prominence of upper lobe arteries but not the veins.
Diffuse interstitial fibrosis: This occurs if the focal reaction was rather generalised.

Gastrointestinal tract
Plain films
Colonic calcification: This is multiple, scattered, visible but non-specific.

Barium meal
Coarsening and irregularity of mucosal fold due to oedema with changes in peristaltic activity more marked in the jejunum.
Stricture: Stricture formation in the ileum simulating Crohn's disease.
Polypoid lesions: Post-inflammatory colonic polyps measuring 1 – 2 cm in diameter seen most commonly in rectum and sigmoid colon.

Barium enema
Ulceration: Mucosal superficial ulcers in the colon shown on double contrast enema.
Mural fibrosis with short segment narrowing: The localised narrowing is frequently observed at the rectosigmoid junction.
Diffuse long-segement narrowing: Diffuse narrowing involving long segment resembling lymphoma is seen in distal colon.

CT scan
CT scan can detect colonic polyps and calcification in the colonic wall. Thickened bowel wall, thickened valvulae conniventes and haustral markings are detected.

Portal venous system
Ultrasound
Hepatosplenomegaly
Portal vein dilatation above 13 mm in diameter due to portal hypertension.
Peripheral fibrosis: Small scattered peripheral hypoechoic foci in up to half of the patients with chronic schistosomiasis. The echo pattern of liver parenchyma is normal.
Thickened gall bladder wall with hyperechoic gall bladder bed.
Thickening of walls of portal channels due to fibrosis.
Rigid tubular portal vein: Appears like clay pipe. This is due to fibrosis of walls of veins and perivascular fibrotic thickenings.
Small echogenic liver due to cirrhosis
Ascites due to cirrhosis
Dilated vascular channels: Vascular collaterals seen as dilated vessels in splenic hilum, gastrorenal, paraumbilical, oesophageal and paraoesophageal and rectal vessels due to portal hypertension.

Barium swallow
Gastric/oesophageal varices: Multiple serpiginous/worm-like filling defects that change position on different films.

Angiography (venography)
Pruning of portal tree: The portal venous capillary and precapillary venous tree are pruned due to fibrotic obstruction.

Portal vein dilatation with collaterals in paraumbilical, splenorenal, gastrorenal and rectal vein due to hepatic fibrosis obstructing the portal emptying of blood to inferior vena cava. Portal hypertension develops.

Spinal cord
Myelography/Spiral CT and MRI
Epidural mass lesion due to granuloma formation.
Subdural mass: Subdural mass lesion due to granuloma formation.
Expanding intramedullary mass due to granuloma in the spinal cord.
Spinal cord compression: Complete block of spinal cord by granulomatous tissue, with paraplegia.
Transverse myelitis: Conus medullaris and cauda aquina are particularly invoved. Inflammatory changes in the whole thickness of spinal cord causing sensory paraparesis and sphincter disturbance.
Small meningeal foci of granulomatous masses

The Brain
Hyperdense masses in the brain: CT scan shows multiple, small, round hyperdense mass lesions in the brain. This is due to granulomatous foci. Histology is required to prove diagnosis.
Features of raised intracranial pressure: Cerebral and cerebellar tumour-like granulomatous mass lesion may be sufficiently large to cause raised intracranial pressure, ventricular obstruction, effacement and contralateral dilatation.

Neuroschistosomiasis
Neuroschistosomiasis is a severe complication of the disease. Inflammatory response of the host to egg deposition in the brain and spinal cord leads to the neurological symptoms. Symptoms of neurological complication of cerebral schistosomiasis include delirium, loss of consciousness, seizures, dysphasia, visual field impairment, focal motor deficits and ataxia. Cerebral and cerebellar tumour-like neuroschistosomiasis can present with increased intracranial pressure, headache, nausea and vomiting, and seizures.

Schistosomal myelopathy
Severe schistosomal myelopathy can provoke a complete flaccid paraplegia with areflexia, sphincter dysfunction and sensory disturbances. Myelopathy (acute transverse myelitis and subacute myeloradiculopathy) is observed as the most common neurological complication of Schistosoma especially S. mansoni infection. The conus medullaris and cauda equina are the most common sites of involvement.

Pulmonary circulation
Plain film features include:
Hilar enlargement: This may occasionally be very large. Generalised disintegration of lung vasculature from fibrosis leads to increase in precapillary pressure and dilatation of hilar vessels.
Right ventricular hypertrophy: This may be so large in advanced cases as to be aneurysmal. It occurs due to arteriovenous communication formed by destruction of pulmonary vessels leading to excessive load on the right side of the heart.
Pulmonary embolism: Chronic pulmonary embolism presenting with very gross dilatation of main and central pulmonary arteries due to emboli.
Pruning of peripheral vessels: The lung fields appear hyperlucent.

Enlarged Azygos vein: Spherical opacity measuring about 1 cm in diameter seen at the right of the carina adjacent to the right bronchus. The azygos vein enlarges as a result of portal hypertension.

(Adam & Dixon, 2008; Dahnert, 2011; Sutton, 1998 and 2003, Palmer & Reeder 2001).

References
1. Umerah BC. The less familiar manifestations of Schistosomiasis of the urinary tract. Br J Radiol 1977; 50:105-109.
2. Carod-Artal FJ. Neurological complications of Schistosoma infection. Trans R Soc Trop Med Hyg 2008;102:107-16.
3. Andrade Filho AS, Queiroz AC, Freire AC, Lima LC, Filho CA, Amado IN, Reis MG, Magalhães IF, Carmo TM. Pseudotumoral form of neuroschistosomiasis: report of three cases. Braz J Infect Dis 2007;11:435-8.
4. Umerah BC. Evaluation of the physiological function of the ureter by fluoroscopy in Bilharziasis. Radiology 1977;124:645-647.
5. Umerah BC. Bilharzial hydronephrosis: A clinic-radiological study. J Urol 1981; 126:164-165.
6. Segun AO, Alebiosu CO, Agboola AO, Banjo AA. Schistosomiasis--An unusual cause of abdominal pseudotumor. J Natl Med Assoc 2006;98:1365-8.
7. Ihekwaba FN. Schistosomiasis of the testis. Cent Afr J Med 1992;38:123-7.
8. Bohrer SP, Lucas AO, Cockshott WP. Roentgenographic features of schistosomiasis in children. Z Tropenmed Parasitol 1971 ;22:177-88.

7.3   RADIOLOGICAL FEATURES OF EXTRAPULMONARY TUBERCULOSIS

Definition
1. Tuberculosis (TB) is an infectious disease caused by *Mycobacterium tuberculosis*. Other strains of mycobacteria like *M. avium-intracellulare, M. kansasii, M. Fortuitum, M. Xenopi* and *M. africanum* may occasionally cause the disease in about 5% of cases.
    The lung is the primary organ of infection.
2. Extrapulmonary TB often results from haematogenous spread of pulmonary TB to other organs and systems.

Radiological imaging modalities
1. Plain radiography – chest, skull, abdomen, skeletal system, neck
2. Ultrasound – skull and brain, abdomen, neck (soft tissue).
3. CT scan
4. Excretory urography
5. Hysterosalpingography
6. Angiography
7. MRI
8. Radionuclide studies
9. Lymphangiography

Features of Extrapulmonary TB
Skull or intracranial calcification
Calcified tuberculosis: Calcified spherical radiodensity with or without surrounding sclerosis. They are seen in people treated for tuberculous meningitis. They are better appreciated with CT scan.
Calcified flakes in basal cisterns: Calcification of basal exudates in the cisterns.
Plaque calcification above the sella turcica
Enlarged vascular grooves

Osteomyelitis
Skull lucencies: These are localised destructive lesions often associated with soft tissue swelling or abscess. It often have irregular margins.
Button sequestrum: This appears as a dense spherical radiodensity within a localised area of lucency in the outer table of the skull. Eosinophilic granuloma and radiation osteitis can also present this appearance.
Puffy tumour with cold abscess: Solitary tuberculous foci associated with fluctuant painful abscess (cold abscess) are termed *puffy tumours*. The bone may have scalloped marin where it may and appears '*eaten away*'at the site of the lesion.

The Brain
Brain tuberculoma: Multiple small round hypo- or isodense lesions. Enhancement occurs after contrast administration on CT scan. There is little oedema or mass effect. Enhancement can be nodular, or fine, or irregular. When the lesions are large, dense ring shadows may resemble pyogenic abscess or glioma.

Using MRI on T_2WI there is high intensity central zone and hypointense periphery. On T_1WI the lesion is isointense. They are commonly found in the posterior fossa and associated with raised intracranial pressure.

Basal exudates: Characteristic small nodules in the healed exudates at the basal cisterns of the brain. Intra-cellular lesions may be seen occasionally with CT scan.

Cerebral infarct: Vasculitis and chronic hypertrophic inflammatory changes cause areas of brain infarction that are hypodense in CT scan.

Dural sinus and cortical venous thrombosis. Best appreciated with sagittal section MRI and venography.

Encephalitis: Gyriform enhancement of cerebral surfaces appearing and disappearing rapidly with variable CT and MRI features.

Cerebral oedema: Diffuse cerebral swelling, patchy enhancement and venous thrombosis.

Hydrocephalus or Raised intracranial pressure: Early affectation of TB meningitis may lead to destruction of arachnoid villi/pacchionian granulations resulting in hydrocephalus and raised intracranial pressure.

The Bones

Haematogenous spread of infection from the lung may occur from primary and later post primary focus. Chest x-ray shows active TB in less than 50%. The bacteria lodge in the spongiosa of bone. Abscess may occur and may become calcified. Abscess may track to the skin through a sinus.

'Bone carries' which means dry rot, may affect any bone and since the disease has very gradual and indolent course, any bone lesion in endemic areas warrants consideration of tuberculosis.

Metaphysis

A common site of involvement with oval or round focus which soon crosses the epiphyseal line. No surrounding sclerosis is seen. Sequestra are small and absorbed by granulation tissue. The initial focus may be sited at the epiphysis. Diaphyseal lesions are rare. Multiple cystic types of lesion are very rare. Slight periosteal reaction may occur if the lesion is subcortical but this lesion is less prominent.

Greater trochanter

Lesions start in the bone or overlying bursa. Lesions are seen which may be deep but are often superficial and difficult to detect. The lesion may be cystic. Involvement of this site is common particularly in the adolescent and young adult.

The Hands

Spina ventosa: Characteristic widening of the medullary cavity and expansion of the affected phalanx of the hand is called spina ventosa.

Tuberculous dactylitis: Osteolysis, infarction with destruction of bony trabeculae of the small bones of the hands and feet may be caused by TB.

Diaphyseal involvement

Multiple pseudocystic lesions resembling multiple abscesses are seen in the diaphysis of long bones. Fusiform local bone enlargement may occur. Abscess cavities within bone resembling simple bone cyst or Brodie's abscess.

The Rib

Widening of rib, erosion of rib, subluxation and destruction may occur individually or in any combination. Adjacent granulation tissue from vertebral TB or abscess may also destroy rib.

Periosteal reaction can occur and may be marked.
Abscesses tracking through intercostal spaces are seen.

The Sternum

Areas of radiolucencies with irregular and ill-defined borders initially. There may be sclerosis of the margins in later stages. Histiocytosis is a differential.

Mastoid region/middle Ear

Well-defined round lesions in bones of the middle ear with chronically discharging sinus. This may be seen in children or adults.

The Mandibles

Part of the mandible including the body, condyle or the whole of the mandible may be destroyed. Radiological signs are worse than clinical signs and healing is not as rapid as in long bones.

The Joints

Major parts are affected especially the hip and knee. One joint is usually affected and multifocal lesions are rare. Epiphyseal plate is attacked and offers little or no resistance to TB. Infection may be synovial or secondary to bone infection.

The Hip

Lesion may arise in the acetabulum, femoral head/epiphysis or metaphysis. Foci may be found in the greater trochanter or ischium. Hip infection is common.
Pointed bird's beak appearance: This may occur due to destruction and flattening of the femoral head.
Protrucio acetabuli: Intrapelvic protrusion of femoral head may occur and this may be unilateral or bilateral.
Fracture of femoral head or neck may occur.
Bone loss: All degrees of bone loss of the femoral head and neck occur
Marked osteopaenia: Marked osteopaenia with upward subluxation of destroyed porotic femoral head and neck leaving part of the head in the acetabulum.

Knee

Joint effusion and *osteopaenia* affecting a variable length of the bones of the joint.
Soft tissue swelling: This could be due to joint effusion, bursitis or tuberculosis arthritis.
Accelerated skeletal maturation, overgrowth and modelling abnormalities.
Bulbous, squared epiphysis: This resembles juvenile rheumatoid arthritis or haemophilia. Later, there is narrowing of joint space with marginal or localized destructive lesion.
Kissing sequestra may occur.
Intracortical cyst resembling degenerative disease.
Soft tissue calcification: At healing, there are extensive surrounding soft tissue calcification and debris.

Shoulder

Humeral head, the glenoid or both may be affected
Large cystic lesion in the humeral head: This resembles osteoclastoma.
Osteopaenia: This can be local or more generalised to the affected are but hardly completely generalised.
Caries sicca. Shoulder involvement by TB with relatively benign course and without pus formation. Small, pitted erosions are seen in the humeral head and may resemble degenerative disease.

Wrist

All carpal bones tend to be attacked in adult whereas in children localised lesion is the rule because children have protective thick articular cartilage responsible for some degree of resistance to spread.

Crowded carpal bones with erosions: With cartilage destruction, the carpal bones become crowded and the destructive foci soon involve adjacent bones even if one bone was initially affected.

Intense demineralization is found throughout the carpus and distal radio-ulnar joint within the confines of the synovium.

Large soft tissue swelling

Kissing sequestra may occur

Intracortical cysts resembling degenerative disease.

Multiple intracortcal cysts affecting several carpal bones and associated with soft tissue swelling. The well-defined nature of the margin of the cystic lesion will prove the benign nature of the lesion as opposed to malignant lesion.

Bones of the hands and feet

Spina ventosa: Multiple cyst-like cavities with associated diaphyseal expansion in the bones of the hands and feet are called *spina ventosa* and signify tuberculous dactylitis.

Sacroiliac joints

Sacroiliac joints involvement occur more in young adult than in children; occasionally it is bilateral.

Sub-articular erosion causes widening of the joint spaces

Abscess formation of the back of the joint and later calcification of pus may occur.

Tuberculosis of the spine is a frequent accompaniment.

The Spine

The spine accounts for about half of all bone TB lesions. Site is mid-thoracic to upper lumbar vertebrae. Upper thoracic and cervical involvements are rare.

Vertebral body involvement occurs at three sites namelyupper and lower disc margins, in the centre and anteriorly under the periosteum.

Erosion of disc substance

Two or more vertebrae are attacked with wedge destruction. CT and conventional tomography often show more extensive lesion than seen on plain film.

Gibbus: Wedge destruction due to anterior body involvement leads to gibbus.

Local angular kyphosis: Due to destruction of anterior part of the vertebral body more than posterior part. Scoliosis may occur.

Abscess: Paravertebral abscesses are seen especially in the thoracic region when they contrast against the radiolucent lung. Abscess may track widely and may become calcified.

Rib-crowding: Collapse of dorsal vertebrae leads to close approximation of ribs in the chest.

Anterior vertebral scalloping: Depression on anterior aspect of the vertebrae due to aortic pulsation transmitted through paravertebral abscess. Aneurysm must be excluded.

Neural arch and pedicle involvement: Sclerosis, destruction, collapse, fracture of the pedicle or neural arches may be unilateral or bilateral. It may occur in one site, multiple sites or a segment.

Ivory vertebra: Dense solitary or multiple vertebrae due to re-ossification in the healing phase after vertebral osteonecrosis.

Vertebra plana: When only one vertebra is affected with conspicuous preservation of adjacent disc even if the body is totally destroyed or flattened. This vertebral body often appears sclerotic and it is reduced in height or flattened.

"Vertebra within vertebra appearance": This is due to reappearance of growth recovery lines.

"Vanishing vertebra": One or more vertebral may be dissolved by the infection and disappear. This is diagnosed by radiography.

Posterior element involvement: This occurs more in the lumbosacral and thoracic regions often with huge abscess.

Amorphous/tear-drop calcification: In paraspinal areas, often anteriorly between L_1 and L_5.

Cervical spine involvement: Dysphagia and paraplegia are complications. More common in Blacks than Caucasians. Erosion of body, posterior elements and collapse may occur.

Atlanto-axial subluxation: From cervical spine involvement or retropharyngeal abscess.

Widening of presacral space: This is due to retropharyngeal abscess, tuberculous cellulitis or tuberculous spnondilitis with pus collection.

Fistula-in-ano

Pseudo-ankylosing spondylitis: Bamboo spine appearance. Some vertebral bodies may show sclerosis. The sacroiliac joint may be involved or normal.

Bridge formation: New bone formation bridging vertebral bodies. Disc space may show alternating narrowing and normality. Bridging may be unilateral or bilateral.

Psoas abscess: This may occur as well as paravertebral or retropharyngeal abscess. It may become calcified.

Spinal cord compression

Gibbus compression: Involvement of spinal cord from gibbus formation and extrusion of granulomatous tissue into the spinal canal may result in paraplegia.

Myelography will demonstrate gibbus as an extradural mass with compression of the cord. CT and MRI are invaluable.

Symphysis pubis

Erosive changes on both sides of the joint with central sequestrum. This is one of the rare sites where sequestrum is found in TB. There can also be marked sclerosis with fusion of the joint for demonstration of this.

The Mediastinum

Unilateral hilar mass: From lymphadenopathy or Ghon's complex.

Paravertebral masses of lymph nodes/mediastinal lymph nodes.

These appear as lobulated multiple round soft tissue masses. They may present with pleural or pulmonary involvement.

Mediastinal lymph node calcification: Healing phase of lymphadenopathy may calcify.

Ghon's focus may also calcify: It may be visible on plain film or CT.

Pleural involvement

Pleural effusion: Fluid in the pleural space and this may be exudative.

Empyema thoracis: Abscess within the pleural cavity due to TB

Pleurisy: Blunted costrophrenic angle or calcified pleurisy minor pleural effusion or empyema or thickened pleura due to previous inflammatory change may calcify.

Retropharyngeal abscess

Retropharungeal abscess: TB of cervical spine or lymph node may caseate and form abscess within the neck in the retropharynx. There is widening of retropharyngeal soft tissue with gas within it. The cervical spine is held in straight orientation.
There may be atlanto-axial subluxation.

Cardiovascular system

Pericardial effusion: Tuberculous exudative pericardial effusion leads to enlargement of the cardiac silhouette. Ultrasound scan will show the echo-free space.
Tuberculoma of pericardium: This appears as well-defined mass with soft tissue consistency. Only histology will prove the definitive diagnosis.

Pericardial tuberculous abscess: This appears as cheesy material with localized bulge of cardiac shape or contour sometimes giving the heart a bizarre shape. There may be associated hilar lymphadenopathy.
Aortitis and Aneurysm: Focal granuloma adherent to the wall of vessels, weakens it and it bulges. When the process reaches the intima, it ulcerates into the lumen. High pressure systemic circulation causes it to form false aneurysm with fibrous and granulomatous wall. Aortic arch and ascending aorta are frequently involved and dissection and rupture may occur.
Abdominal aortic and inferior vena caval aneurysms: These may be involved in the same way as aortitis and aneurysm involve the aortic arch and descending aorta. Degenerative changes in a young patient in areas where TB is endemic and where age is incompatible with such changes suggest TB.
Calcific pericarditis: This results from tuberculous involvement of the pericardium of the heart by medidiatinal or pulmonary tuberculosis. The heart itself is largely spared.

The Neck

Cervical lymphadenopathy: The lymph nodes may be matted together. They are best appreciated with MRI and CT. Histology will prove the diagnosis and differentiate it from lymphoma.

The Oesophagus

Extrinsic filling-defect: Extrinsic filling-defect from compression by mediastinal lymph node. It may also erode into it.
Deep ulcers and fistulas: Due to erosion of mediastinal lymph node into the oesophagus.
Scarring and stricture: This may result and causes dysphagia.
Oesophagitis: M. avium intracellulare may cause oesophagitis, discrete ulcers, scarring, stricture formation and fistulation. They are demonstrated by barium swallow.

Other parts of gastrointestinal tract (GIT)

Gastric outlet obstruction: Mass lesion, tuberculoma or lymph node enlargement in the area of the antrum can cause obstructive mass-effect or lesion with shouldering, filling defect and apple core deformity indistinguishable from lymphoma or carcinoma.
Ulcers: Circumferential ulcers are common in lower ileum and caecum and associated with lymph node enlargement. The ulcers may be large or small and often visualised by appropriate barium studies.

Spasm of ileum and descending colon: This is often caused by transverse ulcers.

Entero-cutaneous fistula

Mucosal irregularity and thickening: Combination of granulomatous infiltration, caseation and fibrosis produces narrowing of bowel lumen and associated mucosal irregularities.

Intestinal obstruction: Healing of ulcers by fibrosis leads to multiple adhesions and sometimes causes intestinal obstruction.

Shortening of the colon

Healing caseating granulomatous lesions in the enlarged Peyer's patches lead to marked fibrosis and results to segmental shortening or diffuse narrowing of bowel with marked shortening of the caecal pole.

Stricture: This may simulate malignancy. They are areas of healing by fibrosis.

Wide patulous ileocaecal valve: (Inverted umbrella sign). This occurs with narrowing of adjacent ileum and rigid caecum. There is also associated oedema.

Intestinal perforation: Erosion of local ulcer into the bowel wall leads to perforation. The ulcer is usually transverse, associated with spasm (more in caecum and ileum) and rapid bowel emptying.

Haemoperitoneum: From bleeding perforated peptic or gastric ulcer.

Pneumoperitoneum: Rupture (perforated ulcer) leads to escape of gas contained in hollow bowels into the peritoneal cavity.

Tuberculoma: Soft tissue mass usually around the caecum in the right iliac fossa. It may be difficult to differentiate from amoeboma, helminthoma, carcinoma, actinomycosis or appendix mass. Histology is diagnostic.

Peritonitis

Exudative peritonitis due to spread of infection. This is highly echogenic fluid which is seen on ultrasound scan.

Omental caking: The omentum is thickened and appears as cake. Masses are seen in the omentum, often irregular masses of soft tissue density which are enlarged lymph nodes.

The Spleen

Splenic abscess may occur.

Tuberculomas of spleen may be small or large and often multiple from disseminated infection.

Calcifications: Tuberculomas may calcify.

Adrenal gland

Multiple granulomas: Small round nodules of granulomas indistinguishable from carcinoma or adenoma except by histology.

Addison's disease: Granulomas may calcify at healing stage and may be the cause of Addison's disease.

Hepatic tuberculosis

From miliary seedings

Granulomas: these are seen as 5–10 mm diameter well-defined areas of parenchymal change.

Multiple oblong hyperechoic areas of innumerable granulomas throughout the liver seen by ultrasound.

Tuberculous abscess: Tuberculous abscess of the liver may occur and is rare. Distortion, contraction and calcification of a segment or a lobe are seen especially in the elderly simulating cirrhosis.

Lymphadenopathy

There is a common affectation of the neck, thorax and abdomen when organs in these regions are involved. They are demonstrated by CT, MRI and barium studies. Histology will prove the diagnosis.

Tuberculous lymphoedema

Lymphoedema: Lymphadenopathy of the lower limbs, genitals, breasts and arm groups of lymph nodes may cause tuberculous lymphoedema.

Racemorse chennels: Obstruction of the lymphatics leads to dilated racemose channels which are bypassing the gland on lymphangiography (using oil-soluble contrast medium).

Filling-defects within lymphnodes: Filling defects are noted in the glands due to caseated debris or necrosis.

Renal tuberculosis

The kidney may be normal or small: A focal cortical loss may occur but the cortex may be normal. The changes can be bilateral or unilateral but when bilateral they are asymmetrical.

Calcification: Punctate area in the parenchyma in mild cases. It occur in one third of cases. The whole kidney may be replaced by calcification.

Autonephrectomy: Non-functional, non-excreting kidney replaced by complete calcified kidney.

Renal abscess: Caseation and abscess formation within kidney noticeable by ultrasound scan.

Fibrosis and atrophy: The kidney may be fibrotic and atrophic.

Renal calculi: This may occur due to calcification of renal granuloma within the calyces. Cavitation. Irregular coalesced cavities which deforms the affected renal calyx simulating renal papillary necrosis. Stricture. Localised areas of proximal dilatation, hydrocalycosis may occur due to stricture of a calyx. *Multiple stricture of renal pelves and ureters* may lead to hydronephrosis. Hydronephrosis due to stricture of renal pelvis, ureter and bladder.

Tuberculoma: Isolated stricture of calyx and ceseating necrosis may form granuloma.

The Ureters

It often follows renal TB and it ulcerates and then heals by fibrosis.

Stricture: Ulceration and healing by fibrosis lead to multiple ureteric strictures.

Cockscrew ureters. Due to multiple ureteric strictures.

Beaded, saw-toothed ureters: Due to multiple areas of stricture and granuloma formation causing filling defects.

Calcification: Solid calcification starting proximally and progressing downwards.

The Urinary bladder

Filling defect due to granuloma simulating polyps.

Thickened bladder wall muscle: Hypertrophy combined with inflammatory tuberculomas.

Bladder wall ulceration (seen by cystoscopy)

Shrunken, scarred bladder with reduced capacity

Bladder wall calcification (rare)

Bladder outlet obstruction: From prostatic TB, prostatic abscess or fibrosis of bladder neck (rare)

The Prostate and Seminal vesicles /vas deferens
Calcification: Solid seminal vesicle and vas deference calcification can occur.
Fistulous communication: This may result.
Stricture formation: it is seen due to fibrosis in healing stage of the disease.
Prostatic abscess: This is occasionally seen in the prostate gland.

The Testes
Multiple, small, round hypodense lesions within testes.
Scrotal granuloma: Well-defined round hypoechoic nodular mass adjacent to the testes due to granuloma. *Reactive hydrocoele is common.*

The Urethra
It appears as filling defects, calcification of the urethra and u*rethral stricture*

Fallopian Tubes
Hydrosalpinx: Dilated fallopian tube seen on HSG (figure 4.21 b and c).
Peritubal adhesion or loculated spillage. It can also result from fimbrial adhesion at the distal end of the tube so that HSG results in spillage which is loculated.
Tubal blockage: Due to stricture, it can be at any position (figure 4.21 a and b).
Beaded tubes: Irregular calibre tube with multiple small filling defects and dilatation at the peripheral end. The tube is obstructed at the fimbrial end (figure 4.21 a and b).
Calcification: Tuberculous pyosalpinx may calcify and this is diagnosed using HSG.

The Uterus
Small, irregular, contracted uterine cavity.
Tuberculous endometritis may result in some degree of adhesion/synaechia.
Granuloma within the uterus may calcify

Breast
Abscess formation
Inflammatory change resembling carcinoma or mastitis.
Lymph node enlargement.

Ovary
Granuloma may simulate ovarian adenoma.

(Adam & Dixon, 2008; Dahnert, 2011; Sutton, 1998 and 2003, Palmer & Reeder 2001).

Reference
1. Engin G, Acunaş B, Acunaş G, Tunaci M. Imaging of extrapulmonary tuberculosis. Radiographics 2000; 20:471-88.
2. Harisinghani MG, McLoud TC, Shepard JO, Ko JP, Shroff MM, Mueller PR. Tuberculosis from head to toe. Radiographics 2000; 20:449-70.
3. Obisesan AA, Lagundoye SB, Lawson EA. Radiological features of tuberculosis of the spine in Ibadan, Nigeria. Afr J Med Med Sci 1977;6:55-67.
4. Baydur A. The spectrum of extrapulmonary tuberculosis. West J Med 1977; 126:253-62.

5. Ogunseyinde AO, Obajimi MO, Ige OM, Alonge T, Fatunde OJ. Computed tomographic evaluation of TB spine in Ibadan. West Afr J Med 2004;23:228-31.

6. Obajimi MO, Jumah KB, Ogoe E, Asiama S, Kaminta A, Brakohiappa E. Computed tomographic evaluation of Pott's disease in Accra. West Afr J Med 2004;23(1):50-3.

7. Umerah BC. Radiological patterns of spinal tuberculosis in the African. East Afr Med J 1977;54:598-605.

8. Okoro EO, Komolafe OF. Gastric tuberculosis: unusual presentations in two patients. Clin Radiol 1999;54:257-9.

9. Tan CH, Kontoyiannis DP, Viswanathan C, Iyer RB. Tuberculosis: a benign impostor. AJR Am J Roentgenol 2010;194:555-61.

10. Ikem IC, Bamgboye EA, Olasinde AA. Spinal tuberculosis: a 15 year review at OAUTHC Ile-Ife. Niger Postgrad Med J 2001;8:22-5.

11. Solagberu BA, Ayorinde RO. Tuberculosis of the spine in Ilorin, Nigeria. East Afr Med J 2001;78:197-9.

7.4   RADIOLOGICAL DIAGNOSIS OF ACUTE APPENDICITIS

Definition
Acute appendicitis is the abrupt-onset inflammation of the vermiform appendix due to infection. It is the commonest acute surgical condition in the developed world and it carries an overall mortality of about 1%.

Problems of diagnosis
Appendicitis is a clinical diagnosis, however the high rate of negative laparotomy findings has naturally pushed for the search for more reliable preoperative imaging diagnosis worldwide. In typical cases, diagnosis is made without radiological investigations. However, in atypical presentation chest X-ray is advocated partly to act as a baseline in case of postoperative complications, to exclude chest conditions that could present in similar way and to show any sign of gas under the diaphragm due to perforation.

Radiological examinations (ultrasound, barium enema or CT examination) are not substitute for a good clinical history and examination, and where the surgeon is confident of the diagnosis there should not be a need for further investigations. However, many conditions clinically simulate appendicitis and may be diagnosed using radiological investigations like plain films, CT scan and ultrasound of the abdomen and pelvis. Ultrasound is advocated in young women with suspected appendicitis in order to exclude some gynaecological and obstetric conditions that simulate appendicitis.

Radiological features
Plain Films
Findings on supine and erect films correspond to the degree of inflammation.

Normal abdominal radiographs
There is normal plain abdominal radiographs at early stages or signs of non-specific gasesous distension.

Signs of intestinal obstruction
Multiple dilated bowel loops with multiple air-fluid levels in keeping with intestinal obstruction. Intestinal obstruction which can be complete or incomplete can occur as several loops of small bowel become matted together from inflammation or stuck to the inflamed appendix making them inflamed, aperistaltic, oedematous and dilated.

Appendicolith
Appendicitis results from occlusion of the appendix lumen by a focus of insipissated faeces with secondary inflammatory response. The appendiceal faecolith may occasionally undergo calcification and become stone called *appendicolith*. About 10% -13% of adult patients with acute appendicitis show appendicoliths while 1% of normal people show appendicoliths. About 5-10% of children with appendicitis show appendicoliths. Its presence indicates appendicitis in 90% of cases and in 75% of these, it is gangrenous. Ileal and caecal fluid levels are found in 50% of patients with appendicoliths.
Compositions of appendicoliths are:
i.   50 % fat or fat derivatives
ii.   25 % inorganic phosphates
iii. 25 % inorganic residue.

Characteristics of appendicoliths are:
a. They are oval in shape
b. They are radiopaque
c. They measure 0.5 - 6.0 cm in diameter.
d. They are frequently laminated.
e. In plain films or CT scans, they can appear as ring calcifications.
f. They are found in the right iliac fossa in a great majority of cases (> 90%).
g. In 50%, appendicoliths are multiple.
h. They cause obstruction of the appendix in about 30%.
i. In CT or ultrasound, they are surround by inflammatory fluid or phlegmon.
j. In ultrasound, they cast distal acoustic shadows.
k. They can be located some distance from the appendix if perforation has occurred.

Differential diagnoses of appendicoliths are:
Phlebolith, ureteral stone, opaque pill, foreign body, calcified mesenteric node, bone island, faecolith or inspissated stool, gallstone (in gallstone ileus it may be found outside the gallbladder).

Abnormalities of terminal ileum and caecum / sentinel loop
Dilated, thickened, oedematous and atonic caecum and / terminal ileum with multiple fluid levels. In addition, if perforation or peritonitis has occurred there may be generalized paralytic ileus. There may be indentation of the caecum at the medial border by abscess that is formed.

Soft tissue mass in the right lower quadrant
Oedematous appendix with surrounding fat and fluid-filled loops of ileum may appear as soft tissue mass. If perforation with abscess formation has occurred, a more clearly defined mass sometimes containing gas may be seen.

Obliteration of soft tissue landmarks
The peri-appendiceal inflammatory response may cause obliteration of lower portion of the properitoneal fat lines on the right lower portion of the psoas outline or the outline of the right obturator or levator ani muscles. The shadows of these muscles may disappear completely in more advanced cases.

Gas–filled appendix
Diseased appendix may be filled with gas and if a gas-fluid level is demonstrated then gangrenous appendix is proven. Gas without fluid level may be seen in normal persons, those with large bowel obstruction and those with paralytic ileus especially if the appendix is high in retrocaecal area.

Pneumoperitoneum
This is evidenced by air under the hemidiaphgragm in an erect chest radiograph and other signs of pneumoperitoneum after the patient has stood or sat erect for at least 10 minutes. Pneumoperitoneum does not usually occur because of the rapidity with which the appendiceal lumen becomes occluded and no longer communicates with the intestinal lumen. And also because the perforated appendix is walled off immediately.

Ascites

Perforated appendix may present with ascites, oedema of the surrounding structures with veil-like opacity in both flanks and also as a result of the resulting peritonitis. This results to a hazy appearance especially in the right iliac fossa.

Fluid in the adnexa and pelvis

Fluid may be seen in the right adnexa and in the cul-de-sac in the pelvis due to reactive fluid from the appendix tracking down to these regions.

Scoliosis concave to the right

The thoraco-lumbar spine may show scoliosis concave to the right due to muscle spasm caused by the appendiceal inflammation in the right iliac fossa.

Lateral displacement of the ascending colon

The ascending colon would be displaced laterally due to right paracolic abscess on plain films. Abscesses in the right paracolic gutter are most likely to originate from appendicitis. However, occasionally they may be due to a subphrenic abscess tracking down toward the pelvis.

Left-sided radiological signs

In situs inversus vicerum with the appendix on the left rather than on the right side, these changes as enumerated above are found in the left side rather than on the right side.

Pneumorrhachis

Gas within the spinal canal. Its presence means well-established gangrenous bowel and it has poor prognostic significance.

Ultrasound Scan

Non-compressible appendix with a diameter of 7 mm or greater

Using a transducer of at least 7.5 MHz frequency, and graded compression techniques with increasing pressure applied in the area of maximum tenderness in the right iliac fossa to displace the bowels, the appendix is demonstrated overlying the psoas muscle. *It is a blind-ending tubular structure, aperistaltic, non-compressible and measuring at least 7 mm in diameter.* It is a highly effective diagnostic tool having a sensitivity of 80-95% and a specificity of 90-95% in both adults and children.

Markedly echogenic non-compressible fat surrounds the appendix

The mesentery and omentum surrounding the blind ending appendiceal structure is echogenic, non-compressible fat.

Fluid / abscess surrounds the tubular structure (appendix)

This is hypoechoic area due to localized abscess from reactive inflammation of varied severity and is seen surrounding the appendix.

Oedematous appendix end/pole

The caecal pole or area is oedematous and hypoechoic due to local inflammation.

Target sign in transverse view

In the transverse view using ultrasound scan, a central hyperchoic structure denoting the appendix is seen with surrounding hypoechoic area due to surrounding oedema or abscess.

Appendix is compressible if perforation has occurred
Non-visualization of the appendix does not exclude appendicitis

Sentinel loop

Ultrasound can demonstrate thickened, dilated and immobile bowels in the right iliac fossa. This is due to local inflammation and oedema of the bowels.

Appendix mass / Complex mass

Appendiceal mass will appear as complex mass in the right iliac fossa on sonography. This is a hyperechoic area with intervening hypoechoic area and adjoining dilated bowels which are aperistaltic and adherent to the hypoechoic mass. *Comet tail sign* due to gas within the abscess is found.

Ascites

Fluid may be seen due to perforation forming ascites, peritonitis.

Abscess in the right iliac fossa

Abscess formed by appendicitis may be found in the right iliac fossa. This is hypoechoic with multiple internal echoes.

Appendicolith

Ultrasound can identify appendicolith within the appendix. This is echogenic, casting distal acoustic shadows.

Increased colour flow due to hyperaemia on Doppler scan

On colour Doppler study, hyperaemia of the appendix is noted.

Small mesenteric lymph nodes are frequently / often noted close to the appendix. Periportal increased echogenicity within the liver is described as a non-specific sign.

Barium Enema

The presence of acute non-perforated appendix is not a contraindication to barium enema which may be the best method to diagnose it.

Irregular indented medial wall of the caecum. This is due to oedema of the caecal pole of the inflamed appendix.

Barium within the appendix

A thin track of barium from the indented ceacal area may point to the incompletely filled lumen of the appendix.

Extrinsic indentation on medial border of caecum/terminal ileum

If perforation or abscess has occured, the caecum or terminal ileum may show smooth or irregular extrinsic pressure deformity.

Other lesions that may show these signs are amoeboma, caecal polyp, post operative appendiceal stump, mucocoele, carcinoma, helmintoma, other adjacent mass lesions.

Diverticulosis

There may be one or multiple diverticula of the appendix found on barium enema and they are associated with appendicitis or perforation.

Appendix tumour

Most of the appendix tumours are carcinoids which arise from the argentaffin cells of the the crypts of Lieberkuhn. About 90% of the carcinoids arise from the appendix and 90% of appendix tumours are carcinoids. They are benign tumours and secrete 5HT. They are small in size and may be demonstrated by ultrasound scan or barium enema where they cause mass indentation or filling-defect. Other benign tumours are leiomyoma, neuroma and fibroma. Malignant tumours consist of adenocarcinoma and lymphoma. Most of these are difficult to diagnose radiologically, are mostly incidental findings in surgery, and are all associated with acute appendicitis which tends to halt the natural cause of the disease and prevent metastasis. The peak age of appendix tumour is 25 years.

Computed Tomography

1. CT scan directly demonstrates periappendiceal inflammation.
2. CT scan shows the appendix measuring greater than 7 mm in diameter
3. There is failure of the appendix to fill with oral contrast agent up to its tip.
4. CT will show air within the lumen of the appendix but this also does not extend up to the tip due to the presence of appendicolith or inflammatory phlegmon.
5. Appendicolith is demonstrated as a hyperdense structure within the hypodense inflamed appendix.
6. Following intravenous contrast injection, there is enhancement of the wall of the inflamed appendix making it appear hyperdense.
7. Other surrounding inflammatory changes seen on CT include increased fat attenuation, fluid, inflammatory phlegmon, caecal thickening, abscess, extraluminal gas and lymphadenopathy.
8. *'Arrow-head' sign*
   The lumen of the caecum can sometimes be seen pointing towards the obstructed opening to the appendix.
9. Other causes of right lower quadrant pain may be seen and CT can be used to recognize if it is of gastrointestinal origin, such as mesenteric adenitis, intussusception, terminal ileitis, diverticulitis, epiploic appendicitis, and typhoid enteritis; or of urogenital origin, such as ureteral stone and urinary tract infection, tubo-ovarian abscess, ovarian torsion, ectopic pregnancy, hemorrhagic ovarian cyst or corpus luteum remnants, etc.
10. In children, CT has an established role in *late-presenting* appendicitis where it conclusively demonstrates localised or multifocal abscesses and is useful in planning radiological drainages for these abscesses.

Magnetic Resonance Imaging

1. *Useful in pregnant patients*: MRI is of great advantage in pregnant patients compared to CT, offering high soft tissue contrast without ionizing radiation. The normal appendix is a tubular structure arising from the caecum, measuring greater than 7 mm in diameter, and is seen filled with air or contrast media.
2. *Enlarged appendix:* In acute appendicitis, the appendix is enlarged, greater than 7 mm in diameter, and not containing air or contrast media.
3. *Signs of peri-appendiceal inflammation:* They are seen and include band-like areas of high signal intensity on T2-weighted images and single-shot fast spin-echo images or fat saturation images.

4. Presence of an appendicolith, seen as an intraluminal low signal intensity focus, confirms the diagnosis.
5. Routine use of gadolinium-based intravenous contrast agents in pregnancy is not allowed.
6. MRI is also useful in identifying other causes of right lower quadrant pain in patients suspected of acute appendicitis such as torsion of ovarian cyst, degenerating pedunculated fibroid, intestinal polyp, etc.

(Adam & Dixon, 2008; Dahnert, 2011; Sutton, 1998 and 2003, Swischuk, 2004; Sanders & Winter, 2006).

References

1. Hernandez JA, Swischuk LE, Angel CA, Chung D, Chandler R, Lee S. Imaging of acute appendicitis: US as the primary imaging modality. Pediatr Radiol 2005;35:392-5.
2. Doria AS. Optimizing the role of imaging in appendicitis. Pediatr Radiol 2009;39 Suppl 2:S144-8.
3. Holscher HC, Heij HA. Imaging of acute appendicitis in children: EU versus U.S.....or US versus CT? A European perspective. Pediatr Radiol 2009;39:497-9.
4. Brown MA. Imaging acute appendicitis. Semin Ultrasound CT MR. 2008;29:293-307.
5. Whitley S, Sookur P, McLean A, Power N. The appendix on CT. Clin Radiol 2009; 64:190-9.
6. Shin LK, Jeffrey RB. Sonography and computed tomography of the mimics of appendicitis. Ultrasound Q 2010;26:201-10.
7. Raja AS, Wright C, Sodickson AD, Zane RD, Schiff GD, Hanson R, Baeyens PF, Khorasani R. N egative appendectomy rate in the era of CT: an 18-year perspective. Radiology 2010;256:460-5.
8. Pacharn P, Ying J, Linam LE, Brody AS, Babcock DS. Sonography in the evaluation of acute appendicitis: are negative sonographic findings good enough? J Ultrasound Med 2010;29:1749-55.
9. Gaitini D. Imaging Acute Appendicitis: State of the Art. J Clin Imaging Sci 2011;1:49.

7.5 RADIOLOGY OF BATTERED BABY SYNDROME (NON-ACCIDENTAL INJURY)

Definition
Battered baby (child) syndrome is the intentional and deliberate infliction of physical, physiological or emotional pain and suffering on a child by a parent or caregiver. It is generally called child abuse and involves a continuum of mistreatment ranging from indifference to the welfare of the child to physical abuse, which is the use of raw force on the child.

It includes the following forms of abuses:[1-3]

1. Neglect; about 60%
2. Physical abuse; about 20%
3. Sexual abuse; about 10% (four times more in girls)
4. Psychological abuse; about 10%

In physical abuse, the syndrome consists of:

1. Subdural haematoma
2. Multiple areas of fracture of long bones at different stages of healing.
3. Multiple bruises / and or burns
4. Evidence of malnutrition, failure to thrive, neglect (on inspection)
5. Associated inconsistencies in history by parents or guardian.

Brief history[1,2,3]
Battered Baby Syndrome (BBS) is also called non-accidental injury or shaken baby syndrome. It is estimated to occur in 2000 children a year in USA alone. Mortality among infants that suffer BBS is estimated at 15-40%; mean is about 20-25% in USA. Intracranial injury is the cause of most of the deaths. Chronic neurological deficits and residual complications include cerebral palsy, mental retardation, blindness and various degrees of cognitive, motor and psychological impairment including depression from some of the chronic disabilities. The child here means any human being under 18 years who is under the authority of his parent or caregiver / guardian. For practical purposes majority of the battered child are under 2 years and a great majority are under 8 years. Females that are involved in sexual abuse may be older.

Mechanism of Injury[1-5]
Bodily injury or physical abuse
The bodily injury (physical abuse) in Battered Baby Syndrome (BBS) is caused by:

1. *Violent and vigorous shaking* of the child causing severe acceleration and deceleration and whiplash injuries in most of the joints, mobile soft tissues and organs of the child including the brain.
2. *Direct blunt trauma* (blow) as the child abuser avoids creating any type of visible abrasion or wound that can lead to the detection of the abuse.
3. The *brain injury results as the child's brain is softer*, contains more water than that of the adult and is thus more prone to injury due to shaking and effects of coup and contre coup.

Physiological abuse
Deliberate malnutrition or starvation including blockade of food from reaching children during war situations.

Psychological violence
Neglect, indifference and emotional deprivation. These are inflicted on the child by parents, caregivers or guardian.

Sexual abuse
This could be by enticing the child with gifts such as toys and clothes and then having various types of advantages on the child after the child's natural resistance is weakened by the want of those gifts. It could also be by intimidation and use of physical power and raw force.

History
This is often very vague. The abuser may be the one giving the history. The relations collectively may withhold the history of abuse. Every form of likely causes of injury may be provided.

Clinical findings
1. Multiple areas of tenderness or tender swellings, bruises or burns.
2. Petechial haemorrhages in the conjunctiva or oral mucosa (the child must be removed from the parent or guardian).
3. Joint pain especially affecting the bones on both sides of the joint.
4. Failure to thrive, poor eating habits, irritability.
5. Injury in the pubic region/external genitalia which may present with dysuria.
6. Haematoma/haemorrhage within the sclera of eye or retina.
7. Vomiting, seizures, difficulty with breathing.
8. Bulging head, tense anterior fontanel, subgaleal cyst.

What are the problems with battered child?
In the USA, alone:[1,2]
a. About 10% of children with cerebral palsy have evidence of abuse.
b. About 10% of children with trauma who are under 5 years have been abused.
c. Battered baby syndrome is the second most common killer in children under 5 years.
d. Head injuries are the most common cause of death in physical abuse followed by intra-abdominal injuries (Figure 6.51 c and Figure 7.51 c).
e. One million children are abused per year while over 3000 die each year from abuse.
f. About 1.22% of children were reported to be abused in USA alone in the year 2000.
g. 44% of the abused children were less than one year showing that the most vulnerable children are the most abused.
h. Parents constituted 77% of the abusers.
i. Females are abused sexually four times more than males.

The figures are worse in developing countries due to the extended family system, poverty, child labour, human trafficking and sexual exploitation for financial gain.

Radiological Diagnosis
Radiological findings necessary for the diagnosis are as follows:[1-5]

1. **Soft tissue injuries**
This is the most common type of injury in child abuse. While performing ultrasound scan, positioning the baby for sonography or radiographic study, the radiologist may notice bruises, scalds, soft tissue swelling, scratch marks, wounds and tenderness in the child, which were never reported or mentioned. It is more commonly discovered by the referring physician but may be detected by the radiologist.

2. **Non-specific lesion**
Bone lesions may be seen on a radiograph done for other conditions that are non- traumatic. This is so as the abuser tries to conceal the history. The following diagnosis may be made because of the concealed history namely spinal dysplasia, bone dysplasia, skeletal dysplasia or growth retardation.

3. **Greater extent of injury than given in history**
Trauma is usually more severe and extensive than suggested from the history. The following may be found in a child who is said to have rolled down the bed.
    i.   Diastatic skull fracture
    ii. Subdural haematoma

4. **Diaphyseal fractures (due to heavy blows)**
This is the second most common type of injury.
    i.   Transverse fractures rather than the usual oblique fracture are seen due to heavy blow in the limbs (Figure 7.51 a and b).
    ii. All other diaphyseal fractures (oblique, transverse, buckle) when alone or with other injuries are highly suggestive of BBS.
    iii. Femoral shaft fracture and fractures at other unusual sites for age.
    iv. Skeletal survey is necessary to check for fractures at other sites (Figure 7.51 a and b).

5. **Metaphyseal-epiphyseal injuries**
    i.   Pathognomonic and most specific diagnostic finding. It is sometimes described as classical metaphyseal lesions (CML).
    ii. Bucket-handle fracture (avulsion corner fracture of type II Salter-Harris fracture). Also called triangular fracture.
    i.   Epiphyseal separation (Salter-Harris type I fracture)
    iv. Multiple or single epiphyseal separation of the Salter-Harris type I fracture.
    ii. Frank metaphyseal fractures with exuberant periosteal reaction. More injuries even at the healing stage of the initial injury.
    iii. Small metaphyseal fractures, microfractures or infractions due to shaking and stretching at the joints.
    iv. Variable periosteal reaction of injuries
    v.   Metaphyseal bony fragments
    ix. Fracture lines are oriented parallel to the physis although it may not extend through the entire width of the bone.

i.   Force generated by vigorous shaking due to the to-and-fro manual movement of the baby held at the chest resulting in whiplash injuries of the metaphysis in children less than 2 years who are unable to control the movement of their dangling limbs.

ii. Majority have no periosteal disruption and no callus formation.

iii. Hypertrophied cartilage.

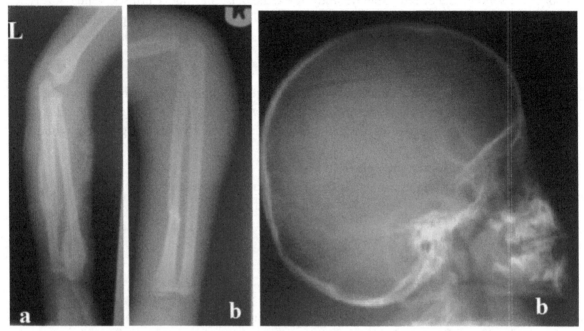

Figure 7.51: Plain radiographs of both radius and ulna in a 7-year old patient showing multiple fractures at different stages of healing (**a** snd **b**), and multiple skull fractures (**c**) in the same patient.

6. Multiplicity of lesions

Injuries occurring in several areas particularly bilateral lesions. Skeletal survey with radiographs of each area of interest taken after positioning for that area is invaluable for detection of abuse. Babygram and poor quality radiographs are the greatest causes of misses in diagnosis of child abuse (Figure 6.51 c and Figure 7.51a, b, c).

7. Fractures at different stages of healing

Repeated trauma causes multiple fractures seen at different stages of healing (hallmark of disease). This is due to repeated injuries and the child continues to cry from pain of the previous injuries.

8. Rib fracture

This is diagnostic and very specific as only large babies weighing 3.3 kg with history of difficult delivery have rib fracture as a result of birth trauma. Rib fractures in a child anywhere but particularly occurring posteriorly and laterally is (specific) strongly diagnostic of BBS. If associated with any of the following injuries the diagnosis is confirmed.

i.   Fracture in diaphysis / metaphysis of bone

ii. Joint effusion or soft tissue swelling anywhere

iii. If the fracture is bilateral particularly if occurring at the same level.

iv. Skeletal survey, oblique view, bone scintigraphy and repeat chest radiography in 2 weeks when callus has started to form helps to confirm the diagnosis.

9. **Follow-up radiographs**
   i.   These show old lesions evident by multiple periosteal reactions even when the initial injuries were not visible or periosteal reactions or callus formation of injuries were not diagnosed at the initial study.
   ii. Multiple growth arrest lines / growth recovery lines
   i.   Calcified haematoma not identified previously
   iv. Periosteal reactions and fractures are more in the long bones of the distal forearms and the legs.
   ii. Multiple fractures with overlying soft tissue swellings in the ribs and skull with attempt at healing / callus formation, periosteal reaction.

10. **Injuries to small bones of hands and feet:** Rare but diagnostic

11. **Unusual type of fracture**
    Any type of fracture is possible in child abuse but the following are almost diagnostic.
    i.   Spiral fracture of the vertebrae.
    ii. Spiral fracture of long bone sometimes extending the whole length of the bone in a child that is not yet walking.
    iii. Sacral injuries / fracture from slamming the child down to sitting position.

12. **Compression fracture of vertebral bodies / spinous processes**
    i.   Due to vigorous shaking causing rapid forceful flexion and extension injuries. Uncommon but diagnostic
    ii. Whiplash injuries

13. **Head injury**
    i.   There may be no external sign of trauma.
    ii.   In neonates and infants aged below 6 months, ultrasound scan through the fontanels may show small linear slit-like cavities at gray-white matter interface due to shearing injuries (pathognomonic) best shown with linear-array transducer.
    iii. Subdural haemorrhage or haematoma (diagnostic with appropriate history)
    iv.   Subarachnoid haemorrhage
    v.   Intracerebral haemorrhage
    vi.   Brain parenchymal injury
          a. Shear injury (axonal injuries, white matter tear and contusion tear)
          b. Cerebral contusion: This is focal haemorrhage within the parenchyma resulting from direct contact forces (Figure 6.51 c).
          c. Cerebral oedema
    vii. Cerebral atrophy or loss of cerebral cortical parenchyma often leads to mental retardation (Figure 6.51c)
    viii. Enlarged ventricles or hydrocephalus
    ix.   Porencephalic cysts or encephalomalacia with cystic changes.
    x.   Epidural haemorrhage or haematoma (rare, more with accidental injuries)
    xi.   Skull fractures
          a. In-bending of the skull bones due to plastic nature of the baby/infant skull.
          b. *Egg-shell or stellate*, linear, depressed fractures.

    c.   Multiple fractures, multiple new and old fractures (specific).

    d.   Fractures that cross suture lines (specific) see Figure 6.51c.

    e.   Bilateral fractures (specific)

    f.   Sutural diastasis greater than 3 mm is associated with abuse.

    g.   Co-existing rib fracture or long bone fracture

14. Generalized cerebral oedema in brain injury

This may be difficult to diagnose apart from the effacement of sulci. However, these important signs help in its diagnosis.

    i.   *Reversal sign:* There is relative high attenuation of basal ganglia, thalami, cerebellum and brain stem on CT compared to the rest of the brain in generalised diffuse cerebral oedema of infants.

    ii.   *Bright cerebra sign:* The reversal sign observed in generalized cerebral oedema in infants is called *bright cerebra sign* on MR imaging.

    iii.   Diffusion-weighted imaging shows areas of ischaemia which may still be persisting when the oedema has subsided and the brain is appearing normal on CT or MR imaging.

15. Visceral injuries

Several types and extents of visceral injuries may exist and these may erroneously be called acute abdomen of idiopathic causes without recognition of the underlying abuse.

    i.   Varied-sized intra-abdominal mass (intramural haematoma, pancreatic pseudocyst)

    ii.   *Acute abdominal crises*

        a.   Bowel or mesenteric oedema, laceration, haematoma, bleeds

        b.   *Liver contusion*, rupture

        c.   *Gas in the portal vein*, portal vein thrombosis

        d.   Intestinal obstruction

        e.   *Bowel rupture* or perforation

        f.   Partial or total intestinal obstruction by haematoma, oedema, laceration.

        g.   *Intussusception:* This is particularly noted. Intramural haematoma may act as lead point for the development of intussusception. Coiled spring appearance is noted on plain radiography.

        h.   Co-existing intrathoracic injuries

        i.   Co-existing multiple skeletal injuries.

16. Pancreatic injury

Various types of pancreatic injuries have been described and include:

    i.   Pancreatic pseudocyst

    ii.   Post-traumatic pancreatitis

    iii.   Transection injuries

    iv.   Intrapancreatic fluid collection

17. Chest injuries

    i. Pleural effusion (due to pleural haemorrhage)

    ii. Pulmonary contusion

    iii. Pneumothorax

    v.   Cardiac laceration

18. Neck injuries

Neck squeezing with pressure on the arterial supply of the brain has been proposed as the mechanism of hypoxic injury to the brain stem that leads to brain tissue hypoxia and damage and various types of injuries. However, specific injuries to the neck have only been described at autopsy and include injuries of cranio-cervical junction, cervical spinal cord system and cervical tissues.

19. Eyes

The findings in the eyes are due to high velocity acceleration and deceleration, vigorous shaking and whiplash type of injuries and shearing injuries. Using high frequency orbital sonography, the following are identified:

i.   Subretinal haemorrhages
ii.   Retinal detachment
iii. Vitreous haemorrhage
iv.   Retinal folds
v.   Retinoschisis (tearing apart of the retina).
vi.   Corneal haemorrhage or haematoma

20. Other injuries

Contusion, laceration and rupture of the adrenal gland, stomach, kidney, bladder, colon, pharynx, oesophagus and the liver have been described and thus may occur.

21. Delay in seeking care

This is a form of child abuse itself and constitutes a great contributor to causes of death in patients with visceral, head and chest injuries, and contribute to high degree of residual neurological sequelae.

22. Lethal signs of strangulation

i.   Major bleeding into the soft tissues of the neck especially muscles, salivary glands, lymph nodes are noted using ultrasound or MR imaging. (The child must be removed from the parent or guardian).
ii.   Subretinal haemorrhages

23. Post-mortem radiography

Radiographs of dead children can show specific signs of abuse at the metaphysis, long bones and other areas. High quality radiographs are required while the body has not been taken to the morgue. Other imaging modalities like ultrasound, CT scan, MR imaging when done as post-mortem studies can accurately elicit signs of abuse necessary for the diagnosis. Thus, minimal invasive autopsy is required to avoid mutilation of the body so that independent pathologists can still perform autopsies without tampering with evidences.

Summary of specificity of radiological findings[4]
High specificity

1.   Classical metaphysical lesion
      (bucket handle or corner-fractures patterns)
2.   Rib fractures, particularly at postero-medial locations
3.   Scapular fractures
4.   Fractures of spinous processes
5.   Fracture of the sternum

Intermediate specificity
1. Multiple fractures, particularly if they are bilateral
2. Fractures at different stages of healing
3. Epiphyseal separation or injuries
4. Vertebral fractures, subluxation
5. Digital fractures or fracture of the digital bones
6. Complex skull fractures

Low specificity but common
1. Subperiosteal new bone formation
2. Clavicular fractures
3. Long bone shaft fractures
4. Linear skull fractures

Differential diagnosis
Rickets, scurvy, birth trauma, sickle cell anaemia, osteogenesis imperfect, accidental trauma-related injuries, congenital insensitivity to pain, iatrogenic injuries-birth injuries, physical resuscitation, developmental variants and Caffey's disease.

(Adam & Dixon, 2008; Dahnert, 2011; Sutton, 2003; Swischuk, 2004; Palmer & Reeder, 2001).

References
1. Radkowski MA. Merten DF, Leonidas JC. The abused child: criteria for the radiologic diagnosis. Radiographics 1983;3: 262-296.
2. Lonergan GJ, Baker AM, Morey MK, Boos SC. Child abuse: radiologic-pathologic correlation. Radiographics 2003; 11:811-845.
3. Uscinski R. Shaken Baby Syndrome: fundamental questions. Br J Neurosurg 2002; 16:217-9
4. Kleinmann PK. The spectrum of non-accidental injuries and its imitators. In: Hodler J, von Schulthess GK, Zollikoffer ChL (eds). Musculoskeletal disease 2009-2012: Diagnostic imaging. Springer-Verlag Italia, 2009-2012:227-152) (227-228).
5. Kivlin JD. Manifestations of the shaken baby syndrome. Curr Opin Ophthalmol 2001; 12:158-63.
6. Umerah BC. (1989). Radiology of battered baby. In: Medical practice and the law, Longman, Ikeja, Nigeria; 97-102.
7. Eregie CO. Child abuse and neglect-a case report. The resident doctor 1987;1:54-56.
8. Carty H, Pierce A. Non-accidental injury: a retrospective analysis of a large cohort. Eur Radiol 2002;12:2919-25.
9. Cox LA. The shaken baby syndrome: diagnosis using CT and MRI. Radiol Technol 1996;67:513-20.
10. Eltermann T, Beer M, Girschick HJ. Magnetic resonance imaging in child abuse. J Child Neurol 2007;22:170-5.
11. Mandelstam SA, Cook D, Fitzgerald M, Ditchfield MR. Complementary use of radiological skeletal survey and bone scintigraphy in detection of bony injuries in suspected child abuse. Arch Dis Child 2003;88:387-90.
12. Demaerel P, Casteels I, Wilms G. Cranial imaging in child abuse. Eur Radiol 2002;12:849-57.
13. Wood J, Rubin DM, Nance ML, Christian CW. Distinguishing inflicted versus accidental abdominal injuries in young children. J Trauma 2005;59:1203-8.

14. Trokel M, Discala C, Terrin NC, Sege RD. Patient and injury characteristics in abusive abdominal injuries. Pediatr Emerg Care 2006;22:700-4.

15. Merten DF, Carpenter BL. Radiologic imaging of inflicted injury in the child abuse syndrome. Pediatr Clin North Am 1990;37:815-37.

16. Gaines BA. Intra-abdominal solid organ injury in children: diagnosis and treatment. J Trauma 2009;67:S135-9.

17. Okeahialam TC. Child abuse in Nigeria. Child Abuse Negl 1984;8(1):69-73.

7.6   ACUTE RADIOLOGY AND ITS ESSENTIAL FEATURES

Definition
Acute Radiology is the radiologist's online and real time response, presence and performance of radiological studies or procedures, reporting the findings and communicating such findings to appropriate clinicians; in critical hyperacute medical and surgical conditions in which the time duration for the opportunity for beneficial medical and surgical interventions is very short.

Origin of the concept
The concept of acute radiology arose from the fact that imaging has become essential to the practice of medicine and is presently at the centre of accurate diagnosis, treatment, referral and patients' outcome across departments. The physical presence of the radiologist in the hospital and his real time presence in the emergency department make a great difference in the prognosis of the patient's condition. In most countries, medical imaging studies has become better, increasing in number and at the same time, it has not become easier. Presently the functions of the radiologist in the hospital include economic gate keeping, public health delivery, patient safety, quality-of-care improvement, information technology and the traditional role of performing procedures and interpreting them. Therefore, the radiologist who is the only person equipped with the long period of training and expertise required for the understanding and accurate practical applications and interpretation of a wide range of imaging studies across wide range of diseases, departments and differential diagnosis, needs to be present at the vital moments and visible to offer his expertise for which he is so highly sought after and regarded.[1-3]

Conditions for practice of acute radiology
1. The time for active response for a beneficial effect in such conditions is in the range of minutes to a maximum of a few hours after the onset of symptoms.
2. There is a well-established effective treatment for the condition, which is available, accessible and acceptable in the country and community.
3. The effectiveness of the treatment is greatest when started very early after the onset of symptoms.
4. The relevant staff and experience for diagnosis and treatment are available in the hospital or community.
5. The medical, surgical and radiology team recognize the critical nature of the conditions.

Major determinants of result of acute radiology within and between the various department and emergency units[1-7]
1. Communication, its effectiveness and clarity within and between the various departments and emergency units.
2. Availability of radiologists, preferably face to face or his access to teleradiology facility and the practicality of his coming in physically, when needed.
3. Nearness and availability of other imaging staff due to availability of on-call sleeping in rooms and restrooms and its nearness to the place of diagnosis and treatment.
4. Availability and functionality of machines, accessories and supplies; genuineness of effective drugs including emergency drugs.
5. Enthusiastic staff with good attitude to emergency. Good attitude gives good result; poor attitude gives poor result.

6. Attitudes of hospital management/government. The hospital management should be responsible for acute medicine/radiology in the provision of basic equipments, accommodation and drugs as well as staff motivation by good habitable sleeping-in rooms, employment of middle level manpower (residents) and remunerations.

7. Co-operation among different specialties, the radiology department, and the effectiveness of such co-operation and communication. Where the staffs are alert to the co-operation, good result will be achieved.

8. Power supply in communities with problems of effective and steady power delivery. This should be of good integrity.

9. There could be errors from request forms/cards as patient conditions may not always guarantee adequate history, (patient must be awake, alert and attentive for good history from patient) and clinical examination. The radiologist should interact with the patient, patient's relations and clinicians to extract more and relevant history in order to focus accurately on the required relevant studies and reduce the number and types of uncessary studies to only those needed for the patient.

10. Security and safety for staff in carrying out treatment in communities experiencing civil strife.

Major problems of acute radiology[1-6]

1. It is mostly done during off-regular hours, at night or other emergency period (including periods of academic meeting, clinical meetings, mortality review, ward rounds, grand ward rounds, departmental meetings, nursing student, medical student or post-graduate medical examinations) when highly trained and adequate number of staff are not available.

2. It is at the centre of time-critical diagnosis for other departments.

3. The other departments depend on it for multi-disciplinary decision-making, treatment and referrals or correlation of their other findings. Without it, these decisions cannot be made accurately.

4. It is at the centre of major acute surgical and medical therapeutic challenges.

5. It at the centre of audit of the performance of various methods of medical or surgical diagnoses, treatments and referrals within and among the departments and hospitals.

6. It is useful for comparing pre-mortem and post-mortem diagnosis.

7. The patients are not usually adequately prepared for the investigation.

8. It is at the centre of litigations involving different departments.

9. Without immediate available imaging, the quality of care is highly compromised and if a radiologist is unavailable, clinicians/technologists may perform the studies or interpretation with poor quality and accuracy, resulting in less favourable patient outcome, documentation and poor medical audit.

Requirements for good practice of acute radiology

1. A good, spacious and functional radiology department with wide entry doors to each room and adequate basic equipment.

2. A good restroom, sleep-in rooms and library for staff. The radiology department should be a home/living room for residents in radiology and from other departments.

3. There should be good and functional imaging modalities.

4. The radiology department should have experienced and motivated radiologists with adequate supporting residents or medical officers.

5. Experienced technologists (radiographers/imaging scientists), darkroom technicians, nurses and maintenance engineers and transport staff (porters).

6. In academic centres, there should be functional, scholarly and progressive residency programme in which the residents have wide knowledge of radiology practice in different countries by spending one to two years in different countries.

7. The radiology resident doctors and the radiologists should live within or near the hospital if effective transport or security is not guaranteed at all times. The department should be guarded as a precious jewel by the availability of radiologists or experienced residents at all times.

What should be done in acute radiology?

1. Whether requested or not, any affordable, accessible and available modality that could elicit or diagnose the condition or answer the questions posed by the patient's condition should be employed.

2. Multiple imaging modalities should be employed when time permits.

3. Multiple staff, residents, and radiologists should be involved in performance of the study, intervention or reporting to reduce errors. The radiologist should increase his visibility by being physically present as it guarantees the quality of the procedure, reports and interactions with his colleagues, bonding with the patient and his self-esteem in the hospital community.

Who should perform acute radiology?

1. The radiologist is at the centre with participation of technologists.

2. The residents doctor with enough experience should assist the radiologist calling him when necessary and at the least doubt.

3. A senior member of the medical or surgical team should be available to ask their real time, online questions which could be answered by altering or modifying the procedure.

4. The radiologist with multi-disciplinary participation of surgeon, physician, gynaecologist and obstetrician.

5. The radiologist should interact with the resuscitating team to know the time available for the patient's studies.

6. The radiologist should show high level of understanding, humility and attention to studies and their interpretations, technical details and to the points raised by the patient, patient's relations and clinicians to achieve good success.

The most important aspect of acute radiology[1-4]

1. Human lives are on the balance and require action in minutes to save them.

2. The radiologist is the central focus and should understand this, and also know what should be done, what he is doing and the critical need of his presence, judgement, actions, reports and timely communication of reports to the referring clinician.

3. Online presence of other specialists in the radiology department to ask their real time questions at the time the patient is in the radiology department is critical to solving multiple problems at the same time.

4. While reporting imaging studies in acute setting, the radiologist must avoid *"Instant Happiness Syndrome"* which means the unconscious practice of ending the search for more abnormalities when an obvious abnormality is found.

5. Other technologists (radiographers/imaging scientists) and relevant radiology staff like nurses and orderlies should be present.

6. Co-operation is required among radiology staff and with the management of the hospital and other staff in other departments to put in place and use what is available in the most advantageous manner.

Duties of the radiology managers for effective practice of acute radiology
1. Generation of adequate political priority for radiology departments in the presence of hospital managers.
2. Adequate servicing of radiology equipment and maintenance of service agreements.
3. X-ray machines and other imaging modalities should be functional at all times since they have medico-legal qualities.
4. Drawing up of practical protocol for some cases that are seen in acute radiology call duty period to maintain high standard and reduce inter-operator variability in studies.
5. Make simple protocol for effective communication between residents and radiologists, and between radiology department and the requesting department including mode of telephone calls and writing, collecting and communicating reports.
6. Adequate, conducive call-duty rooms and rest rooms for staff. The radiology department should be a living house comfortable for staff and patients.

Responsibilities of the radiologist in acute radiology
The radiologist is responsible to
1. *First the patient*: This involves accurate timely diagnosis, treatment or interpretation of her condition using the least expensive, most non-invasive and safest modalities.
2. To his staff: There should be good quality and integrity of input from the department to other departments and the hospital in general. The various departments should view the result from radiology department as dependable by the consistent contribution of the radiologist in ensuring that what goes out of the department is the best that can be achieved with available manpower and facilities.
3. *The referring clinician*: He should answer the queries of the referring physician to clarify the diagnosis and ease patients' management and improve his knowledge for future referrals.
4. *Second, the employer/hospital*: His real time presence or that of adequately trained senior resident doctors will increase his value as seen by the employer. The radiologist or his dependable senior registrar should be highly visible in the hospital.
5. *The community/government*: The overall value of a radiologist is by doing what others cannot do, and in making a difference especially in high quality interpretation and input in non-routine procedure. These can best be appreciated when done as a clinician with human interface rather than as a remote reporter in teleradiology.

Responsibilities of the radiologist to the patient
1. Neither the radiologist nor his staff should embrace a responsibility for which they have not been trained and permitted by law. Therefore, to carry out his functions accurately, the radiologist should be there online and real time.
2. He should determine the type and number of investigations to be used for the condition acting quickly and sending back the patient as fast as possible to referring department for prompt implementation of his report.
4. He should ensure that detailed clinical examinations with good clinical practice and bed side diagnostic tests are used before radiology to avoid unnecessary radiological investigations, not

only for reducing costs but also for preventing adverse effects of unnecessary and unwarranted application of ionising radiations.

5. The radiologist is functioning as a consultant-in-charge and also as consultant to consultants from other departments and not as an adviser in imaging management and interpretation. Therefore, high level of versatile knowledge is the cornerstone of the driving force for accurate management of acute radiology.

Conclusion: Acute Radiology is a major aspect of emergency medicine and surgery and most often determines the public-perceived image of the hospital. It should involve many different specialists co-operating while the other disciplines should be available to clear their doubts, give ideas and ask their real time questions for differential diagnosis in which the radiologist is at the centre of time-critical diagnosis and intervention.

References

1. Mann FA, Gean AD, Kazerooni EA, Roger LF. An overview of Acute Radiology. Radiographic 1999, 19:1319-1322
2. Fries JW. Night Radiology. AJR Am J Roentgenol 1985:145: 109-1092
3. Heilman RS. Practice corner. It's 10:00 pm: do you know where your radiologist is? Radiographics 1999;19(5):1178.
4. Hoffman RB. Heeding the call: radiologists in the emergency department. AJR Am J Roentgenol 2001;177(1):253-4.
5. Mueller CF, Yu JS. The concept of a dedicated emergency radiology section: justification and blueprint. AJR Am J Roentgenol 2002;179(5):1129-31.
6. Craig O. Emergency radiology. II. Medical emergencies. Postgrad Med J 1967;43(504):625-38.
7. Eze KC, Marchie TT, Eze CU. An audit of ultrasonography performed and reported by trainee radiologists. West Africa Journal of medicine 2009; 28 (4):275-261.
8. Berlin L. Standards for radiology interpretation and reporting in the emergency setting. Pediatr Radiol 2008;38 Suppl 4:S639-44.
9. Branstetter BF 4th. Are residents' on-call errors worse than the alternatives? J Am Coll Radiol 2005;2(10):870-1.
10. Rogers LF. Heeding the call: radiologists in the ED (Emergency Department). AJR Am J Roentgenol. 2000;175(5):1213.
11. Hunter TB, Taljanovic MS, Krupinski E, Ovitt T, Stubbs AY. Academic radiologists' on-call and late-evening duties. J Am Coll Radiol 2007;4(10):716-9.
12. Carmichael JH. Out-of-hours radiology. Br J Radiol 1988;61(722):175-6.
13. McDonald JM, Berbaum K, Bennett DL, Mullan B. Radiology residency call: residents' perceptions of the on-call experience. J Am Coll Radiol 2005;2(11):932-8.
14. DeFlorio R, Coughlin B, Coughlin R, Li H, Santoro J, Akey B, Favreau M. Process modification and emergency department radiology service. Emerg Radiol 2008;15(6):405-12.
15. Saket DD. The provision of emergency radiology services and potential radiologist workforce crisis: is there a role for the emergency-dedicated radiologist? Semin Ultrasound CT MR 2007;28(2):81-4.

7.7 OVERVIEW OF JUSTIFICATIONS FOR THE EMERGENCE OF RADIOLOGICAL MINIMALLY INVASIVE AUTOPSY

Definition
Autopsy has been defined literally as the art of examination of the dead body "to see with one's eyes" in order to identify and establish the cause and manner of death.

Aims and Objectives
1. To determine the cause and manner of death.
2. To evaluate the vitality and nature of the sustained injuries.
3. To develop forensic reconstruction of the incidence based on the findings.

Usefulness of autopsy
1. To establish the cause of death.
2. It is essential in medical education.
3. It helps in the identification of new or changing disease pattern.
4. It is important in the evaluation of new therapies.
5. It is used to produce accurate vital statistics.
6. It is used for epidemiological survey and to advise public health policies
7. It is used to assess the quality of medical practice.
8. To reassure family members about the cause of death (to segregate natural deaths from murder and suicide), inherited or infectious diseases.
9. It is used to protect medical staff, health institutions and insurance oraganisations against false liability claim.
10. It is use in medico-legal identification of diseased persons
11. It is use in medico-legal identification of offenders

Methods used in autopsy
There are four main methods used in autopsy, viz:
1. Conventional (traditional, destructive) autopsy.
2. DNA profile analysis.
3. Toxicological analysis
4. Radiological minimally invasive or non-invasive autopsy.
5. Verbal autopsy.

Only the conventional method is common. Verbal autopsy is newly developed. The other methods involve the use of high technological equipment and are not readily available even in the developed countries. However, they greatly enhance the accuracy of results as they are objective and are not observer- or performer-dependent.

Tools used in conventional autopsy
1. Verbal description.
2. Conventional two-dimensional photography.
3. The use of scalpel to dissect the body.

Practical importance of autopsy to patients and hospital[1-5]

1. Over 40% of the autopsies reveal substantial information about the patient's condition beyond what was known antemortem.
2. Post-mortem findings provide information that would have changed the management had it been available antemortem in 10-13% of the cases.
3. Seventy five percent (75%) of antemortem undiagnosed conditions are treatable and often curable if they were accurately diagnosed before (class one diagnostic error), e.g. infection, infestation and malignant diseases.
4. Autopsy is the final and most important quality control method to establish and maintain a strong quality assurance programme in the hospital.

Major disadvantages of conventional autopsy[1-3]

1. Observer dependence. Documentation is in an unintentional subjective manner.
2. Findings that are not identified, elicited, or searched for are not documented and therefore irretrievably destroyed if the body is cremated.
   The brain in not examined in over 15-20% of autopsies in the UK alone.
3. Foreign bodies may be shifted during dissection from their original positions leading to inaccurate or conflicting reports.
4. Very low rate of acceptance by family members, cultures and religious bodies (mostly due to deep-rooted believe in reincarnation and life after death). Such group includes Jewish, Christians, Moslems communities and adherents of African traditional religions.
5. Distortion of the body preventing accurate repeat examination by independent pathologists. In the UK, the body is not inspected by the pathologist before opening and removal of organs by the technologist in over 30% of the cases effectively destroying body surface evidences and accurate localisation of foreign objects.
6. Lack of adherence to standard methods by performers. In over 20% of the cases the state cause of death after autopsy is questionable and in over 25% of the autopsies, the result is deemed poor and unacceptable in the UK.

Reasons for the present decline or low rate of autopsy

1. Failure to give permission by relations because they perceive it as mutilating the body and that the dead patient has suffered enough.
2. Lack of awareness of the usefulness or value of autopsy by relations and physicians.
3. Religious obligations. Prompt burial of the dead by the Muslims within 24 hours and within 14 days by some Christian denominations.
4. Failure to request for permission by physicians as they feel that autopsy is unnecessary.
5. High sense of autonomy towards the integrity of the individual by modern society who feel that permission should have been obtained from the person before death.

Factors that led to the emergence of radiological minimally invasive autopsy[1,2]

The application of conventional autopsy done without high technological tools have been very subjective, frequently resulting in conflicting reports by different pathologists in high profile murder cases involving the police and highly placed individuals. There are very low rates of hospital-based autopsies today reported at 0-13% in 2009 compared to 70% in the 1960s. The very low autopsy rate today are probably due to the earlier-stated reasons. In order to continue to achieve very high rate of autopsy because of the practical importance of autopsy, attempts were made to develop a method of autopsy that will circumvent those major factors that contribute to low autopsy rate. Radiological non-invasive autopsy was then considered. In over 85% of bodies initially examined by radiological modalities, the radiologist provides a cause of death, that was accepted by the Coroner without conventional autopsy.

Development of radiological autopsy[1,2]

1. The first X-ray was used as evidence in law court in 1896 only a year after the discovery of x-ray by Rontgen in 1895.
2. The first CT scan image forensic application in gunshot injury to the head was used in 1977.
3. The first high technological three-dimensional radiological autopsies were performed in the early 1980s.
4. MR imaging for full post-mortem identification of diseased person was first used in 1990.
5. The first MR microscopy for histology was in 1990 (Dirnhofer et al, 2006).

Methods used in radiological non-invasive, virtual autopsy (Virtopsy) or minimally invasive autopsy (MIA)

1. Body documentation and analysis using plain films, CT, MR imaging and microradiology.
2. 3D body surface documentation of evidences. This may involve the use of forensic photogrammetry and 3D optical scanning.
3. Workstation with volume rendering tool to manipulate the data.
4. The data set contains high-resolution 3D colour-encoded documentation of body surface and 3D volume documentation of the interior of the body.

Basic equipment for radiological autopsy

1. Plain radiography (preferably digital radiography).
2. CT scanner. (Multisection or multislice CT).
3. MR imager. (MR imaging of the whole body).
4. CT fluoroscopy for placement of biopsy needle.
5. Micro-CT system. This should be capable of imaging 3D volume with isotropic resolution from 10-100 μm and for samples with diameter of 1-40 mm.
6. MR microscopy.
7. Photogrammetry-based 3D optical scanner. This document images in three dimensional planes.
8. Very high resolution (100-200 MHz) ultrasound scanner for histological identification of tissue in situ without cutting the body (future development).

Advantages of radiological non-invasive or minimal invasive autopsy[1-4]

1. Non-mutilation of the body and therefore consent will not be a problem.
2. Digitally acquired data could be reconstructed in any form whenever new questions arise and the needed information obtained.
3. The objective image can be sent to other experts for a second opinion without distortion.
4. New information can be collected by repeat of the procedure with minimal or no alteration from the previous imaging.
5. Objective accurate non-invasive documentation of the exact location and shapes of foreign bodies, bullets, holes or defects in the body without distortion.
6. Observer-independent documentation of the interior of the body.
7. Observer-independent documentation of the body surface

8. No forensic findings are destroyed or distorted as they would be by the destructive technique used in conventional autopsy.
9. By manipulating the data set with volume rendering (VR) tool at a workstation, one can perform virtual autopsy anytime, anywhere.

Applications for Identity detection[1-5]

Identification of bodies and persons

It is preferable that bodies be identified before imaging studies. However, imaging can identify and establish the identity of the unidentified body. Traditional accurate post-mortem identification of the body is done with.

1. DNA testing profile.
2. Finger printing
3. Identification using dental records.

DNA testing is very expensive and time-consuming and therefore not commonly used even though it is very accurate. Finger printing and dental status identification are more commonly employed. Imaging is invaluable in dental status identification.

Dental status identification using radiological imaging

1. An initial antemortem cranial CT data obtained can be used to reconstruct projections of the teeth for comparison with the data of dental profile obtained post-mortem.
2. Post-mortem dental images can be created and compared with the antemortem dental records.
3. The restoration material (dental filling, bridges, artificial teeth) that was used in the patient can be accurately ascertained on the post-mortem CT data and correlated with the antemortem dental records of suspected missing persons.

Other parameters for accurately identifying a person radiologically

1. Endoprosthesis of the shoulder, hip, knee, spine or elsewhere in the body (artificial pacemaker, vena cava filters, aneurysm prosthesis, and bypass surgery catheters) can be used in whole body CT of the body to identify the patient and exclude or confirm a suspected person without conventional autopsy.
2. Mobile CT machine for post-mortem data acquisition can be used in mass casualties such as natural disasters (earthquakes, tsunami, hurricanes) and air crashes for disaster victims identification.
3. CT and MR post-mortem imaging can help in identification of human and animal remain of past cultures without disturbing or distorting them thus providing evidence of age, gender, dating as well as the disease or injury suffered by the deceased.

Disadvantages of radiological minimally invasive autopsy

1. It is high-technology-based.
2. It requires very expensive equipment
3. It requires extra training of highly qualified manpower, two specialist areas, and more personnel including the radiologist, radiographer and the pathologist for accurate interpretation of findings.
4. It requires regular power supply and may not be easily practiced in rural areas of developing countries due to lack of, or poor power supply.
5. The hi-tech and expensive equipment that are required may further deplete the foreign exchange of technologically less developed countries leading to serious economic burden for poor developing countries.

References

1. Dirnhofer R, Jackowski C, Vock P, Potter K, Thali MJ. VIRTOPSY: Minimally invasive imaging-guided Virtual Autopsy. Radiographics 2006; 26: 1305-1333. Weustink AC, Hnink MGM, van Dijke CF, Renken NS, Krestin GP, Oosterhuis JW. Minimally invasive autopsy: an alternative to conventional autopsy. Radiology 2009; 250:897-904.

2. Thali MJ, Braun M, Buck U, Aghayev E, Jackowski C, Vock P, Sonnenschein M, Dirnhofer R. VIRTOPSY--scientific documentation, reconstruction and animation in forensic: individual and real 3D data based geo-metric approach including optical body/object surface and radiological CT/MRI scanning. J Forensic Sci. 2005;50:428-42.

3. Daramola AO, Banjo AA. Autopsy as a tool in the prevention of maternal mortality. Niger J Clin Pract 2009 Dec;12:457-60.

4. Diegbe IT, Idaewor PE, Igbokwe UO. Autopsy audit in a teaching hospital in Nigeria--the Benin experience. West Afr J Med 1998;17:213-6.

5. Soleman N, Chandramohan D, Shibuya K. Verbal autopsy: current practices and challenges. Bull World Health Organ 2006;84(3):239-45.

6. Fottrell E, Byass P. Verbal autopsy: methods in transition. Epidemiol Rev 2010;32(1):38-55.

7.8 PRINCIPLES OF RADIOLOGICAL MINIMALLY INVASIVE AUTOPSY AND IMPORTANT FINDINGS

Definition
This is the use of non-invasive radiological imaging modalities to arrive at the aims and objectives of autopsy, taking advantage of the objectivity, data archiving and retrieval capabilities of computer technology while not tampering with the original source (the body).

Aims and objectives of radiological minimally invasive autopsy
Determination of the cause and manner of death
Determination of the presence and nature of any sustained injury
Forensic reconstruction of the incidence
Determination of important medico-legal issues

Cause and manner of death
The cause of death specific to certain organs can be identified irrespective of the manner of death (suicide, accident, homicide, iatrogenic, natural disaster).

Systemic findings[1-4]

Identification of physical parameters
1. In hypothermia, areas of bleed within the musculature of the body core are typical findings.
2. In patients with sharp force trauma, major blood loss at the site of injury, pale internal organs and subendothelial areas of bleed indicate that the bleed was lethal.
3. The blood loss in fatal haemorrhage can be quantified by post-mortem measurement of the cross sectional areas of major blood vessels to find out the volume of blood remaining in the body. This can be subtracted from the normal blood volume to determine the blood loss.
4. The weight of the organ can also be estimated using cross-sectional volume imaging. By multiplying the volume by the tissue density factor of the organ (1.05g / mol for liver) the weight can be estimated.

Vitality of the sustained injury
The aim is to elucidate and document the sequence of injury and death in forensic pathological investigation. The question is "Was the injury sustained before or after death?" The forensic radiologist aims to demonstrate the forensic findings that occur only with intact metabolism, consciousness, respiration (cutaneous emphysema, aspiration) and circulation (fatal haemorrhage, air and fat embolism). These findings are called *forensic vital reactions*

Hanging
Vital reactions help to uncover simulated suicidal hanging covering up some kind of homicide. They are uncovered as follows.
1. Bleeding at the insertion of sternocleidomastoid muscle or soft tissue structures of the neck prove that circulation was intact and preserved at the onset of strangulation.
2. Strong breathing attempts (of a living person) against the occluded airway cause alveolar ruptures and subsequent mediastinal emphysema. Absence of this means simulated suicide.
3. Soft tissue emphysema ascending into the neck is a continuation of the mediastinal emphysema in (2) above and means that hanging was not simulated. Absence of this means simulated suicide.

Trauma

Aspirated materials (blood, gastric contents, soot) means ongoing ventilation at the time of the trauma. Extensive soft tissue emphysema in blunt trauma means ongoing respiration/ventilation (however, it is important to consider the possibility of gas production following decomposition). Active swallowing of foreign materials means that the victim was alive at the time of occurrence of the incidence.

The Brain

The findings in trauma in post-mortem imaging are the same or similar in ante-mortem imaging. MR provides an anatomical overview of the brain in-situ without distortion. This is very important and useful when advanced putrefaction makes conventional autopsy of the brain impracticable. A major drawback is that very small lesions less than 5 mm cannot be identified with the current technology. However, improvement in technology is offering prospects of overcoming this.

The heart and related injuries

There is accurate, detailed 3D visualization of the intact heart. Embolized air from cranial trauma (gunshot wound of the head and neck, stab wound of the neck) which is a very common cause of heart-related death can be seen which is not available using conventional autopsy. Right ventricular failure from venous air embolism is shown.

Cardiomyopathies and chronic heart diseases

Chronic cardiac diseases like cardiomyopathies and valvular heart diseases are identified. Cardiac injuries resulting from suicide and homicide causing cardiac tamponade and haemothorax are identified using imaging.

Myocardial infarction

Postmortem MR imaging can demonstrate myocardial infarction undisturbed and permits estimation the age of an infarction based on the signal intensities of infracted tissues. Three or higher telsa cardiac MR imaging can demonstrate cardiac deth by showing myocardial injuries and infarction that are not visible on conventional autopsy examinations.

Pneumothorax is identified using post-mortem imaging and this cannot be identified using conventional autopsy unless the chest is opened under a water bath. Imaging is the gold standard for showing pneumothorax as the lesion is preserved for subsequent independent examiner. Even when a body is opened under a water bath, to demonstrate pneumothorax, the lesion is authomatically destroyed during the procedure and thus unavailable for independent study group to comfirm or refute the earlier findings.

Pulmonary oedema

This is similar to ante-mortem imaging findings. Pulmonary oedema is seen in toxicological deaths and cardiac deaths. The lungs show internal livores due to interval-dependent overlap of blood sedimentations in the dorsal parts of the lung. They are not focal pneumonias.

Pneumonias

Pneumonias have similar appearance in antemortem CT and pulmonary hyper-attenuation and hypersensitivity on MR is shown.

Emphysema aquosum
Drowning manifests as emphysema aquosum and retrosternal touching of the upper lobes and also fluid is seen within the gastrointestinal tract indicating conscious drowning process.

Pulmonary embolus
Pulmonary embolus can be seen within the major vessel using MR imaging or CT scanning with an adjacent consolidation. Virtopsy is superior to conventional autopsy in the detection of air-embolism. Detection of embolus in smaller vessels is abysmally low.

Blood vessels
Dissecting aortic aneurysm can be shown clearly by both CT and MR imaging These imaging modalities can illustrate the presence of old clot, old, calcified intimal flap and calcified margins of the aneurysm and thus differentiate ruptured spontaneous aneurysm from ruptured traumatic aneurysm or aortic transection.

Bone fractures
CT scan and MR imaging often show fractures that are not identifiable with conventional autopsy. In many cases imaging can prove if the fracture occurred with intact circulation in which case there will be associated haemorrhage to the surrounding structures close to the site of the fracture.

Vertebral fracture
Post-mortem MR imaging of vertebral column can differentiate between antemortem and post-mortem vertebral fracture and thus confirm or rule out simulated injury. If the injury was antemortem, there will be bone marrow oedema which will be absent in post-mortem vertebral fracture.

Subcutaneous emphysema
Virtopsy can detect subcutaneous emphysema better than conventional autopsy and thus comfirm trauma during life and intact respiration.

Death by asphyxia
Imaging can detect asphyxial death in a manner that is unavailable through conventional autopsy. Even though the superficial signs of strangulation and mild subcutaneous lacerations that could be a pointer to the diagnosis are not recorded by imaging, but it can detect food bolus obstruction the airway. Even when the obstruction is dislodged before death, it can identify pieces of foreign material in the lung, and mutidetector CT can be used to analyse the respiratory and mastication apparatus.

Tumours and metastases
Both MDCT and MR imaging can clearly demonstrate tumour masses, bone marrow, vessel or nerve involvement by metastasis and tumour invasion into different tissues and organs without disturbing the affected structures. These allows for study of antemortem tumour behaviour and also exclude other causes of death in a patient with previously undiagnosed tumour lesions or metastasis with history of fall or traumatic imaging findings.

Forensic reconstruction of the incidence[1-3]
The direction of impact
The direction of force causing bone fracture can be assessed by analysis of the fracture system.

Messere wedge: The base of a wedge-shaped fracture piece indicates the direction of force.

Force of impact: The grade of contusion of the fatty subcutaneous tissue indicates the force of impact and sometimes the direction.

i. Tangential directional impact (rolled over by car). This is more likely when there is destruction of fatty tissue with formation of subcutaneous cavity in which blood and liquefied fat collect. The subcutaneous cavity is detected in imaging due to sedimentation of blood and formation of fluid levels within the cavity.
ii. Whether head injury is caused by fall to the ground or by blow to the head. Imaging can answer the question by showing typical skull comminuted burst fracture system. A fall will show comminuted burst fracture while a blow will show local impression and ring fracture due to the shape of the fist, hammer, axe or any other weapon used.

Entry and exit wounds
1. Cone-shaped (with outward bevelling) defects shows the direction in which the projectile passed through the skull.
2. Old fracture will stop at previously formed ones (Puppe's rule) showing the chronological order of fracture occurrence.

Automobile driver or airplane pilot can be identified in mass casualty
The specific injury can tell who was steering the vehicle or who the pilot was.
1. Cutaneous marks from seat belts or dash board injuries on the lower legs can help to ascertain the person who was sitting in the front.
2. Specific palmar injuries can indicate who the pilot in a plane crash was. Fracture, haematoma of the hand, palmar soft tissue injuries and bleeding caused by the control lever of the plane are elicited.

Medico-legal issues
Post-mortem CT can help to document the following important findings:
1. Correct or incorrect positions of tubes, catheters, probes; forgotten artery forceps, gauze materials or drains.
2. It can identify dislodged prosthesis, heart valves, venous filters or pulmonary embolization by cements, catheter, or other intra-arterial prostheses.
3. Vertebroplasty with cement may result in cement embolization of the IVC and the pulmonary artery leading to death. These are identified by CT or MRI.
4. Gossypibomas can be more easily diagnosed particularly if the retained swab lodge in difficult to reach sites.

Specific forensic findings with different applications[1-5]

Application of conventional imaging procedures
1. *Heat epidural:* This is seen in burned patients and corpses. It indicates epidural haematoma caused by epidural heat. It does not indicate antemortem injury.
2. *Putrefaction:* This begins 2-3 days after death and smell due to accumulation of gas within the vascular system, body cavities and soft tissues is the earliest finding. Putrefaction can destroy

forensic findings obtained at autopsy and post-mortem imaging if the body is not preserved for independent study groups.

3. *Intracranial pathologies on MRI:* Even in severe putrefaction when conventional autopsy may not elicit anything due to decomposition and liquefaction of brain structures, MR imaging can exclude major intracranial pathologies and intra-axial bleed.

Application of minimally invasive technique

1. *Angiography:* Post-mortem angiography can allow for visualization of vessels, stenosis, minor vascular injuries, occlusion and aneurysm. However, there are some drawbacks to its performance. Hindrances to post-mortem angiography are:
   i.   Stagnancy of the circulation.
   ii. Venous injection with arterial distribution is not possible.
   iii. Pumps must be used since the heart is no longer functioning.
   iv. Sedimentation of cellular blood components and clots influences the distribution of contrast.
   v.   Putrefaction and vulnerable vessels of pancreas and intestines disallow system angiography.
   vi. Putrefaction gas within the vascular system causes filling defects.

2. *Aspiration of body fluid* under image guidance for DNA, toxicological or other forensic analysis. Such body fluids include urine, bile, blood, CSF, effusion, ascites, gastric contents, synovial fluid, etc.

3. *Minimally invasive image-guided tissue biopsy* to obtain tissue in the region of pathology for histological examination.

Application of microradiological techniques

High-resolution CT (Micro-CT) and MR microscopy (micro-MR) provide images with extremely high spatial resolution to analyze tissues in which the resolution of conventional CT and MR is considered too low.

Micro-CT can answer questions in osteoporosis and other bone conditions.

MR microscopy is useful in.

i.   Soft tissue injuries and blood vessels changes in vessel occlusion.
ii. Phenotyping, pathology and toxicological analysis.
iii. Electrical injuries pattern of the skin.
iv. Specific ophthalmic findings that may indicate battered baby syndrome or shaken baby syndrome.
v.   It yields maps of tissue morphological features and tissue composition.
vi. Whole body CT or MR imaging will show the areas of soft tissue injuries, fractures and haematoma in battered baby syndrome, assault and violent traumatic death.

Image-guided biopsy

This can be used to obtain specimen for histological examination and therefore reduce sampling errors since the area of the disease is visualized and biopsied. Tissue architectural pattern is preserved and tissue distortion associated with conventional autopsy and sectioning for histology is avoided. Advanced graphic software and 3D data collection can help multi-planar reformatting of the histology images.

Three dimensional (3D) colour–encoded surface scanning

With conventional photography, 3D objects are displayed in two dimensions, which occasionally are insufficient for forensic and scientific analysis. This is overcome by surface encoded surface scanning in several ways.

1. 3D documentation of the formed injury on the body (skin, bone)
2. 3D documentation of the weapon (injury-causing instrument) that presumably was used.
3. Morphological fingerprint: 3D data set in a so-called patterned injury is called morphological fingerprint.
4. The documentation is independent of the perishability of the wound finding (biological decomposition in deceased person, healing in living person).
5. The suspected weapon can be documented three-dimensionally.
6. Since the 3D models are real database, their sizes and dimensions calibrated, the suspected weapon used can be confirmed or excluded on the basis of their conformity to the formed injury.
7. Weapons that turn up months or years after autopsy was performed can be linked to the patterned injury on the body after the weapon is scanned and attempts at correlation made with the 3D space.
8. Small bite wounds can be correlated with the dentition of possible offenders.
9. The patterned injury in the body of road traffic accident victims can be correlated with the scanned dent in the body of the vehicle.

Fusion of cross-sectional and 3D surface scanning

Radiological markers (multi-modality markers) can be placed in the bodies. These serve as fixed points to help to correlate surface injuries with underlying injuries elicited by 2D cross- sectional imaging. One or two markers must be placed in the foot and if possible the head for accurate measurements. Specific 3D software programs are used to fuse the images.

1. It is possible to merge the photogrammetric data set for smaller injury with radiographic reconstructed image of skin and soft tissue. Visible radiographic markers are used to correlate the data set. Geometric anatomic fusion process is possible without radiographic markers if the wound is located in anatomically stable region.
2. The 3D optical surface scan can be merged with radiological data set. This is used in two main areas.
   i. Analysis of large, widespread or complex injuries on the body surface.
   ii. In cases where whole body documentation is necessary.

Real database 3D forensic reconstruction of incidence[1,2,3]

1. With CT data concerning the skeletal joints and fractures in the deceased patient, it is possible to rearrange the positions of the extremities and of the entire body.
2. An incident can be investigated on the basis of real data and reconstructed with animation to answer many real life questions.
3. The method can be used for forensic purposes in both living and dead people.
4. Dynamic development of patterned injury (morphologic fingerprint) is possible.
5. Matchability and linkability of patterned injury to injury-causing instrument can be evaluated months or years after the body has been buried.
6. This method can be used for forensic purposes in both the living and the dead persons.
7. Real 3D database documentation can open up a new area of scientific reconstruction and animation.
8. It improves the quality of forensic science in terms of accuracy, precision, variability and objectivity ideal as a method of choice for court room procedures.

It also shows mortal changes of strangulation, which are:
1. Major bleeding into muscles of the neck.
2. Major bleeding into the salivary glands.
3. Major bleeding into the lymph nodes.

In conventional autopsy, the changes of life-threatening strangulation are:
1. Temporary loss of consciousness.
2. Unconscious urination.
3. Increased pressure or sensitivity to the neck.

All of the above findings are subjective. The only objective findings are:
1. Petechial haemorrhages within the conjunctiva due to congestion (which are however, not pathognomonic).
2. Petechial haemorrhages within the oral mucosa due to congestion (which are also not pathognomonic).

All these must be shown on the day or a few days from the day of the injury otherwise, the evidences may be lost. Real database 3D reconstruction can show the objective evidence, and at the same time preserve the evidence for objective analysis any time.

Sonographic autopsy of dead foetuses and babies
Using different types of appropriate transducers, post-mortem sonography is capable of providing autopy findings that is agreeable with conventional autopsy in about 88-95% in both sensitivey and specificity.

Virtual skeleton for age and sex determination
Multidetector CT scanning and image reconstruction and soft tissue subtraction techniques can bring out the skeleton which will help in age and sex determination. Also by looking at the vertebrae for degerative changes and the dentitions as obtained by the MDCT, close to 100% accuracy is achieved even without destruction of the body allowing for future independent assessment.

Limitations of radiological minimum invasive autopsy
a. Ischaemic heart diseases are not shown by the presently available methods unless angiography of coronary and of the intracranial vessels are performed.
b. Virtopsy is inferior to conventional autopsy at the detection of intra-tissue haemorrhage and fat embolism.
c. Imaging tends to misdiagnose pulmonary embolism, bronchopneumonia and intestinal infarction because the changes in the affected organs following death alter the imaging findings leading to both false negative and false positive findings.
d. Since the body is prepared and wrapped in a waterproof container before being brought o the radiology department and scanning, if angiography and aspiration of body fluid or biopsy is not done where the body is exposed, the smell, colour, texture, height, surface and scarification marks may not be recorded by the radiological pathologist leading to loss of vital physiological information.
e. Imaging findings of some post-mortem events may vary from their antemortem appearances so that radiologists need additional training in the interpretation of post-mortem images. Such confusing findings are putrefaction, gas in small vessels, ducts and heart chambers.

f. The fear that pathologists may have reduced importance may arise. Everyone is still in his own area but only multi-departmental collaboration between clinicians, radiologists and pathologists is needed as already done in diagnosis and treatment of other diseases, for the improvement that is expected to be obtained from radiological minimal invasive autopsy.

g. Since it is technologically-based, it may be very financially challenging to implement in economically emerging countries in terms of equipments, manpower and legislation. The cost of MRI and CT alone may be greater than the cost of conventional autopsy. A dedicated CT and MRI may be required in order not to interfere with daily job for patients needing these services in the hospital.

References

1. Dirnhofer R, Jackowski C, Vock P, Potter K, Thali MJ. VIRTOPSY: Minimally invasive imaging-guided Virtual Autopsy. Radiographics 2006; 26: 1305-1333.

2. Weustink AC, Hnink MGM, van Dijke CF, Renken NS, Krestin GP, Oosterhuis JW. Minimally invasive autopsy: an alternative to conventional autopsy. Radiology 2009; 250:897-904.

3. Thali MJ, Braun M, Buck U, Aghayev E, Jackowski C, Vock P, Sonnenschein M, Dirnhofer R. VIRTOPSY--scientific documentation, reconstruction and animation in forensic: individual and real 3D data based geo-metric approach including optical body/object surface and radiological CT/MRI scanning. J Forensic Sci 2005;50:428-42.

4. Bolliger SA, Thali MJ, Ross S, Buck U, Naether S, Vock P. Virtual autopsy using imaging: bridging radiologic and forensic sciences. A review of the Virtopsy and similar projects. Eur Radiol 2008;18:273-82.

5. Ozkalipci O, Volpellier M. Photographic documentation, a practical guide for non professional forensic photography. Torture 2010;20:45-52.

6. Reynolds A. Forensic radiography: an overview. Radiol Technol 2010;81:361-79.

GENERAL REFERENCES

1. Adam A, Dixon AK (Eds). Grainger's and Allison's Diagnostic Radiology: a textbook of medical imaging. Churchill Livingstone Elsevier, Philadelphia, USA; 2008.
2. Behrman RE, Vaughan VC. Nelson's textbook of paediatrics (19th Edition) Philadelphia, WB Saunders Co. 2011.
3. Chapman DS, Nakielnyly R. Aids to Radiological Differential diagnosis. 5th Edition, London. WB Saunders 2009.
4. Chapman S, Nakielny R. A Guide to Radiological procedure. 3rd Edition, London, Bailliere Tindall; 2001
5. Dahnert W. Radiology Review Manual. 7th Edition Baltimore, USA, Williams and Wilkins. 2011.
6. Hodler J, von Schulthess GK, Zollikoffer ChL. Musculoskeletal diseases 2009-2012:Diagnostic imaging (syllabus IDKD 2009-2012). Springer-Verlag Italia, Milan 2009.
7. Holder J, von Schulthess GK, Zollikoffer ChL. Diseases of the brain, head and neck, spine: Diagnostic imaging and interventional technique (syllabus IDKD 2008). Springer-Verlag Italia, Milan 2008 (syllabus IDKD 2008).
8. Juhl JH, Crummy AB, Kuhlman JE, Paul LW (Eds). Paul and Juhl's Essentials of Radiologic Imaging. Lippincott Williams & Wilkins; Baltimore, 7th edition; 1998.
9. Kreel L, Thornton A. Outline of Medical Imaging (Vol. I and II) Oxford. Butterworth/ Heinemann. 1992.
10. Ozonoff MB. Paediatric orthopaedic Radiology. (2nd Edition) Philadelphia, WB Saunders Company, 1992.
11. Reeder MM, Palmer PES. Radiology of tropical diseases with epidermiological, pathological and clinical correlation. Philadelphia, Lippincott Williams & Wilkins, 2001.
12. Sanders RC, Winter TC. Clinical Sonography: a practical guide. 4th Edition; Philadelphia, Lippincott, 2006.
13. Sutton D. Textbook of Radiology and imaging. 7th Edition. London, Elsevier Science Limited 2003. Vol. I and II.
14. Sutton D. Textbook of Radiology and imaging. Sixth Edition. London, Churchill Livingstone 1998. Vol. I and II.
15. Swischuk LE. Imaging newborn, infant and young child. Philadelphia, 5th edition, Lippincott Williams and Wilkins, 2004.

INDEX

Printed in the United States
By Bookmasters